Drugs and Pharmacology for Nurses

S. J. Hopkins PhD FRPharmS

Honorary Consultant Pharmacist
Addenbrooke's Hospital, Cambridge

TWELFTH EDITION

CHURCHILL LIVINGSTONE
EDINBURGH HONG KONG LONDON MADRID MELBOURNE NEW YORK AND
TOKYO 1995

CHURCHILL LIVINGSTONE
Medical Division of Pearson Professional Limited

Distributed in the United States of America by Churchill Livingstone Inc., 650 Avenue of the Americas, New York, N.Y. 10011, and by associated companies, branches and representatives throughout the world.

First edition 1963
Second edition 1965
Third edition 1966
Fourth edition 1968
Fifth edition 1971
Sixth edition 1975
Seventh edition 1979

Eighth edition 1983
Ninth edition 1986
Tenth edition 1989
Eleventh edition 1992
    Reprinted 1993
Twelfth Edition 1995

ISBN 0-443-05249 2

British Library Cataloguing in Publication Data
A catalogue record for this book is available from the British Library.

Library of Congress Cataloging in Publication Data
A catalogue record for this book is available from the Library of Congress.

The
publisher's
policy is to use
**paper manufactured
from sustainable forests**

Produced by Longman Singapore Publishers (Pte) Ltd
Printed in Singapore

Contents

Preface

In this 12th edition, much new material has been inserted and the arrangement of certain sections has been altered, whilst retaining the successful format of the previous editions. The book provides a guide to the actions and clinical applications of a very wide range of currently available drugs, but is not intended to be a manual of nursing practice. Although originally intended exclusively for nurses, *Drugs and Pharmacology for Nurses* has achieved a wider readership amongst many others concerned with the use of medicinal substances.

Changes made to this edition

Many of the introductory paragraphs to sections have been revised and extended to indicate the principles of drug usage.
  Monographs on recently introduced drugs include:

- notes of new antibiotics and other antibacterial agents
- anti-cancer drugs, including a highly interesting plant product – paclitaxel
- new types of anti-epileptics
- cardiac drugs
- blood-lipid lowering agents
- drugs for the relief of the respiratory distress syndrome of premature babies
- selective serotonin re-uptake inhibitors in the treatment of depression
- an enzyme product that offers a new approach to the symptomatic relief of cystic fibrosis.

  Boxes entitled 'Points about...' provide brief summaries of the most important aspects of certain groups of drugs.
  Also included in this edition are references to important papers on certain new drugs. These references are mainly to journals that

are likely to be accessible to nurses, and are clearly highlighted in the text.

Approved and brand names

An extensive list of approved and brand names is given in Appendix II, including many drugs over and above those referred to specifically in the text. Approved names can be used by any manufacturer, but a brand name refers to the product of a single maker, so the same drug may be available under more than one brand name, which can sometimes be very confusing.

Mixed products, because of their multiplicity, are referred to only occasionally, however, the official names for certain widely prescribed mixed products have been listed on page 590. The use of mixed products has met with some disapproval, as the dose of each constituent is fixed. For patients on multiple therapy, however, they have the great advantage of reducing the number of tablets to be taken daily, thereby minimising the risks of confusion. The omission of any drug is merely a reflection of the wide range now available.

Dose ranges

When a dose range is given, the lower dose is often an initial dose, to be increased according to need and response.

Dosages given to children and the elderly should be lower than for others. In the young, the ability to metabolise drugs may not be fully developed, and overdose may easily occur. In the elderly, impaired renal function may reduce adequate elimination of a drug, so a reduced dose may be necessary to prevent accumulation of the drug to possibly toxic levels.

Side-effects

The references to side-effects are for guidance only, as their nature and frequency vary widely with both drug and patient. An exhaustive list of side-effects, including those rarely encountered, would be more confusing than helpful.

A general warning is given here that many potent drugs will impair car driving and similar activities, and that no drug should be given during pregnancy without consideration of the risks involved. The absence of any such warning later in the book does not mean that the drug is free from such risks.

Nurses can play an important role in detecting side-effects, as they are in frequent contact with patients, and any unanticipated side-effect that the nurse might observe should always be reported without delay.

Symbols and abbreviations used

New drugs that are currently under surveillance by the Committee of Safety of Medicines for the detection of adverse reactions are distinguished in the text by a black triangle ▼.

Drugs that are available only on prescription (the POM group, which includes most potent drugs) are distinguished in the main references by the sign §; Controlled Drugs (CDs, or drugs of addiction) are identified by a bold star *.

The abbreviation BNF refers to the British National Formulary, and BP to the British Pharmacopoeia.

Medical and pharmacological terms

A small glossary is included as Appendix V. For an explanation of other medical and pharmacological terms used in the text, nurses are advised to consult a reference book, such as the Churchill Livingstone Nurses' Dictionary.

Thanks are again due to those readers who have kindly suggested additions and alterations.

Cambridge 1995   S. J. H.

Note on drug dosages and nurse-prescribing

The doses given in this book are for guidance only as, although great care has been taken, the possibility of error remains, and it is the responsibility of the users of the book to obtain confirmation of dose and other information from official publications such as the British National Formulary (BNF) and Martindale's Extra Pharmacopoeia, or from the Data Sheet issued by the manufacturer of the drug concerned. When possible, the information leaflets included in the package inserts of many drugs should be consulted to confirm that there have been no changes in the use and dose of the drug concerned.

Drug administration, nursing reponsibilities and nurse-prescribing

The prescriber is responsible for the accuracy of his prescriptions, but nurses are largely responsible for the day-to-day administration of drugs. Before giving any drug to a patient, every care should be taken to be certain that the right drug is being given in the right doses to the right patient, and that the label on the medicine has been checked against the prescription. The golden rule is simple — READ THE LABEL. Unless the label conveys the required information in full, the product should be rejected until confirmation has been obtained. Drug names can be confusing at times, but even genuine belief that the prescribed drug is being given in the prescribed dose is no substitute for certainty of knowledge. It is sometimes said that safety could be increased by having drug labels and containers distinguishable to some extent by shape and colour, but if conditions make it difficult to check the accuracy of a label, then it is the conditions that require modification, not the label.

Nurses are not always helped by the fact that the amount of drug in an injection or present in a topical preparation may be expressed as a percentage. Many doctors, as well as nurses, have difficulty in translating percentages into the equivalent amount of substance per millilitre, or know that a 10 ml ampoule of a 5% solution contains 500 mg of the drug. It is worthwhile remembering that a 1% solution contains 10 mg/ml, as with that in mind, the amount in a 0.1% or 10% solution can be calculated without difficulty. At the end, however, nurses must accept the fact that they, like doctors and pharmacists, are responsible for any errors they may make.

Nurse-prescribing

The authority to prescribe has long been restricted to registered medical practitioners. Nurses, however, by the nature of their training and their close contact with patients are uniquely placed to assess the need for a limited range of drugs for minor illness. There has been increasing pressure for official recognition of the contribution that a certain amount of nurse-prescribing could make to the National Health Service, and that pressure has resulted in the setting up of some Nurse-Prescribing Demonstration Centres to prepare Community Nurses to prescribe from an agreed formulary that will include non-opioid analgesics, piperazine, laxatives, desloughing agents, skin antiseptics and stoma care products. The setting up of these Centres is a long-overdue recognition of the increasingly important part that nurses play in medication and patient care. It may well be that the limited prescribing authority now given to nurses will lead eventually to still wider responsibilities for nurses by extending the range of the present limited formulary. Few will doubt that nurses will rise to the new challenge of nurse-prescribing.

1

Introduction

DRUGS AND PHARMACOLOGY

Drugs or medicines are substances used for the treatment of illness, and pharmacology is the study of the mode of action of such agents. Medicines of some sort have been used since the dawn of history, but Hippocrates (c. 400 BC) was one of the first medical writers, and has been called the 'Father of Medicine'. Treatment was then empirical and directed towards symptomatic relief, and that approach to illness persisted until the latter part of the 19th century, when advances in pharmacology gradually began to place therapeutics on a scientific basis. Since then developments have occurred with increasing rapidity, and the physician now has at his command an almost bewildering range of therapeutically active substances. That range includes vegetable drugs, mineral salts, animal products, antibiotics and synthetic drugs.

The subject of therapeutics is one of expanding horizons, which can fascinate by its immense potentialities, and perplex by its apparent anomalies, but a few simplifying generalizations can be made. Thus all drugs may be divided into a few main groups according to their origin, i.e. vegetable drugs, mineral salts, animal products and synthetic drugs — or they may be classified according to their pharmacological action. Some synthetic drugs may be grouped according to their chemical structure.

Crude or vegetable drugs

This is the oldest group, and includes various leaves, roots, seeds and barks. The main action of a vegetable drug is often due to a single constituent or active principle, which may be an alkaloid such as atropine, or a glycoside such as digoxin. Alkaloids can combine with acids to form salts, e.g., atropine sulphate, codeine phosphate, but glycosides contain an active fraction combined with a sugar. Alkaloids and other active principles have virtually replaced preparations of crude drugs as their action is more consistent and reliable. The importance of vegetable drugs has declined with the development of synthetic drugs, but their potential is not yet exhausted, as shown by the recent introduction of an anticancer agent obtained from the Pacific Yew, and many plant products still await full investigation for medicinal activity.

Mineral salts

These are metallic compounds such as sodium chloride (common salt), potassium chloride, sodium bicarbonate, ferrous sulphate and calcium gluconate. Some mineral salts are of very great physiological importance, and are constituents of certain intravenous solutions used to restore the electrolyte balance of the body.

Animal products

This group once enjoyed considerable popularity, as indicated by the witches' scene in *Macbeth*, but few products of animal origin are in use today. Those few that remain in use are of importance therapeutically, as the group includes drugs such as hormones and heparin. Bio-engineering techniques have led to the production of some hormone products in quantity and purity.

Synthetic drugs

Synthetic drugs form the most important group of modern therapeutic agents. Representative compounds are antihypertensive agents, tranquillizers, antidepressants, analgesics, spasmolytics, antibacterial agents, angiotensin-converting enzyme inhibitors and hypoglycaemic agents.

Antibiotics

Antibiotics can be described as antimicrobial substances produced during the growth of certain fungi and associated organisms, although many antibiotics in current use are semisynthetic derivatives. The first of this remarkable group of substances to be discovered was penicillin (p. 111).

ADMINISTRATION, ABSORPTION AND DISTRIBUTION OF DRUGS (Figs 1.1 and 1.2)

Before a drug can have any systemic pharmacological action it must reach the receptor site at which it acts, in an active form, and at an effective concentration, but the route of administration, degree of absorption, distribution, metabolism and rate of excretion are important factors in modifying the ultimate response to a drug (Fig. 1.1). The various forms of drug presentation are referred to on page 21, but as most drugs are absorbed from the gastrointestinal tract the oral route is the most common and convenient form of drug administration. Absorption takes place mainly in the small intestine, where the lining villi offer an enormous area for absorption, but it may be modified by several factors. The presence of food may enhance the absorption of drugs such as propranolol and phenytoin, yet reduce the absorption of isoniazid and the tetracyclines. A few drugs such as captopril, digoxin and rifampicin are better absorbed on an empty

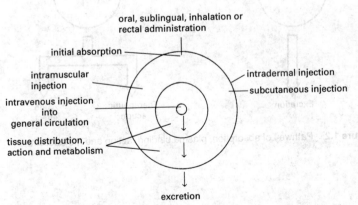

Figure 1.1 Drug administration, absorption, distribution and excretion.

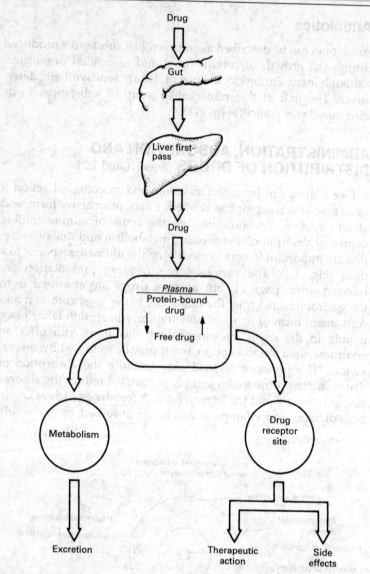

Figure 1.2 Pathway of absorption, plasma binding, action and metabolism.

stomach. Some drugs, represented by certain antibiotics and hormones, may be broken down by gastric acid or digestive enzymes, and so never reach the small intestine, and are therefore inactive if given orally.

When a drug finally reaches the small intestine, absorption largely depends on its ability to cross the cell membrane. Initially there will be a relatively high concentration of the drug outside the cell, so in most cases the drug will pass into the cell by passive diffusion to equalize the concentration, but with some drugs, lipid solubility is a dominant factor governing absorption. Cell membranes have a lipid or fatty layer, so drugs that are not lipid-soluble will not pass readily across the cell membrane, and absorption may be insufficient to give a systemically effective plasma level. That explains why some water-soluble drugs such as the antibiotic gentamicin must be given by injection. The degree of ionisation also plays a part in drug absorption, as only unionised compounds are lipid-soluble.

Occasionally, the absence of absorption is desirable, as a drug may be required that has a local action on the intestinal tract, as exemplified by the use of salazopyrin in the treatment of ulcerative colitis.

Lipid solubility

Lipid solubility also influences drug penetration into the central nervous system, as few drugs pass easily into the brain because of the presence of the blood–brain barrier. The capillaries that supply the brain are surrounded by closely-packed lipid-containing cells (the glial cells) which, together with the choroid plexus, function as a barrier through which drugs must pass. Lipid-soluble drugs can penetrate the barrier with relative ease, but many others are not sufficiently lipid-soluble to pass through the barrier and exert a central effect. In certain infections, however, such as meningitis, the efficiency of the barrier is reduced, and penicillin, for example, which does not normally reach the CNS, may then pass from the circulation via the barrier to reach the brain.

Lipid solubility also influences the duration of action of lipid-soluble drugs such as the intravenous anaesthetic thiopentone. Thiopentone has a short action, not because it is readily metabolized, but because it is rapidly removed from the circulation by temporary storage in body fat and muscle. Lipid solubility may also be linked with side-effects. Propranolol is lipid-soluble and may reach the brain and cause sleep disturbances, whereas atenolol, being poorly soluble in lipids, has little central activity.

First-pass metabolism

Following absorption, drugs pass via the portal vein, which drains the small intestine, into the liver. Some drugs may then pass directly and unaltered into the circulation, but many undergo some degree of metabolic change by liver enzymes of which cytochrome P450 is one of the most important. In consequence of that hepatic metabolism, only part of the dose of an absorbed drug may eventually reach the tissues to have a therapeutic effect. With a few drugs, such as glyceryl trinitrate and lignocaine, hepatic metabolism and breakdown is virtually complete, so those drugs are inactive orally simply because they never reach the general circulation. First-pass metabolism is therefore of considerable importance, and explains to some extent the differences between oral and injection doses of certain drugs, and why, in liver disease, larger than normal amounts of a drug may escape hepatic metabolism and reach the circulation. In such cases, an adjustment of dose may be necessary to avoid an excessive response or accumulation of the drug.

Occasionally, a genetic factor is involved in drug metabolism. Some drugs are modified in the liver by the enzyme acetyltransferase with the formation of acetylated derivatives. Some individuals are slow acetylators, others are referred to as fast acetylators. The former may develop side-effects associated with an increased plasma concentration of the drug, and should be given lower doses than fast acetylators (see isoniazid, p. 154).

Enzyme induction

Many drugs are metabolized and inactivated by liver enzymes, but some have the ability to induce the further production of such enzymes. Such enzyme induction may have a knock-on effect by increasing the breakdown of other drugs that may also be given, and require an adjustment of dose to maintain the response. Rifampicin is an example of an enzyme-inducing drug, and combined use may lead to a reduction in the plasma levels of propranolol, cimetidine, phenytoin and other drugs.

Distribution and uptake

After drugs have been absorbed and passed through the liver, their distribution is effected via the circulation and is followed by uptake by the storage tissues and receptor-sites before further metabolism and excretion occurs. Uptake can be modified by many factors, including the degree of lipid and water solubility, and the extent of plasma and tissue binding. In a few cases uptake is selective, as iodine is preferentially taken up by the thyroid gland for the production of thyroxine.

Most drugs are carried in the circulation either in the free state, or as a plasma protein–drug complex, with acidic and neutral compounds binding to albumin, and basic substances to glyco-proteins. The degree of firmness of plasma binding is of consider-able importance. Only the free drug is active, and can penetrate cells or act on receptor sites, and so is responsible for the pharma-cological effects, and as the free drug is metabolized or excreted, part of the plasma-bound drug is released. The plasma–drug complex is not lipid-soluble, and it cannot penetrate cell membranes, so plasma binding therefore functions as a storage as well as a transport mechanism. The degree and firmness of plasma binding, and the rate of metabolism and excretion of the free drug are reflected in the dose and duration of action of a drug. Plasma binding is also of considerable importance in some cases of combined therapy (see Drug Interactions, p. 9).

Drug metabolism and plasma binding

Apart from any first-pass metabolism, many drugs are metabolized by combination with endogenous substances such as glucuronic acid or sulphate, and converted into water-soluble compounds that are excreted in the urine.

In some cases, such drug metabolism can be of clinical impor-tance. Some antibacterial agents are metabolized and excreted in the urine in an inactive form, and so are useless against infections of the urinary tract. On the other hand, some drugs may be inactive as given, but are metabolized into active derivatives and are referred to as 'pro-drugs'. Chloral hydrate, for example, is broken down after absorption to trichlorethanol, to which the sedative action of chloral is due, and bacampicillin also functions as a pro-drug, as it is metabolized to release the active antibiotic ampicillin.

After absorption, many drugs become bound to a varying extent to protein binding sites, but the degree and firmness of the binding is variable. When two or more drugs are given together, the drug with the greatest affinity for a binding site will displace a drug with a lower affinity, so the plasma level of the displaced drug will rise. The oral anticoagulant warfarin can be displaced from its binding sites by a variety of other drugs, so its anticoagulant effect is potentiated, and an adjustment of dose may be necessary. In practice, the increased plasma level of the displaced drug is often transient, as other factors such as increased metabolism and elimination come into play. Patients at most risk from drug reactions are the elderly, and those with impaired renal or hepatic function.

In a few cases, the action of two drugs may be complementary, and increase the response. Such combined action is referred to as synergism, represented by the action of carbidopa and levodopa in parkinsonism (p. 254) and clavulanic acid in augmenting the action of amoxycillin (p. 125).

Excretion of drugs

Most absorbed drugs are excreted in the urine, either unchanged or as a conjugated metabolite, such as glucuronide. A few are also excreted in the bile. Renal excretion is of considerable importance, as any reduction in the glomerular filtration rate will reduce excretion, and may require a reduction in dose to avoid an undesirable rise in the plasma levels of the drug. Gentamicin is an example of a drug requiring a dose reduction in renal impairment, with monitoring of the plasma levels of the antibiotic to avoid toxicity. It should be remembered that the kidneys excrete a concentrated filtrate as urine, and are therefore open to the full action of any potentially nephrotoxic drug.

It is sometimes possible to modify drug excretion by combined therapy. Probenecid promotes the excretion of urates by inhibiting re-absorption by the tubules, and so probenecid is useful in the treatment of gout. Yet it has the opposite effect of reducing the tubular excretion of penicillin, and probenecid is occasionally given to increase the plasma level of penicillin in conditions such as infective endocarditis when high and sustained plasma levels of the antibiotic are required.

Drugs that are excreted in the bile may be re-absorbed to some extent by the entero-hepatic circulation, and so have an extended action, as with some very long-acting sulphonamides. A few drugs, such as paraldehyde, are excreted in part by the lungs; others are excreted by sweat glands, and may cause skin irritation.

Drug interactions

The introduction of new and powerful drugs and the widespread use of multiple therapy has increased the risk of drug interactions, which may occur at almost any stage from absorption to excretion, and may result in either a reduction of activity or a potentiation of effect. Iron salts and simple antacids form insoluble complexes in the gastrointestinal tract with tetracyclines, and cholestyramine similarly reduces the absorption of digoxin and warfarin by the formation of an insoluble complex. In other cases, the administration of two or more drugs together may lead to an increase in effect, sometimes with potentially serious consequences. The monoamine oxidase inhibitors, by preventing the breakdown of endogenous pressor amines such as noradrenaline, potentiate the action of pressor drugs. They may also cause an unexpected hypertensive episode if a food such as cheese, broad beans or yeast extract is taken in any quantity, as such foods contain relatively large amounts of the pressor agent tyramine.

Very occasionally a drug reaction can be exploited. Disulfiram is sometimes used in the treatment of alcoholism, as if it is given in association with even a small amount of alcohol, it causes nausea and vomiting, the so-called disulfiram or Antabuse reaction, which discourages further intake of alcohol. It should be noted that a similar reaction may occur if alcohol is taken with drugs such as metronidazole and cephamandole.

A more specific enzyme-associated reaction that is of clinical value is the inhibition of xanthine oxidase by allopurinol, which reduces the formation of uric acid, and is used in the treatment of gout.

It is worth bearing in mind that occasionally a reaction has been traced to a herbal medicine that the patient has been taking in addition to the prescribed drugs.

Appendix I gives some notes on drug interactions, but the range is so wide that the list is not exhaustive and some reactions are rare. It should be noted that if a reaction occurs with one type of drug, a similar reaction may occur with other drugs of the same type, e.g. clofibrate potentiates the action of oral anticoagulants, and a similar potentiation may occur with related hypolipidaemic agents.

Mode of action

The mode of action of many drugs is still far from clear. A few, such as the simple antacids, have a direct chemical action, but most important drugs act by modifying cell activity in some way. A cell is a highly complex structure, and drugs may act by inhibiting enzyme activity, or interfere with metabolic functions by acting on a cell receptor site. Receptors are specific points on cell surfaces capable of binding with certain endogenous substances such as adrenaline, or with exogenous drugs. Such binding sets in train a series of changes, many of which are still imperfectly understood, that finally results in a pharmacological response. The general term for receptor-binding substances is 'ligand', and ligands that evoke a response are termed 'agonists'. Ligands that inhibit a response are 'antagonists'. It should be remembered that receptors are not static points, as their number and functional activity vary with drug treatment. Continuous exposure to an agonist may lead to an internalization of receptors, and so reduce their activity, a process known as 'down-regulation'. That may show up as tolerance to a drug, whereby an increased dose may be required to produce the same effect, although tolerance may sometimes be due to an increased metabolic breakdown of the drug in the body. Many receptors have been identified, as well as some sub-types of receptors and the closer the relationship between a drug and the receptor it acts upon, the more specific is the subsequent response. The relationship can be compared to some extent with that between a lock and a key, as both receptor and agonist or antagonist must 'fit' together. The position is complicated as some ligands may have a dual action. Thus although the beta-adrenoceptor blocking agents, represented by propranolol, have as a class a depressant action on cardiac activity, some members of that class may also have limited cardiac stimulant properties, and are referred to as partial agonists. Such beta-blockers have what is described as an 'intrinsic sympathomimetic action'. That difference may sometimes have a clinical advantage, as a partial agonist, whilst exhibiting the main activity of the beta-blockers generally, may cause less bradycardia than the full antagonists represented by propranolol (p. 190).

Very few drugs have in fact a single specific action, and side-effects may be mediated by an action on receptors other than those concerned with the desired clinical response. Thus the tricylic antidepressants, which have a main action on receptors in the central nervous system, may cause dryness of the mouth by inhibiting the action of acetylcholine on the cholinoreceptors. Table 1.1 gives examples of some receptors, agonists and antagonists.

Idiosyncrasy, hypersensitivity and skin reactions

The normal therapeutic response to a drug can be anticipated from experience, but as patients do not react to drugs with

Table 1.1 Receptors

Type	Sub-type	Agonists	Antagonists
Adrenoceptors (see also p. 186)	a/b	noradrenaline, adrenaline	labetalol
	a_1	phenylephrine	indoramin, prazosin
	a_2	clonidine	phentolamine
	a_1/a_2		phentolamine
	b_1	dopamine, dobutamine	atenolol, metoprolol
	b_2	salbutamol and related drugs, dopexamine	
	b_1/b_2	isoprenaline	
Cholinoceptors		acetylcholine, carbachol	anticholinergic/ muscarinic agents
Dopamine receptors		dopamine, dopexamine, bromocriptine	phenothiazines
GABA receptors		GABA, benzodiazepines, baclofen, vigabatrin, zopilcone	flumazenil
Histamine receptors	H_1	histamine	antihistamines
	H_2	histamine	cimetidine and other H_2 antagonists
Opioid receptors		morphine and related drugs	naloxone, naltrexone
Serotonin receptors		serotonin	cyproheptadine, ketanserin, methysergide

machine-like precision, some individual variation in response is not uncommon. However a patient may occasionally exhibit a markedly unusual response to a drug, and such a reaction is known as an idiosyncrasy.

These reactions may be associated with a genetic abnormality, such as the rare aplastic anaemia associated with chloramphenicol, or the haemolysis that sometimes follows the use of the antimalarial drug primaquine. The methaemoglobinaemia that may occur with the sulphonamides and other drugs is also linked with an enzyme deficiency.

Hypersensitivity to drugs is much more serious. It is usually allergic in nature, and is of the antigen–antibody reaction type, indicating that the patient has become sensitized to the drug, so that subsequent treatment evokes undesirable effects. Nurses should always ask patients about any previous drug reactions before giving a drug for the first time.

Aspirin, for example, may precipitate a severe asthmatic attack in hypersensitive patients, especially those with a history of allergic disease. Penicillin may sometimes evoke a hypersensitivity reaction, which can then occur with any other penicillin derivatives and extend to cross-sensitivity with the related cephalosporins. Many other drugs can occasionally cause a similar reaction, which is linked with the release of histamine, and manifested by bronchospasm and cardiovascular collapse (anaphylactic shock) (p. 233).

Other hypersensitivity reactions that may occur include skin reactions, blood dyscrasias and the so-called 'drug fever'. Drug-induced fever may occur with anticholinergic agents in high doses, with antitubercular drugs, cytotoxic agents, methydopa, nitrofurantoin, penicillamine and many others. Fever may also occur if systemic treatment with corticosteroids is withdrawn too rapidly.

Disturbances of the blood-forming system such as aplastic anaemia, agranulocytosis and haemolysis may also be the result of a drug reaction. Desensitization to some drugs such as penicillin, can sometimes be achieved by an extended course of injection treatment, commencing with very low doses of the offending drug, but the method is not without risk (p. 431).

Skin reactions

Drug-induced skin reactions may take different forms. Urticaria and erythematous eruptions are relatively common, and appear to be linked with the release of endogenous substances such as histamine. Not all drug-induced skin reactions are serious, but a change in medication is usually necessary. A more severe morbilliform rash may follow treatment with ampicillin and the related amoxycillin, bacampicillin, and pivampicillin. It is more likely to occur in patients with glandular fever (infectious mononucleosis), and chronic lymphatic leukaemia. It is not regarded as a true penicillin allergy in such patients. The Stevens–Johnson syndrome (*Erythema multiforme*) is a much more serious skin reaction with blistering and mucosal lesions.

A few drugs occasionally cause photosensitivity, an abnormal skin reaction associated with exposure to light. Drugs known to cause photosensitivity include the tetracyclines, nalidixic acid, phenothiazines and chloroquine. Care should be taken to avoid sunlight particularly at midday, and to use a sun-screen preparation that is effective against the entire ultraviolet spectrum (p. 545).

Side-effects and adverse reactions

Hypersensitivity reactions to drugs must be distinguished from side-effects. Few drugs have a clear-cut and selective action on a particular organ of the body, and a side-effect is an unwanted pharmacological response that cannot be separated from the main action of the drug, although a side-effect may sometimes be reduced by an adjustment of dose. Thus, many antihistamines cause an often unwanted drowsiness, and the few that do not probably fail to penetrate the blood–brain barrier.

Another example is morphine, a powerful analgesic by virtue of its depressant effect on the sensory area of the brain but it also has a stimulant effect on the vomiting centre. That stimulation is the cause of the nausea and vomiting that may follow an injection of morphine, and which is a potential post-operative danger.

Other side-effects of drugs include the dryness of the mouth and disturbances of vision that may occur with atropine and other anticholinergic drugs, and the drug-induced symptoms resembling Parkinson's disease that may result from extended treatment with tranquillizers of the phenothiazine type. In a few cases, the localized application of drugs may reduce side-effects. A case in point is the administration of small doses of corticosteroids and bronchodilators by aerosol inhalation in the treatment of asthma. By the use of such inhalation therapy, many of the undesired other systemic as well as the side-effects of the drugs can largely be avoided. Another example is the use of drug-containing skin patches.

Adverse reactions may be more serious, and drug-induced blood dyscrasias are among the more common drug reactions. Such reactions include neutropenia (a reduction in the number of circulating neutrophils); agranulocytosis (a complete absence of neutrophils); aplastic anaemia, which follows suppression of all bone marrow functions; thrombocytopenia (a reduction in the blood platelet count). Haemolytic anaemia is less common, and involves the destruction and lysis of the red cells at a rate greater than the compensatory rate of red cell production. In many cases these reactions are reversible on withdrawal of the offending drugs, but they should never be given again as the patient may have become sensitized. Many drugs have been associated with the development of blood dyscrasias from time to time and a few are listed in Table 1.2.

Screening of new drugs

A new drug is always subjected to exhaustive and prolonged tests before its clinical use can be considered. Such tests are first carried out in animals to assess activity, potency and toxicity, and only after satisfactory studies is a new drug used in carefully controlled clinical trials. There is always some difficulty in relating results in animal trials to the response likely to be obtained in the clinical situation, and in spite of exhaustive tests, some side-effects may not become apparent until a new drug is used therapeutically, and sometimes for a considerable time. Hepatic reactions for example, are often difficult to detect because of the low incidence of such reactions. In this field nurses can and do play an important part in noting and reporting any unusual or

Table 1.2 Drugs that may cause blood dyscrasias

ACE inhibitors	anticonvulsants	cytotoxics	heparin
allopurinol	antimalarials	diuretics	NSAIDs
antibacterials	antithyroids	gold salts	psychotorophics
			rifampicin
			sulphonylureas

unanticipated response to either a new or established drug, as they spend much more time with a patient that the investigating doctor. The Committee on Safety of Medicines keeps certain new drugs under intense surveillance, and requires any adverse reaction to be reported on the 'Yellow Cards' provided by the Committee. Those drugs currently under such surveillance are indicated by an inverted triangle thus ▼.

The dose of drugs

The optimum dose for a drug is high enough to elicit the desired therapeutic effect, yet not high enough to cause unwanted side-effects. The margin between those doses is sometimes referred to as the therapeutic window, and with some drugs such as digoxin, the window is narrow and requires careful adjustment of dose (Fig. 1.3). In such cases, a measurement of the plasma level of the drug may be necessary to avoid overdose.

Drugs that have a long elimination half-life, such as digoxin, are sometimes given initially as a loading dose to obtain a high tissue up-take, followed by correspondingly low maintenance doses. The accepted range of dose used clinically is thus a compromise, and the dose prescribed may also vary to some extent with the weight and sex of the patient. The doses of a few very potent drugs are based upon body surface area. Renal or hepatic damage may delay excretion, and require a reduction in dose to avoid toxic

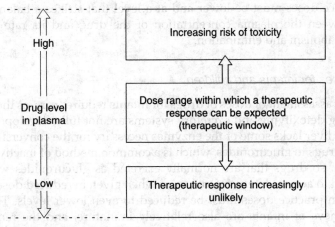

Figure 1.3 Diagram of therapeutic window.

effects. In other cases, tolerance to a drug may be acquired, and a larger dose may be necessary to obtain the same response. The dose may also vary according to the condition to be treated. Some tranquillizers, for example, that have anti-emetic properties are given in much larger doses for psychiatric conditions than when used for the treatment of nausea and vomiting.

The route of administration also influences the size of dose given. Doses by injection are usually smaller than those given orally, and intravenous doses smaller than those given by intramuscular injection. Administration by injection has the advantages of evoking a rapid response and of eliminating the problems of absorption and first-pass loss in the liver. Intravenous injections, however, are not free from risks, as all the injected drug reaches the systemic circulation immediately, and the organs with high blood flows, such as the heart, kidneys, lungs and brain are exposed to high concentrations of the injected drug, with a corresponding increased risk of toxic effects. As a rule, intravenous injections should be made slowly to reduce the risks of immediate side-effects, and sometimes intravenous infusion of a dilute solution of the drug is preferred.

In all cases, whatever the route of administration, frequency of dose is important, and with long-acting drugs, care must be taken to avoid over-dosage, otherwise the drug may accumulate in the body and increase the risk of toxic reactions. On the other hand, in some cases a relatively high dose of a drug may be required initially to obtain the required response, but subsequent maintenance doses must be lower and at a level that strikes a balance between the plasma concentration of the drug and its rate of metabolism and elimination.

Doses for infants and children

The assessment of doses of drugs for infants requires care, as their drug detoxifying and excretory systems are not fully developed. The liver lacks some of the enzymes necessary for the conversion of drugs to glucuronides, which is a common method of inactivation, so drugs that are normally excreted as glucuronides will tend to accumulate in infants, even when given in reduced doses; so in practice doses must be reduced to even lower levels. The kidneys of infants are also relatively immature, and the renal excretion of drugs may be delayed; so again, doses must be reduced to avoid toxicity, and sometimes monitoring of the drug plasma level may be necessary to control dosage

Further care is necessary in infants that are seriously ill as the risks of reactions to drug treatment correspondingly increases. Care is also necessary with locally applied drugs, such as corticosteroids, as the skin of infants is thin and may allow excessive absorption to occur and cause highly undesirable systemic effects.

In general, proportion-to-age-weight doses of drugs that have a wide margin of safety are often used, but doses based on skin surface area are more satisfactory. The problems of dosage are also increased because very young children have a higher metabolic rate than adults, and in some cases they may require higher doses than body-weight might suggest. In older children, hepatic metabolism of drugs may sometimes be more rapid than that of adults, as epileptic children, for example, can tolerate relatively high doses of anticonvulsant drugs.

Doses for the elderly

Increasing age brings with it a deterioration of the glomerular filtration rate, a reduction in renal blood flow, and a general loss of renal efficiency. Those changes can result in drug accumulation, so the elderly require adjustment of drug dose no less than young children. With age, the CNS also becomes more sensitive to a wide range of drugs, and even small doses of sedatives may cause confusion. In addition, cardiovascular reflexes become impaired, and the compensatory mechanisms that normally prevent any fall in blood pressure when getting up quickly may fail, and the elderly may experience attacks of dizziness. Postural hypotension may occur with diuretic and antihypertensive therapy. Acute infections can also cause a temporary but significant reduction in plasma proteins levels, and so alter the concentration of protein-bound drugs with unexpected effects on target organ response. Confusion may also occur as a result of over-medication, as multiple therapy increases the risks of drug reactions as well as that of accidental overdose. In general, drug treatment for the elderly should be kept as simple as possible, and dosage times should be linked with some recurring factor, such as a favourite television programme, to improve patient compliance with treatment.

Drugs in pregnancy and lactation

In pregnancy, drugs may cross the placental barrier and affect the fetus, a fact that was highlighted by the thalidomide disaster. Many antibiotics, and drugs which influence the central nervous system, may pass into the fetal circulation and as fetal enzymes and renal excretory mechanisms are poorly developed, the metabolism of such drugs is correspondingly slow, and their effects may be prolonged.

For many drugs, there is insufficient evidence to be certain that they are harmless to the fetus, especially during the first trimester of pregnancy, and ideally no drug should be given during pregnancy unless its use is essential, and balanced against the risks involved. The absence of such a warning about any drug referred to in the text does not imply, and must not be taken to imply, that the drug can be given during pregnancy.

Similar caution is necessary during lactation, as many drugs appear in breast milk. Although the amount of drug actually received by the breast-fed infant may often be clinically insignificant, that is not always the case (Table 1.3). A few drugs may also affect the milk flow. The dopamine antagonists metoclopramide and domperidone are said to improve lactation by stimulating the production of prolactin, whereas bromocriptine, a dopamine agonist, is used to suppress lactation. On rational grounds, iodine compounds should be avoided during breast feeding, as an excessive amount of iodine in breast milk could cause thyroid disturbance in the infant, although the actual risk of an excessive amount of iodine appearing in the breast milk may be slight. The risks of adverse drug reaction in infants can be reduced by avoiding breast feeding when the drug–milk level is likely to be high, usually 2 hours or so after oral administration, by using drugs with short half-lives, and avoiding long-acting products.

Presentation of drugs and patient compliance

There are three main stages in the treatment of illness: diagnosis, prescription of treatment and compliance by the patient with that treatment. Yet many patients fail to collect their prescribed medicines, and some who collect them do not take them; so unless patients comply with treatment, diagnosis and prescrip-

Table 1.3 Drugs that should be avoided in breast feeding. The following notes are a general guide only, as in many cases information is scanty. It should be assumed that if a drug of a certain class is listed, related drugs may have a similar pattern of excretion. The omission of any drug does *not* imply that it is suitable for use during breast feeding, as such use remains the responsibility of the prescriber

Drug	Problem
amiodarone	An iodine-containing anti-arrhythmic drug. There is a theoretical risk that it could cause thyroid disturbance
androgens	Could cause masculinization of female and precocious development in male babies; could suppress lactation
aspirin	May cause Rey's syndrome (see p. 102); impairs platelet function in high doses
atropine	Anticholinergic effects
benzodiazepines	Extended use could cause lethargy and weight loss
bromocriptine	May suppress lactation
calcitonin	Best avoided; may inhibit lactation
carbimazole	May depress thyroid function
chloramphenicol	An antibiotic that could cause 'grey baby' syndrome, with vomiting, cyanosis and collapse, as well as bone marrow toxicity
colchicine	Has cytotoxic properties
corticosteroids	Large doses could depress adrenal function
cyclosporin	Best avoided; may appear in breast milk
cytotoxics	Could depress bone marrow function
doxepin	May cause sedation and depress respiration
ergotamine	Could cause ergotism
ethosuximide	Could cause excitability
ganciclovir	Is teratogenic and best avoided
gold	Idiosyncratic reactions and rash
indomethacin	Appreciable amounts in breast milk, risk of neuropathy
isoniazid	Theoretical risk of convulsions
isotretinoin	Is teratogenic and best avoided
lithium	May cause lithium toxicity with cyanosis, neonatal goitre
meprobamate	Appreciable amount in breast milk; may cause drowsiness
metronidazole	Best avoided; may appear in breast milk
nalidixic acid	Avoid in G6PD deficiency
nitrofurantoin	Avoid in G6PD deficiency

Table 1.3 *(cont'd)*

Drug	Problem
oestrogens	May suppress lactation and cause feminization of male infants
phenindione	Risk of haemorrhage in vitamin K deficiency
phenolphthalein	May cause diarrhoea
progestogens	May suppress lactation
sulphonamides	May possibly cause kernicterus in jaundiced infants, and haemolysis in G6PD deficiency
sulphonylureas	Could cause hypoglycaemia
sulpiride	Best avoided; appreciable amounts in breast milk
tetracyclines	Best avoided; theoretical risk of tooth discoloration
thiazide diuretics	Large doses may suppress lactation
vitamins A and D	Best avoided; risk of hypercalcaemia with high doses of vitamin D

tion writing are virtually a waste of time. Nurses can help by educating patients on the importance of treatment; tactful questioning may reveal non-compliance, and much has been done to increase the acceptability of drugs by improvements in presentation. The main point about drug presentation is that whatever method is used, the activity of the drug must be maintained, and successful formulation requires a wide knowledge of the chemistry, pharmacology, solubility, stability and activity of drugs. Even the choice of a suitable container is of considerable importance in ensuring that a product will retain its stability. The term 'bioavailability' is sometimes used to indicate that different formulations of a drug may affect the eventual release and availability of the contained drug after it has been administered.

 Griffith S A 1990 A review of the factors associated with patient compliance and the taking of prescribed medicines. British Journal of General Practice 40: 114–116

Many preparations of drugs now on the market exhibit considerable ingenuity in the means employed to increase acceptability or prolong the action of the drug, but basically the preparations of drugs used in therapeutics can be divided into three main groups — i.e. oral preparations, injections and applications. Each group may be further subdivided, and examples of most forms of presentation will be found in the British National Formulary (BNF).

Oral preparations

Tablets. One of the most satisfactory and reliable forms of oral medication. They have the great advantage over liquid medicines of affording an accurate dose. A few tablets, notably those containing glyceryl trinitrate, are designed to be placed under the tongue, to promote the absorption and reduce the breakdown of the drug, but many tablets are coated to improve stability and appearance, and contain additives to ensure disintegration and absorption in the intestinal tract.

In cases where the drug is a gastric irritant or is broken down by gastric acid, a so-called 'enteric' coating may be used. Such coating is designed to permit the tablet to pass unchanged into the intestine. Some long-acting tablets contain the drug in the interstices of a porous plastic core, from which the active compound is slowly leached out as the tablet passes along the alimentary tract.

It should *not* be assumed that different sustained-action tablets, although containing the same amount of a drug, will all release the drug at the same rate, or that they are necessarily bio-equivalent, or interchangeable, as different formulations may be used by different manufacturers.

Nurses should always advise patients to take tablets and capsules in a standing or sitting position, and with adequate fluid, to avoid delay in oesophageal transit. Such delay may cause oesophageal damage, and has occurred with some non-steroidal anti-inflammatory drugs, with slow-release potassium preparations, and with other drugs including some antibiotics. Such precautionary measures are of general application, and the risks will not be referred to again when discussing individual drugs.

Channer K S, Virjee J 1992 Effect of posture and drink volume on the swallowing of capsules. British Medical Journal 285: 1702

Nurses should also warn patients that long-acting tablet products should be swallowed whole, not chewed or divided by cutting, otherwise the extended action of the product will be lost. Some standard tablet products, on the other hand, have a 'split line' to facilitate the administration of divided doses.

Capsules. Small containers made of hard gelatin, resembling a cylindrical box with a very deep lid. They are useful as a means of administering bitter drugs, and are popular as containers for orally-active antibiotics. Flexible gelatin capsules are also used occasionally, particularly for small doses of unpleasant liquids such as chlormethiazole. Capsules should be swallowed whole, with water, and no attempt should be made to open or split a capsule. Most capsules are now sealed to prevent such manipulation.

Mixtures. Mixtures are aqueous solutions or suspensions of drugs in water, together with flavouring or suspending agents. They were once the most popular form of drug presentation, but have been largely replaced by tablets and capsules.

Mixtures, however, are still of value in selected circumstances, and it is worth noting that some are still described in the BNF. The standard dose of mixtures in the BNF is 10 ml, and Kaolin and Morphine. Mixture is a familiar example.

Elixirs and syrups. Flavoured and sweetened solutions or suspensions of drugs, often suitable for administration in small doses to children. Some oral antibiotic products are presented as elixirs or syrups.

Emulsion. A term applied to mixtures of oils and water, rendered homogeneous by the addition of other substances known as emulsifying agents. Liquid Paraffin Emulsion is an example of an oil-in-water emulsion and contains methyl cellulose as the emulsifying agent.

Linctus. A sweet, syrupy preparation of a drug used in the treatment of cough, e.g. Codeine Linctus, Simple Linctus.

Tinctures. Tinctures are alcoholic solutions of the active principles of crude drugs.

Inhalations

Modern oral aerosol inhalers represent a valuable method of administering drugs such as bronchodilators or corticosteroids in a form that permits rapid absorption of small doses with reduced

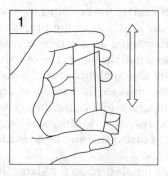

Remove the cover from the mouthpiece and shake the inhaler vigorously.

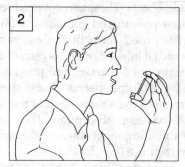

Holding the inhaler as shown, breathe out gently (but not fully) and then immediately...

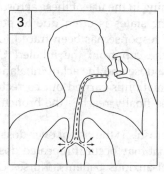

Place the mouthpiece in the mouth and close your lips around it. After starting to breathe in slowly and deeply through your mouth, press the inhaler firmly, as shown, to release Ventolin and continue to breathe in.

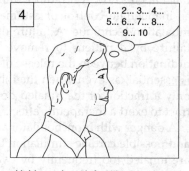

Hold your breath for 10 seconds, or as long as is comfortable, before breathing out slowly.

5

If you are to take a second inhalation you should wait at least one minute before repeating steps 2, 3 and 4.

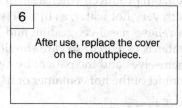

After use, replace the cover on the mouthpiece.

Figure 1.4   Diagram to indicate the use of an aerosol inhaler. (Reproduced by kind permission of Allen and Hanburys Limited, Greenford.)

side-effects. These aerosol products contain the drug in a metered-dose pressurized container, with an inert gas as the propellant. When used correctly, a dose is discharged as a very fine spray, which if inhaled orally, is carried deep into the lungs. The effectiveness can be markedly improved by the combined use of aerosol 'large volume spacers'. These spacers increase the amount of drug reaching the airways and at the same time reduce the dosage loss by systemic absorption. They are readily available, and every asthmatic patient should be aware of their value and be instructed in their use (Fig. 1.4).

The area of lung surface available for absorption is so large that the response to an inhaled dose may be almost as rapid as that following an injection. Such devices permit a patient to give himself a dose at a time of need when a rapid response is essential. Patients however require training in the use of these aerosols, as inadequate control of asthmatic states is often due to poor inhalation technique. A failure of response has been traced to a failure by a patient to remove the cap from the inhaler! Co-ordination between the release of a dose and the act of inhalation is essential, as even when the inhalation is carried out correctly, only a fraction of the inhaled dose finally reaches the bronchial tract to exert a therapeutic effect.

A danger with bronchodilator aerosols is the risk of over-dosage and possible cardiac stimulation that may occur if repeated doses are inhaled too frequently by over-anxious patients. Nurses can play a valuable part by giving explicit instructions to patients about the proper use of aerosol inhalation devices. It should be noted that sodium cromoglycate, when used for the *prophylactic* treatment of asthma, is given by oral inhalation of the dry powder.

The term 'inhalation' also refers to the steam inhalation of the volatile constituents of such products as Compound Tincture of Benzoin produced when a small amount of the product is mixed with very hot water, as in a Nelson inhaler. The method is used to relieve nasal congestion and liquefy sputum, but really hot water is essential, so care should be taken by nurses to protect themselves and the patient by avoiding both spillage and direct contact of the hot container or its contents with the skin.

Injections

An injection is a sterile solution or suspension of a drug intended for parenteral administration. It may be prepared for administration by intramuscular, subcutaneous or intravenous injection, or less frequently by intra-articular or intradermal injection. The intramuscular route is employed for most injections, as absorption is fairly rapid and even potentially irritant solutions of drugs may be tolerated by this route. Subcutaneous injections are absorbed more slowly, and may be less well tolerated.

The rate of response to an injection can sometimes be modified. The addition of adrenaline to local anaesthetic solutions such as lignocaine delays absorption and extends the action by constricting adjacent blood vessels, and an extended action can occasionally be obtained by giving a drug by intramuscular injection as an oily solution. (*Oily solutions must always be given by intramuscular injection.*) In other cases, a greatly prolonged action can be obtained by injecting the drug in a chemically modified form. Fluphenazine decanoate, for example, which is used in chronic schizophrenia, has a long action that permits dosing at intervals of 4–6 weeks.

Drugs which are too irritant to be given intramuscularly can often be given in dilute solution by slow intravenous injection or by intravenous infusion.

Intrathecal injections are occasionally employed when the drug concerned does not penetrate the blood–brain barrier easily, and direct injection into the CSF is necessary, as in the treatment of meningitis. Intra-articular injection refers to the injection of a solution or suspension of a drug into a joint. In ophthalmology, a few drugs may occasionally be given by subconjunctival injection.

Some vaccine products are given by subcutaneous injection, but intradermal injection is used mainly for diagnostic agents.

Injections are best supplied as ampoules, which are sealed glass containers containing a single dose. Multiple-dose containers are also used but are less satisfactory. All solutions supplied in multiple-dose containers must contain a preservative to guard against the risk of accidental bacterial contamination of the contents.

Rectal preparations

The rectal route of administration of drugs remains largely unexploited, although it has the advantages of largely avoiding first-pass metabolism, permits medication during nausea and vomiting, and is an alternative to an injection in unconscious patients.

Suppositories. Solid products, torpedo or cone-shaped, for rectal administration. They contain an active drug in a base that melts at body temperature. As absorption from the rectal mucosa is slow, the contained drug has an extended action. Indomethacin suppositories for example are used at night to reduce morning stiffness in arthritic patients. Glycerin (glycerol) suppositories on the other hand have a simple laxative action and are used in the treatment of constipation. Pessaries, or vaginal suppositories, are formulated to have a local effect on the vaginal tract. Suppositories are normally inserted via the pointed end, but a recent paper suggests that retention is more certain if the blunt end is inserted first.

 Walker R 1992 The correct insertion of rectal suppositories. British Journal of Pharmaceutical Practice 4: 8–10

Enemas. Solutions administered per rectum as (a) laxatives or (b) retention enemas. Laxative enemas include soft soap solution, now used infrequently, and sodium phosphate or magnesium sulphate solutions. These latter solutions are available as prepacked disposable products, and have a laxative effect by distending the bowel. Oxyphenisatin and docusate sodium enemas are used mainly for bowel clearance before radiological examination or surgery.

Retention enemas include arachis oil for softening impacted faeces; magnesium sulphate, occasionally used to increase the water content of the bowel to produce a temporary lowering of intracranial pressure; prednisolone and salazopyrin, used to reduce inflammation in ulcerative colitis.

Preparations for local application

Conventional products for application to the skin can be divided into the following main groups.

Creams. These are semi-solid emulsions, and differ from ointments in containing a high proportion of water, e.g. Aqueous Cream and Hydrocortisone Cream.

Liniments. Thin creams or oily preparations of drugs, intended for application to the skin to relieve mild pain, as pain can be relieved to some extent by rubbing the skin with a mildly irritant product. A number of proprietary products for the relief of rheumatic and other pain are formulated on that basis.

Lotions. Solutions or suspensions (shake lotions) of drugs for application to the skin, wounds or mucous membranes, e.g. Calamine Lotion and Aluminium Acetate Lotion.

Ointments. Semi-solid preparations mainly used for application to dry skin lesions. Most ointment bases contain soft paraffin, often with other agents such as emulsifying waxes or wool fat. Wool fat, also known as lanolin, may cause a sensitivity reaction with some patients.

Pastes. Stiff ointments, often containing a large amount of zinc oxide, e.g. Zinc Oxide and Salicylic Acid Paste.

Absorption from the skin

Many preparations for application to the skin have a local or protective action. The skin is not an inert barrier, and has a multi-layer structure, and some locally applied drugs, such as some anti-inflammatory corticosteroids, are taken up by the stratum corneum, from which slow diffusion of the drug into the lower layers of the skin takes place. Systemic effects from such locally applied steroids are not common, but may occur if large areas of inflamed skin are so treated, or if occlusive dressings are used. In such cases significant amounts of the drug may reach the circulation via the dermal capillaries to cause systemic side-effects, particularly where children are concerned.

On the other hand, the value of the skin as a means of drug administration which in the past has been largely overlooked, is now being exploited, as shown by the development of a skin patch for the transdermal absorption of glyceryl trinitrate for the treatment of angina. The patch includes a drug-containing reservoir and a rate-controlling membrane. Release and absorption of the contained glyceryl trinitrate occurs at a steady rate, and the virtually complete metabolic destruction of the drug that occurs after oral administration is avoided (Fig. 1.5).

Similar skin patches are available for replacement therapy in the menopause, and nicotine patches to assist those wishing to give up the smoking habit.

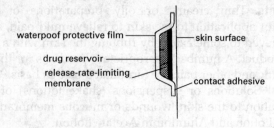

waterpoof protective film — skin surface

drug reservoir

release-rate-limiting membrane

contact adhesive

Figure 1.5 Diagram of glyceryl trinitrate skin patch.

Liposomes

New or more effective ways of administering drugs are under investigation as alternatives to conventional therapy, and one of these developments is the use of liposomes. Liposomes can be described briefly as very small vesicles, bounded by layers of phospholipids, glycolipids or other substances according to the method of manufacture. Small quantities of a drug can be encapsulated in these liposomes, and the method is a new concept in drug administration.

The advantages of a liposome-entrapped drug include the use of smaller doses, a decrease in toxicity and rapidity of degradation, and the possibility of achieving a localized effect on a target organ or tissue. The use of liposomes containing drugs has already been tried out in the treatment of cancer, and liposome-entrapped corticosteroids have been used by intra-articular injection in the treatment of rheumatoid arthritis. The method has been adopted for the presentation of amphotericin in the treatment of fungal infections (p. 165) and further developments can be expected.

2

Sedatives, hypnotics and anaesthetics

Drugs which depress some part of the central nervous system represent one of the largest and most important groups of therapeutic agents. They include hypnotics, sedatives, tranquillizers, antidepressants, anticonvulsants, narcotics, anaesthetics and analgesics. This chapter deals with sedatives and hypnotics, with merely brief notes on general anaesthesia.

SEDATIVES AND HYPNOTICS

Sedatives, now often referred to as anxiolytics, are drugs that reduce mental activity, and thus predispose to sleep, whereas hypnotics are sleep-inducing drugs. There is no sharp distinction between the groups, as small doses of some hypnotics have useful sedative properties and large doses of anxiolytics promote sleep.

The mode of action of drugs that depress the central nervous system, and so have a sedative or hypnotic action, is highly complex and not clearly understood. It is considered that many such depressants act on the cortex and the reticular formation of the brain, which receives stimuli such as light, noise and pain, as well as internal stress factors such as anxiety and emotion. Stimulation of the reticular formation leads to cerebral cortex arousal and wakefulness, and CNS depressants may act by depressing such activity, or they may have a more direct action on the cerebral cortex involving gamma-aminobutyric acid (GABA p. 32).

Sedatives and hypnotics are in general unspecific depressants of the CNS. They are widely used in the treatment of insomnia due to anxiety and stress, but before they are given, it should be remembered that simple measures, such as adequate physical relaxation and absence of stimulants will often promote sleep. Many drugs can also cause sleep disturbances, for example, most beta-blockers and steroids. In some cases, such side-effects may be reduced by avoiding evening administration. Experienced nurses are often in a better position to assess a patient's need for sedation than is the visiting doctor.

It should be borne in mind that although drug-induced sleep may appear to resemble natural sleep, the two are far from being identical. Natural sleep has two main phases, referred to as the orthodox or slow-wave phase, and the paradoxical or REM (rapid eye movement) phase. Hypnotic drugs may suppress the REM phase, and also influence the orthodox phase. The latter plays an important part in the growth and restoration of body tissues, but the REM phase is linked with the restorative activities of brain tissue.

Thus both sedatives and hypnotics should be regarded as drugs for short-term treatment only, as tolerance and dependence may occur with extended use. They may cause confusion in the

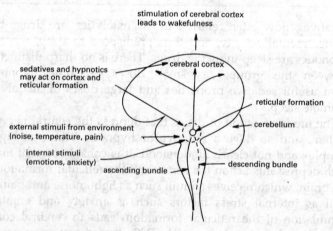

Figure 2.1 Diagram of central nervous system and points of action of some CNS depressants.

elderly, who are more susceptible to the action of such drugs and whenever possible, the cause of the anxiety and insomnia should be sought. Insomnia is often associated with depression, and treatment of the depression may indirectly relieve the insomnia. Similarly, when insomnia is due to pain, measures should be taken to relieve the pain before giving an hypnotic.

Drug dependence

Sedatives and hypnotics may cause drug dependence with extended use. The condition is such that the patient has a strong desire to continue taking the drug, often in increasing doses, and the development of withdrawal symptoms occurs if the drug is withdrawn. Such symptoms include apprehension, anxiety, dizziness, tremor, tachycardia and insomnia. Later symptoms include hallucinations. Abrupt withdrawal should be avoided, as otherwise severe withdrawal symptoms may be precipitated suddenly.

Points about hypnotics

(a) Hypnotics should normally be given about 20–30 minutes before going to bed to give time for absorption. The exceptions are zolpidem, which has a rapid action and is taken immediately before retiring, and the antihistamines diphenhydramine and promethazine. Their onset of action is slow, and they should be given about 2 hours before retiring.

(b) Low initial doses, especially in the elderly.

(c) Treatment should be limited to 2–3 weeks, and preferably intermittent, as on alternate nights or one night in three.

(d) The onset of drug-induced sleep may be followed by a deterioration of a patient's condition.

(e) If dependence has occurred, withdrawal must be carried out slowly to avoid the sudden onset of withdrawal symptoms.

BARBITURATES (Table 2.1)

The barbiturates have long been used as hypnotics and sedatives, but their use has declined markedly in recent years following the introduction of the less toxic benzodiazepines. They are still used to a limited extent in the treatment of severe intractable insomnia but repeated doses are cumulative, and tolerance and dependence may occur. Abrupt withdrawal may result in rebound insomnia and severe withdrawal symptoms. Tolerance is linked with the induction of liver enzymes (p. 5), which increases the risks of reactions with other drugs, including alcohol. Coma and death have occurred from alcohol–barbiturate-induced respiratory depression. Many authorities now consider that the barbiturates have no place in modern therapy. The following barbiturates are still available, but prescriptions must now comply with the Misuse of Drugs Regulations (CD).

Table 2.1 Barbiturates

Approved name	Brand name	Dose
amylobarbitone	Amytal	100–200 mg
amylobarbitone sodium	Sodium Amytal	100–200 mg
butobarbitone	Soneryl	100–200 mg
quinalbarbitone sodium	Seconal Sodium	100–200 mg
amylobarbitone sodium quinalbarbitone sodium }	Tuinal	100–200 mg

---

Points about barbiturates

(a) Barbiturates are used only in severe and intractable insomnia.
(b) Warn patients of the combined effects of alcohol.

BENZODIAZEPINES

The benzodiazepines are a widely used group of drugs, as some are hypnotics, but others have anxiolytic or tranquillizing properties, depending to some extent on the dose (see diazepam, p. 60). The ideal hypnotic should evoke a condition resembling normal sleep, and of adequate duration, yet it should not have any residual hangover effects or risk of dependence. That ideal drug still awaits discovery, but some benzodiazepines have certain advantages over older drugs.

Benzodiazepines (BZs) have a selective action on the central nervous system, and appear to act by augmenting the effects of the neurotransmitter GABA (gamma aminobutyric acid). GABA inhibits excitability by binding to specific GABA-receptors in the cerebral cortex. Some specific BZ-receptors have also been identfied that seem to be coupled with the GABA-receptors in some way to form a GABA/BZ-receptor complex in the cerebral cortex. The benzodiazepines thus appear to have an hypnotic action mediated by an inhibition of neuronal response to stimulation. As a group, the BZs have a wide margin of safety with reduced side-effects, and are often regarded as first-choice drugs for the short-term treatment of the more severe forms of insomnia. Those BZs listed in Table 2.2 exhibit a range of hypnotic activity, as some have a short action and are therefore of less value when early awakening is a problem, and others have a long action with which some daytime sedation may be experienced. Car-driving ability and similar activities may be impaired, of which patients should be warned. The benzodiazepines have few side-effects, but an occasional paradoxical response is a varying degree of excitement and aggression. They do not induce the production of microsomal enzymes by the liver, so reactions with other drugs are less likely. Dependence on the benzodiazepines is a risk, and they should not be used continuously for more than 4 weeks.

Withdrawal symptoms may occur with any BZ, but are more common after extended treatment, or after high doses, and result in a syndrome of rebound insomnia, anxiety, tremor and loss of appetite. Rapid withdrawal should be avoided, as a toxic psychosis with convulsions may be precipitated.

The use of benzodiazepines and other supplementary agents in anxiety and tension states is referred to on page 158.

Points about benzodiazepines

(a) Normally for short-term treatment.
(b) Drowsiness is a side-effect—warn patients about car-driving.
(c) Alcohol may have additive effects and should be avoided.
(d) Withdrawal of treatment should be slow.

Table 2.2 Benzodiazepine hypnotics

Approved name	Brand name	Dose
flunitrazepam[b]	Rohypnol	0.5–1 mg
flurazepam[b]	Dalmane	15–30 mg
loprazolam[a]	Dormonoct	1–2 mg
lormetazepam[a]		0.5–1 mg
nitrazepam[b]	Mogadon	5–10 mg
temazepam	Normisan	10–60 mg

[a] Short-acting hypnotics.
[b] Long-acting hypnotics.

Nitrazepam § (dose: 5–10 mg)

Brand name: Mogadon §

Nitrazepam is a long-acting benzodiazepine hypnotic used mainly when some degree of daytime sedation is tolerated. Induction of sleep begins within 30 minutes, and any subsequent arousal and return to sleep tends to follow a natural pattern. Nitrazepam is given in doses of 5–10 mg, but the smaller doses should be used in the elderly and the full response may not be seen immediately in patients who have been receiving barbiturates.

Adverse effects include hangover, dreaming with nightmares, and paradoxically, agitation and aggression have been noted with some patients. As with all benzodiazepines, care is necessary in respiratory disease and in renal or hepatic impairment.

Temazepam § (dose: 10–30 mg)

Brand name: Normison §

Temazepam is a short-acting benzodiazepine hypnotic of value in the elderly, to whom doses of 5–15 mg should be given. Cumulative effects in standard doses are not common, but some daytime sedation may occur if high doses are given for severe insomnia.

Zolpidem §

Brand name: Stilnoct §

The benzodiazepines bind to a group of BZ-receptor sites. Zolpidem, although not a benzodiazepine, is referred to here as it binds selectively to a subgroup of BZ-receptors, and is used in the short-term treatment of insomnia. It has a rapid action, and is given in doses of 10 mg immediately before retiring, and in doses of 5 mg for the elderly, and in hepatic or renal impairment. Side-effects are drowsiness, dizziness and gastrointestinal disturbances. Unlike the benzodiazepines, zolpidem has no anticonvulsant or muscle relaxant properties.

Benzodiazepine antagonist:

Flumazenil § (dose: 100–400 micrograms by intravenous infusion)

Brand name: Anexate §

Some benzodiazepines are used for their sedative effects in intensive care units, and also as supplementary agents in anaesthesia. The subsequent reversal of those effects is often desirable, and a new benzodiazepine antagonist for that purpose is flumazenil. It acts as a competitive inhibitor at BZ-receptor binding sites, and following intravenous injection it brings about a rapid reversal of the hypno-sedative effects of the benzodiazepines, and a return of spontaneous respiration and consciousness in anaethesized patients.

The use of flumazenil requires care, as the action of the drug is relatively brief, and the sedative effects of the benzodiazepine may return within a few hours, when further flumazenil treatment may be required. Flumazenil is given by slow intravenous injection or infusion in an initial dose of 200 micrograms, followed by 100 microgram doses at 1 minute intervals as required. If drowsiness recurs, further doses of 100–400 micrograms hourly should be given, adjusted to individual need and response. Care should be taken not to arouse patients too rapidly, as they may become agitated. It is contraindicated in epileptics who have received extended treatment with a benzodiazepine. The possibility of using flumazenil in the treatment of benzodiazepine overdose, and controlling the symptoms of acute benzodiazepine withdrawal is under investigation.

Sanders L D et al 1991 Reversal of benzodiazepine sedation with the antagonist flumazenil. British Journal of Anaesthesiology 66: 445–453

OTHER HYPNOTICS AND SEDATIVES
Chloral hydrate § (dose: 0.5–2 g)

Brand name: Noctec §

Chloral hydrate is an old drug that is useful when a mild and safe hypnotic is required. It is rapidly absorbed, and metabolized to trichloroethanol, to which the sedative action is finally due. It may be given as Chloral Mixture (500 mg/5 ml) in doses of 5–20 ml, but as chloral hydrate has some gastric irritant properties, the mixture should be well diluted with water. The mixture may be given to children of 6–12 years in doses of 5–10 ml. Chloral is a useful sedative for infants, and may be given as Chloral Elixir Paediatric in doses of 5 ml (well diluted) to infants up to 1 year of age. Chloral hydrate cannot be formulated as a tablet, but it forms a stable complex with betaine, which is present in Welldorm tablets, each equivalent to 414 mg of chloral. The compound breaks down rapidly in the stomach to release the active drug. A derivative of trichloroethanol is also available as Triclofos Elixir (500 mg/5 ml).

Chlormethiazole § (dose: 192–384 mg)

Brand name: Heminevrin §

Chlormethiazole is a short-acting hypnotic of value in the elderly, especially when some agitation is present, as it has little hangover action. It is given in doses of 192–384 mg as capsules or syrup at night, and doses of 192 mg may be given three times a day for restlessness, agitation and confusional states. Dependence may occur with extended treatment.

Chlormethiazole is also used under hospital control to treat acute withdrawal symptoms in alcoholics. Such treatment requires care, and resuscitation facilities must be available, as severe respiratory depression may occur.

Chlormethiazole is also used intravenously in the treatment of status epilepticus (p. 75).

Side-effects of the drug include sneezing, headache and gastrointestinal disturbance.

Paraldehyde (dose: 5–10 ml, well diluted)

Paraldehyde is a colourless liquid with a characteristic odour. It is excreted in part by the lungs, and gives an unpleasant odour to the breath. It is a safe hypnotic, as it causes little respiratory depression, but it is now used mainly in status epilepticus (p. 80).

As a hypnotic it is given in doses of 5–10 ml orally, well diluted, or by deep intramuscular injection. Doses of 5–10 ml, diluted with arachis oil or saline, may also be given rectally.

Side-effects include gastric disturbance and rash. Paraldehyde decomposes on storage, especially in partly-used bottles, with the formation of toxic breakdown products. Any discoloured paraldehyde, or that having an odour of acetic acid must be rejected.

Points about paraldehyde

(a) Use glass syringe for injections, as the drug has a solvent action on most plastics.
(b) Deep intramuscular injection to avoid excessive pain.
(c) Not more than 5 ml per injection.
(d) Vary the injection site.
(e) Discoloured drug must not be used.

Promethazine (dose: 25–75 mg)

Brand names: Phenergan, Sominex

Some anthistamines, of which promethazine is an example, have a sedative action of value in mild insomnia, and are useful in reduced doses for daytime sedation.

Promethazine is given in doses up to 50 mg at night for mild insomnia in adults. It is also useful as a hypnotic for children in doses of 15–20 mg for those of 1–5 years of age, and 20–25 mg for the 5–10 year group.

Side-effects, such as dry mouth and blurred vision, are those of the antihistamines in general (p. 434).

Trimeprazine § (dose: 3–4.5 mg/kg)

Brand name: Vallergan §

Trimeprazine has an action similar to that of promethazine, although it is used mainly in the relief of pruritus (p. 535). It is also useful as a pre-operative sedative for both adults and children, and is then given $1\frac{1}{2}$–2 hours before operation.
Dose: 3–4.5 mg/kg; children 2–4 mg/kg.

Zopiclone § (dose: 7.5–15 mg)

Brand name: Zimovane §

Zopiclone represents a new class of hypnotic agents, chemically unrelated to others in current use. It acts in a manner similar to that of the benzodiazepines by modulating the action of the neurotransmitter GABA, but has a different receptor binding site. Zopiclone is indicated for the short-term treatment of insomnia, including early awakening, and for the insomnia secondary to psychiatric disturbances. It initiates sleep rapidly, does not reduce REM sleep, and has little residual hangover action. It is given in doses of 7.5–15 mg at night, with initial doses of 3.75 mg for the elderly.

Side-effects of zopiclone are similar to those of many hypnotics, but are usually less common, the most frequent side-effect being a bitter or metallic after-taste.

 Tyrer P 1990 Zopiclone. British Journal of Hospital Medicine 44: 264–265

GENERAL ANAESTHETICS

These vary widely from simple gases to complex organic chemicals, but fall easily into two main groups — those given by inhalation, and those given by intravenous injection. The mode of action of general anaesthetics on the central nervous system is still far from clear and their diverse chemical structure suggests that they do not all act on identical receptor sites. They all act by depressing the CNS and produce unconsciousness, analgesia and muscle relaxation. The ideal anaesthetic would be rapidly effective, metabolically inert, and be eliminated without delay. No single drug has all the required properties, and in practice anaesthesia is often induced by an intravenous drug, and maintained by an inhalation anaesthetic, together with muscle relaxant and other supplementary drugs. Injected drugs reach the brain by crossing the blood–brain barrier, and recovery takes place as the drug is temporarily taken up by body tissues for subsequent elimination. Inhalation anaesthetics reach the brain after being taken up by the blood from the alveolar space, and recovery occurs as the concentration of the drug in the brain subsequently falls.

Surgical anaesthesia is characterized by loss of both consciousness and pain, and an adequate degree of relaxation of muscle. Three main stages are recognized. Stage I — a stage in which the perception of pain is reduced, or almost suppressed, but the patient is still conscious, although very detached. Stage II — a very variable stage in which consciousness is lost, but irrational acts of an excited nature can occur. This stage is not common with intravenous anaesthetics. Stage III — surgical anaesthesia. In this stage the irregular breathing of Stage II becomes steady, reflexes are abolished, and a progressive muscular relaxation occurs as anaesthesia deepens. The depth of anaesthesia is controlled according to surgical needs.

The speed of induction of anaesthesia varies with the nature of the anaesthetic. A slow induction occurs when a volatile anaesthetic such as ether is taken up extensively by the blood, as subsequent diffusion into the brain is secondary to the saturation of the blood with the anaesthetic. Recovery from a highly blood-soluble anaesthetic such as halothane is correspondingly delayed, as the blood acts as a reservoir from which the anaesthetic is slowly released.

Before the introduction of muscle relaxants, adequate relaxation could be achieved only by full anaesthesia, with undesired toxic side-effects. Now, by suitable premedication and the use of relaxants, a relatively light plane of anaesthesia is often adequate, thus reducing shock and trauma, and enabling major operations to be carried out in the elderly that were once considered impossible. In all cases, before general anaesthesia is carried out, the effects of any drugs that the patient may already be receiving should be reviewed.

A rare but very serious occurrence during inhalation anaesthesia is malignant hyperthermia or hyperpyrexia. It appears to be triggered off in susceptible patients by anaesthetic drugs, usually halothane and suxamethonium. It is a genetically determined condition, linked with a sudden increase in the concentration of calcium in muscle cells. Early tachycardia with hyperventilation may occur, followed by skeletal muscle rigidity and hyperthermia. Pulmonary oedema and renal failure are later symptoms.

The specific therapy is the *early* intravenous injection of the skeletal muscle relaxant dantrolene, which inhibits calcium movement in muscle cells, and brings about muscle relaxation, a reduction of the raised body temperature, and a decrease in heart rate. Treatment should be commenced immediately the syndrome is diagnosed with the intravenous injection of dantrolene sodium in a dose of 1 mg/kg, repeated according to response up to an average total dose of 2.5 mg/kg, although total doses of up to 10 mg/kg have been given. Care must be taken to avoid extravasation. The oral use of dantrolene for prophylaxis in susceptible patients may be of value and the drug is then given in a dose of 5 mg/kg 24 hours before surgery.

Ward A et al 1986 Dantrolene: a review of its properties and therapeutic use in malignant hyperthermia. Drugs 32: 130–168

INHALATION ANAESTHETICS
Chloroform

A clear heavy liquid with a characteristic odour. It is of historical interest as one of the first inhalation anaesthetics, but is now rarely used.

Cyclopropane

Cyclopropane is an inflammable gas, and is supplied in orange-coloured cylinders. It is a non-irritant, volatile anaesthetic, for use in closed-circuit apparatus, as it forms an explosive mixture with air and oxygen. It is used mainly for induction. Cyclopropane causes little hypotension, and recovery is rapid, although some restlessness and postoperative vomiting may occur. It causes some respiratory depression which may lead to cardiac irregularities, and adrenaline and related drugs should therefore be avoided during cyclopropane anaesthesia.

Ether (diethylether)

A clear, colourless, inflammable liquid. Although it has a wide margin of safety, both induction and recovery are slow, and postoperative nausea and vomiting are common. The vapour forms an explosive mixture with oxygen, and ether is now used much less frequently.

Halothane

Brand name: Fluothane

A clear colourless liquid with a chloroform-like odour. It is a volatile anaesthetic of high potency with which induction is smooth and rapid and the incidence of postoperative vomiting low. It is often used with nitrous oxide–oxygen mixtures from calibrated vaporizers. It has the advantages of not being inflammable, or forming explosive mixtures with air or oxygen, but it may cause hypotension, respiratory depression and cardiac arrhythmias. Severe liver dysfunction and jaundice have occasionally followed halothane anaesthesia, and the drug should not be given to patients with liver damage. Repeated exposure within 3 months should be avoided, and halothane should never again be given to a patient who has had unexplained jaundice or pyrexia after halothane anaesthesia.

Enflurane

Enflurane is a widely used volatile anaesthetic of the halothane type. It has the advantage of causing less hepatotoxicity, as it largely escapes metabolism, so, unlike halothane, it can be used when repeated anaesthesia is required. It is usually given in association with nitrous oxide–oxygen anaesthesia from a calibrated vaporizer. Enflurane may cause some respiratory depression, but side-effects such as ventricular dysrhythmias are uncommon. Desflurane § (Suprane §)▼ is a new low-potency inhalation anaesthetic. Cough, laryngospasm and increased secretions are side-effects.

Nitrous oxide

The oldest and safest of the inhalation anaesthetics. It is a gas at ordinary temperatures, but for anaesthetic purposes it is compressed and supplied in blue cylinders. It is used for the induction and maintenance of anaesthesia, usually as a 50–70% nitrous oxide–oxygen mixture, often in association with other anaesthetic agents. Combined or sequential use may permit lower overall dosage.

In weaker concentrations it produces analgesia without anaesthesia, and Entonox, a 50% mixture of nitrous oxide and oxygen, can be given by self-administration from suitable apparatus for obstetric analgesia. Entonox also has applications in changing painful dressings, and in first-aid ambulance work. Theatre nurses should remember that prolonged exposure to nitrous oxide may cause a megaloblastic anaemia by an alteration of vitamin B_{12} activity. It is of interest that a mixture of nitrous oxide and xenon, one of the rare gases of the atmosphere, is under investigation as an anaesthetic.

INTRAVENOUS ANAESTHETICS

Intravenous anaesthetics are rapidly-acting drugs used mainly for induction, although they may be used alone for short operations. They are highly lipid-soluble, and cross the blood–brain barrier rapidly, with an arm–brain circulation time of 15–20 seconds. With these agents, the induction phase characteristic of inhalation anaesthesia is absent, and surgical anaesthesia occurs very quickly without excitement. Because of their potency and variations in individual response, overdose with cardiorespiratory depression may occur, and the use of these drugs requires care.

The sodium salts of some short-acting barbiturates, represented by thiopentone, were the first to be used as intravenous anaesthetics. Aqueous solutions of these drugs are very alkaline, and great care must be taken that none of the intravenous injection solution escapes into the surrounding tissues, as any such leakage may cause severe tissue or nerve damage. If accidentally injected intra-arterially instead of intravenously, severe and extremely painful arterial spasm is caused, followed by thrombosis which may lead to subsequent gangrene.

Thiopentone sodium §

Brand name: Intraval sodium §

Thiopentone sodium is a widely used intravenous anaesthetic, suitable for the induction of general anaesthesia, and for short duration anaesthesia in minor surgery. It is given as a freshly prepared 2.5% solution, in doses of 100–150 mg, with further doses at intervals if anaesthesia is to be prolonged. A 5% solution is also used occasionally, but it is more likely to cause venous thrombosis. It is sometimes given by continuous intravenous infusion as a 0.2–0.4% solution.

Thiopentone is used mainly for the induction of anaesthesia as it has little muscle relaxant action, and specific muscle relaxants may be required for major surgery. These should be given separately. It produces some fall in blood pressure, and care is necessary in patients with hypertension, cardiac disease or impaired liver function. Respiratory depression is common and, although relatively transient, may be severe. Recovery from thiopentone anaesthesia is usually rapid, as the drug is quickly removed from the circulation by temporary storage in the tissues, but its subsequent metabolism is slow, and some residual sedative action may persist for 24 hours.

Methohexitone sodium §

Brand name: Brietal §

The action of methohexitone sodium is similar to that of thiopentone sodium, but it is less irritant to the tissues, and recovery of consciousness is more rapid. It is useful for minor procedures in out-patient and casualty departments. Dose 50–120 mg initially as a 1–2% solution with maintenance doses of 20–40 mg at intervals of 4–7 minutes, according to response. For more prolonged anaesthesia, combined treatment with other agents is necessary.

Etomidate §

Brand name: Hypnomidate §

Etomidate is a short-acting non-barbiturate intravenous anaesthetic, used chiefly for induction. It is given in a dose of 300 micrograms/kg initially, and supplementary doses can be given at intervals of 6–10 minutes for short operations, or maintained for longer periods by other anaesthetics. Etomidate has no analgesic properties, and pre-medication is necessary to prevent pain on injection, and undesirable muscle movement during anaesthesia.

Ketamine §

Brand name: Ketalar §

This synthetic compound has an unusual type of anaesthetic–analgesic activity. It is given by slow intravenous injection in doses of 1–2 mg/kg, repeated according to need and response. A slower onset of action and a longer effect can be obtained by the deep intramuscular injection of the drug in doses of 4–10 mg/kg. It is used mainly for anaesthesia in children, but it is also used for induction of anaesthesia and its analgesic properties are of value in the management of patients with severe burns requiring skin grafts. Vivid dreams and hallucinations may occur during the recovery period, but may be reduced by premedication with droperidol in doses of 0.1 mg/kg by intramuscular injection, or by the intravenous injection of diazepam in doses of 100–200 micrograms/kg. Ketamine is also used as a supplementary analgesic in severe pain no longer responding to very high doses of opiates.

Points about ketamine
Great care must be taken not to disturb a patient recovering from ketamine anaesthesia—may cause vivid dreams and hallucinations.

Midazolam §

Brand name: Hypnovel §

Midazolam has some of the properties of diazepam, but it is used mainly for induction in doses of 200–300 mg/kg intravenously, given over 2.5–3 minutes with the patient in the supine position. Its use requires care, as the full response may be sudden, and respiratory depression and severe hypotension may occur. Continuous control of cardiac and respiratory functions are necessary with midazolam, and ready access to resuscitation facilities are essential. Midazolam is also given for premedication to produce sedation and amnesia, and is then given in doses of 7–10 micrograms/kg by intramuscular injection.

Propofol §

Brand name: Diprivan §

Propofol, or di-isopropyl phenol, is a liquid, and following intravenous injection it has an anaesthetic action similar to that of thiopentone. It is used for the induction and maintenance of anaesthesia for periods of up to 1 hour. Dose 2–2.5 mg/kg initially, with maintenance doses of 0.1–0.2 mg/kg per minute as required.

Side-effects during anaesthesia include mild hypotension, transient apnoea and bradycardia, but recovery is usually uneventful. Propofol is supplied as an emulsion, which should not be mixed with other drugs. The emulsion may cause some pain during injection, but unlike thiopentone, extravascular injection does not cause local tissue damage.

As with other intravenous anaesthetics, care is necessary in respiratory, cardiovascular or renal impairment.

Involuntary movements or convulsions may occur more frequently with propofol than with thiopentone.

Anaphylactic reactions have also been reported, and emergency treatment should be available. Occasionally, recovery of consciousness may be delayed, and an adequate period of recovery must be allowed before any day-patient who has received propofol is allowed to go.

LOCAL ANAESTHETICS

Local anaesthetics are drugs that prevent the transmission of impulses along sensory nerves, so that the impulse does not reach the central nervous system to be felt as pain. They function as cell membrane stabilizers by displacing calcium ions from their membrane sites, and so prevent the transient increase in ionic permeability that is linked with nerve impulse conduction. Small nerve fibres that convey painful stimuli are more sensitive than large fibres to such blockade, so sensory impulse conduction in such fibres can be inhibited whilst larger nerve fibres remain unaffected. As a group, local anaesthetics are of considerable importance, and can be divided into those compounds which are applied to the mucous membranes, and those which are injected. The distinction is not complete as some compounds can be used both topically and by injection. Some are used to produce regional anaesthesia by intraspinal or epidural injection.

Most local anaesthetics are used as water-soluble salts, and are of little value when applied to the unbroken skin, as they are not absorbed. Only lipid-soluble bases are so absorbed, but one product suitable for anaesthesia of the skin contains a mixture of lignocaine and prilocaine in an emulsified form as Emla. It is used to produce local anaesthesia before needle puncture and is applied under an occlusive dressing for 1–2 hours. It is of great value when children require repeated injections or venous cannulations. Minimum amounts should be used on infants, as methaemoglobinaemia has occurred after repeated daily use.

Lignocaine § (lidocaine)

Brand name: Xylocaine §

Lignocaine is one of the most active and widely used of the local anaesthetics, as it has a rapid, intense and prolonged action. It is widely employed in dentistry as a 2% solution: in infiltration and regional anaesthesia 0.25–0.5% solutions are used, often with a vasoconstrictor such as adrenaline (1–200000) to localize and extend the action, which may then last for about $1\frac{1}{2}$ hours. Such combined solutions should not be used for anaesthesia of fingers or toes, as the vasoconstrictor action may cause local tissue damage.

Side-effects of lignocaine include hypotension and bradycardia; depression of cardiac function may cause cardiac arrest. The central action may cause agitation and convulsions, and care is necessary in epilepsy. Reduced doses should be given to the elderly, and in hepatic impairment. Lignocaine is contraindicated in myasthenia gravis.

Lignocaine is well absorbed when applied to mucous membranes, and is used topically as ointment (5%), eye drops (2%) and throat spray (4%). A gel containing 2% lignocaine is used as an urethral anaesthetic before instrumentation. (The use of lignocaine in the treatment of cardiac arrhythmias is referred to on p. 181).

Bupivacaine §

Brand name: Marcain §

Bupivacaine is characterized by its extended duration of action. It is used to obtain a prolonged regional anaesthesia by nerve block, and is given by injection in doses of 2 mg/kg, up to a total dose of 150 mg, with or without added adrenaline. Further doses of up to 50 mg, may be given at intervals of 4 hours or more according to need and response. Bupivacaine is also used in doses of 10–20 mg for spinal anaesthesia, and it is given by continuous epidural injection for prolonged analgesia during labour.

Side-effects are similar to those of lignocaine.

Other local anaesthetics of interest are **prilocaine** (Citanest 0.5% and 1%), resembling lignocaine in action and uses: **oxybuprocaine** (Benoxinate 0.4%), **amethocaine** 0.5% and **proxymetacaine** (Ophthaine 0.5%) are used in ophthalmology.

Points about local anaesthetics

(a) Action may be further localized by adrenaline or noradrenaline:
(b) Such mixed injections should not be used for anaesthesia of the extremities (fingers, toes, ears, nose), as vasoconstriction of end arteries may cause tissue damage and gangrene.

Cocaine*

Cocaine is the alkaloid obtained from coca leaves and is the oldest of the local anaesthetics, but it has now been largely superseded by safer drugs. It still has a limited place in ophthalmology, as it dilates the pupil of the eye as well as producing anaesthesia. It is used as a 2–4% solution, often in association with homatropine (p. 523).

Procaine hydrochloride (novocaine)

Procaine hydrochloride was once the most widely used of the less toxic cocaine substitutes, but it has now been replaced by lignocaine. When injected as a 1–2% solution, anaesthesia is rapidly produced, and such solutions were widely employed for infiltration anaesthesia in minor surgery, regional nerve blocks, and in dentistry. Procaine is not absorbed through mucous membranes, and so is useless for surface anaesthesia.

Benzocaine

Benzocaine is virtually insoluble in water, and is used for surface anaesthesia by local application as ointment (10%) or dusting powder. It is the anaesthetic constituent of various antiseptic lozenges. Suppositories of benzocaine (500 mg) are used for painful haemorrhoids.

Spinal and epidural anaesthesia

Bupivacaine and some related drugs are used by intraspinal and epidural injection to produce a localised anaesthesia and for a full consideration of the subject the standard textbooks of anaesthesia should be consulted. Briefly, anaesthesia of the thoracic structures and the lower limbs may be obtained by injecting specially prepared local anaesthetic solutions into the spinal fluid. Such solutions are injected below the first and second lumbar vertebrae to avoid injury to the spinal cord. The area of anaesthesia can be controlled by using solutions that are lighter or heavier than the spinal fluid, and positioning the patient so that the solution flows over the appropriate nerves. Disadvantages of the method include the high risk of infection by bacteria reaching the cerebrospinal fluid, and the fall in blood pressure that often occurs.

Epidural anaesthesia is carried out by injecting the anaesthetic solution into the space outside the dura. It is free from many of the disadvantages of intraspinal anaesthesia, and is often preferred in obstetrics.

3

Tranquillizers, antidepressants, anticonvulsants and stimulants

TRANQUILLIZERS OR ANTIPSYCHOTIC DRUGS

This section refers to a highly varied group of drugs of widely different chemical structure, with a more than merely tranquillizing action, used in the treatment of anxiety, schizophrenia and other forms of mental illness. Temporary anxiety and depression is a natural reaction to an emotional stress, and in normal individuals the mental balance is soon restored. In psychotic and psychoneurotic patients this balance is markedly disturbed, with severe anxiety, tension, agitation or mania as the result.

For many years there was no specific treatment for psychiatric conditions, but the introduction of the major tranquillizers derived from phenothiazine, represented by chlorpromazine, marked a great advance in the treatment of some forms of mental illness, particularly schizophrenia. Other drugs with a more specific action on certain tissues of the brain have also been discovered, and selective antidepressant drugs such as **amitriptyline** (p. 65) are widely used.

The chlorpromazine-type drugs (Table 3.1) are described as antipsychotic or neuroleptic drugs, and less accurately as major tranquillizers. They act mainly on the subcortical tissues of the brain, including the reticular formation, and interrupt neurotransmission by a blocking action on the central dopamine recep-

Table 3.1 Phenothiazine-derived neuroleptics

Approved name	Brand name	Oral daily dose range	Dose by injection
chlorpromazine	Largactil	75–300 mg	25–50 mg i.m., 6–8 hourly
fluphenazine	Moditen	1–20 mg	
fluphenazine	Modecate		12.5–100 mg i.m., monthly
loxapine	Loxapac	20–100 mg	
methotrimeprazine	Veractil Nozinan	25–200 mg	12.5–25 mg i.m., or i.v. 6–8 hourly
pericyazine	Neulactil	10–75 mg	
perphenazine	Fentazin	8–24 mg	5–10 mg i.m., 6 hourly
prochlorperazine	Stemetil	15–50 mg	12.5–25 mg i.m., 8–12 hourly
promazine	Sparine	50–400 mg	
thioridazine	Melleril	30–600 mg	
trifluoperazine	Stelazine		1–2 mg i.m., 6–8 hourly

Note: Those phenothiazine derivatives used mainly as anti-emetics are referred to on page 332.

tors of which D_1 and D_2 are important sub-groups. The differences in the action and side-effects of the various antipsychotic drugs has been ascribed to differences in the degree of selectivity of the drug–receptor relationship.

They are used therapeutically in a wide range of severe psychiatric conditions, including schizophrenia, acute and chronic psychoses, mania, agitation and anxiety. Some have other forms of central activity, and auxiliary effects include the potentiation of anaesthetics and analgesics. They may also bring about a reduction in the perception of and reaction to pain that may be of value in terminal illness, and most members of the group have useful anti-emetic properties.

Side-effects of these powerful drugs are linked with their action on the dopamine and other receptors, which are present in the extrapyramidal (nigrostriatal) tissues as well as in the reticular formation and the limbic system. They function as dopamine antagonists, and the blockade of dopamine and related receptors results in a varying degree of parkinsonism-like (extrapyramidal) symptoms. Such symptoms can be relieved to some extent by a reduction of dose, or the administration of an antimuscarinic agent used in the treatment of parkinsonism (p. 254) such as procyclidine. Such agents should not be given prophylactively, as they may cause tardive dyskinesia.

Other side-effects include hepatic dysfunction and cholestasis, haemolytic anaemia, agranulocytosis and other blood dyscrasias, rash and contact dermatitis. Hypotension and a lowering of body temperature may occur, particularly in the elderly, and care is necessary with patients over 70 years of age. Hormonal disturbances such as galactorrhoea are occasional and troublesome side-effects, and with prolonged use in high doses, lens opacity and pigmentation of the cornea may occur. A rare but severe reaction with hyperthermia is referred to as the neuroleptic malignant syndrome. It requires immediate withdrawal of the causative drug and treatment with dantrolene (p. 40).

All these chlorpromazine-like drugs have a basically similar action, but they can be classified broadly into three groups. Group I includes those drugs with a marked sedative action and moderate anticholinergic and extrapyramidal side-effects, such as chlorpromazine, promazine and methotrimeprazine. Group II compounds are less sedating, and have fewer extrapyramidal side-effects, but the anticholinergic activity is increased, as with pericyazine, pipothiazine and thioridazine. Group III drugs, represented by fluphenazine, perphenazine, prochlorperazine and trifluoperazine, have reduced sedative and anticholinergic activity, but are more likely to induce extrapyramidal symptoms than group I or group II drugs. Some esters, such as fluphenazine decanoate, have a depot effect when injected, and are useful for maintenance therapy. With such long-acting products it is usual to give an initial test dose. In all cases, withdrawal of treatment should be slow to avoid a relapse.

Points about antipsychotics

(a) Warn patients about the sedative effects, and the increased risks of car-driving and machine-related activities.
(b) Tablets to be swallowed whole with water to avoid skin contact.
(c) Avoid over-exposure to direct sunlight.
(d) They may cause hypotension — advise patients not to stand up or get out of bed quickly.
(e) Advise patients of the need to continue treatment and consequences of abrupt withdrawal.
(f) Warn patients that parkinsonism-like side-effects may occur, and should be reported.

Chlorpromazine § (dose: 75–300 mg daily; 25–50 mg by *deep* intramuscular injection)

Brand name: Largactil §

Chlorpromazine was the first of the potent antipsychotic drugs. It has a powerful calming action on aggressive schizophrenic patients, and on those exhibiting acute behavioural disturbances. It is also valuable in the short-term treatment of acute anxiety. Chlorpromazine is also used as a pre-operative sedative, as it reduces apprehension, and by potentiating the subsequent response to anaesthesia, it permits the use of a lower dose of anaesthetic. Chlorpromazine is useful in the supplementary treatment of painful terminal disease, as it not only reduces nausea and vomiting, but brings about an emotional reduction in the awareness of pain, and augments the action of narcotic analgesics. It is occasionally useful for the control of intractable hiccups.

The initial oral dose of chlorpromazine is 75 mg daily, increased as required, with maintenance doses of 75–300 mg daily, but in some severe psychotic conditions larger doses, sometimes up to 1 g daily may be required. In acute conditions, and in emergencies when a rapid action is necessary, the drug may be given by *deep* intramuscular injection in doses of 25–50 mg, repeated as required after 6–8 hours, but transfer to oral therapy should be made as soon as possible. Chlorpromazine may also be given as a 100 mg suppository, and rectal therapy is useful when a slower but more prolonged action is required.

Side-effects. Mild side-effects, such as dryness of the mouth / and drowsiness, may occur, or paradoxically, insomnia, and extrapyramidal symptoms may develop. Other side-effects of chlorpromazine are those common to many antipsychotic drugs as already indicated. Chlorpromazine may also cause skin sensitisation and care should be taken to avoid to all contact with solutions of the drug.

Loxapine §▼(dose: 20–100 mg daily)

Brand name: Loxapac §▼

Loxapine is a new antipsychotic drug of the chlorpromazine type, with similar actions and uses and side-effects. It is given in acute and chronic psychoses in doses of 10–25 mg twice a day, slowly increased over 7–10 days if necessary up to 100 mg daily. Larger doses have been given but a daily dose of 250 mg should not be exceeded. Reduced doses are advisable in the elderly.

Related phenothiazine-derived tranquillizers

Many potent antipsychotic drugs related to chlorpromazine are available. They all have a basically similar action, but changes in chemical structure may be reflected in a reduced dose or a more selective action, or when given by injection, they may provide a long-term depot effect. Promazine for example is a less potent drug, used mainly for the control of agitation in the elderly; thioridazine is a powerful antipsychotic drug that unlike chlorpromazine has no anti-emetic properties; and methotrimeprazine has increased analgesic-enhancing potency of value in terminal illness. Available products are listed in Table 3.1.

BUTYROPHENONES AND OTHER POWERFUL ANTIPSYCHOTIC AGENTS

The butyrophenones and pharmacologically related compounds represent an important group of potent antipsychotic agents of value in the treatment of schizophrenia. Although they differ chemically from the phenothiazine derivatives represented by chlorpromazine, they resemble those drugs classified as group III (p. 51) in having reduced sedative and anticholinergic side-effects, but being more likely to induce extrapyramidal symptoms. Table 3.2 (p. 59) indicates the range of drugs available, and the following notes refer to some individual compounds.

Haloperidol § (dose: 1.5–20 mg daily; 2–10 mg by intramuscular injection)

Brand names: Serenace §, Haldol §, Fortunan §, Dozic §

Haloperidol is a butyrophenone and has some of the actions, uses and side-effects of chlorpromazine, but it is effective in smaller doses. It is used mainly in the control of severe schizophrenia, mania and paranoid psychoses, and in the treatment of behavioural disturbances. Haloperidol is also used in the supplementary short-term treatment of severe anxiety, and in the control of nausea and vomiting.

In psychoses, haloperidol is given in doses of 1.5–20 mg daily, although in very severe and resistant conditions doses of 100 mg daily or more may be required. For the rapid control of acute conditions, haloperidol may be given by intramuscular injection in doses of 2–10 mg or more according to the severity of the condition, with supplementary doses of 5 mg hourly as required. Lower doses are usually adequate in elderly and debilitated patients.

Haloperidol decanoate is a derivative that is given by deep intramuscular injection when a long-acting depot effect is required. Following a test dose of 6.25–12.5 mg, doses of 50 mg are given at intervals of 4 weeks. The response is variable, and subsequent increases in dose and interval are based on individual need. Haloperidol is also used in the short-term treatment of some non-psychotic emotional disturbances such as severe anxiety when other drugs have proved unsatisfactory, and it is then given in doses of 500 micrograms twice daily.

Side-effects of haloperidol are basically similar to those of chlorpromazine, and although extrapyramidal symptoms may be more severe, hypotension is less likely to occur. With long-term treatment, some patients may develop symptoms of tardive dyskinesia, and exhibit the involuntary movements of the tongue, mouth etc. characteristic of that condition.

Benperidol § (dose: 0.25–1.5 mg daily)

Brand name: Anquil §

Benperidol is a butyrophenone with some of the properties of haloperidol, but it is used only in the management of aberrant sexual and antisocial behaviour. Its value in such conditions has yet to be confirmed.

Clozapine § (dose: 25–450 mg daily)

Brand name: Clozaril §

Clozapine is an antipsychotic drug which differs from conventional agents which block dopamine receptors in both the limbic and striatal areas of the brain. Clozapine has an action that is mediated by a selective blockade of certain dopamine and serotonin receptors in the limbic system, and may bring about an improved balance between dopaminergic and serotoninergic neurotransmission. Clozapine is indicated in schizophrenia resistant or not responding to other neuroleptic drugs, and is given as an initial dose of 12.5 mg once or twice daily, slowly increased over 2–3 weeks up to 300 mg daily.

By its selective action, clozapine has a low incidence of extrapyramidal side-effects, but it may cause some initial drowsiness. Clozapine may cause severe neutropenia that may lead to a fatal agranulocytosis, and routine blood monitoring is *essential*. Prompt withdrawal is usually followed by a return of the neutrophil count to a more normal level in about 2 weeks. At present, the use of the drug is restricted to patients registered with the Clozaril Patient Monitoring Service (CPMS), so that treatment may be withdrawn if necessary.

Finkel M J, Schwimmer J L 1991 Clozapine — a novel antipsychotic agent. New England Journal of Medicine 325: 518–519

Droperidol § (dose: 15–100 mg daily; 5–10 mg by injection)

Brand name: Droleptan §

Droperidol is a butyrophenone of value in the control of agitation in acute psychoses, and of aggression in brain-damaged patients. It is given in doses of 25–100 mg daily, or 5–10 mg by intramuscular or intravenous injection at intervals of 4–6 hours as required. Droperidol is also used for pre-operative sedation in doses of 2.5–10 mg by intramuscular injection 30–60 minutes before operation. Droperidol also has some anti-emetic properties, and has been used, sometimes by continuous intravenous infusion, during cancer chemotherapy.

In association with a potent narcotic analgesic such as **fentanyl** or **phenoperidine**, droperidol is used to induce a state of neuroleptanalgesia, a condition characterized by a detachment from and an indifference to the environment, whilst the ability to communicate is retained. Such a state is desirable when an operative procedure must be carried out during which the patient must be co-operative, yet free from pain and anxiety. For neuroleptanalgesia droperidol is given in doses up to 15 mg by intravenous injection.

Side-effects of droperidol are similar to those of haloperidol.

Fluspirilene § (dose: 2–20 mg by deep intramuscular injection)

Brand name: Redeptin §

Fluspirilene is an antipsychotic drug chemically related to haloperidol and has similar actions and uses. Following injection it has a prolonged action extending over 7 days, and so is of value in the treatment of schizophrenic patients unwilling to accept or co-operate with oral therapy.

Fluspirilene is given by deep intramuscular injection in doses of 2 mg weekly initially, rising by increments of 2 mg weekly up to a maximum of 20 mg weekly as required.

Side-effects include restlessness, sweating and extrapyramidal symptoms. The latter usually occur some 6–12 hours after injection, and may subside after 48 hours. Subcutaneous nodules may appear at injection sites if treatment is prolonged.

Pimozide § (dose: 2–20 mg daily)

Brand name: Orap §

Pimozide is chemically related to the butyrophenones, and is used in the control of both acute and chronic schizophrenia. In acute conditions, treatment is usually commenced with doses of 2–4 mg daily, increased as required at weekly intervals up to a total of 20 mg. Exceptionally, a starting dose of 10 mg may be necessary. In chronic conditions, and when apathy is present, smaller doses may be adequate. Pimozide is also useful for the short-term supplementary treatment of severe anxiety, and is then given in doses of 2–4 mg daily.

Side-effects of pimozide are basically similar to those of chlorpromazine. Ventricular arrhythmia is an occasional side-effect, and it is now recommended that an ECG should be carried out before beginning pimozide treatment, and periodically in patients receiving doses of 16 mg or more daily. Care is necessary in depression, epilepsy and parkinsonism, as pimozide may aggravate the symptoms. It is contraindicated in patients with a history of cardiac arrhythmias.

Risperidone §▼ (dose: 6–10 mg daily)

Brand name: Risperdal §▼

Risperidone is a recent addition to the range of drugs for the treatment of schizophrenia. It resembles clozapine in its pattern of activity, as it has a high and selective affinity for serotinin $5-HT_2$ and dopamine D_2 receptors as well as some lower affinity for $alpha_1$-adrenoreceptors. Unlike many other antipsychotic agents, risperidone appears to relieve both the positive symptoms of schizophrenia such as hostility and delusions, and the negative symptoms of apathy and withdrawal. It is given in doses of 1 mg twice a day, increased over 2–3 days to 3 mg twice a day according to response, up to 4 mg twice a day. Doses over 10 mg daily are more likely to increase extra-pyramidal symptoms than improve the response. Some hypotension may occur, mediated by the alpha-receptor blockade, and require adjustment of dose.

Side-effects include headache, insomnia, agitation and dizziness, but extra-pyramidal effects are usually mild and reversible with adjustment of dose or supplementary treatment with an anticholinergic drug. Unlike clozapine, risperidone does not appear to cause agranulocytosis, and routine blood monitoring is not necessary.

Sulpiride § (dose: 400 mg–2.4 g daily)

Brand name: Dolmatil §, Sulpitil §

Sulpiride is unusual in having a bimodal action, as it has both neuroleptic and antidepressant properties. It is used in acute and chronic schizophrenia in doses dependent to some extent on the condition. In chronic states associated with apathy and depression, initial doses of 400 mg twice daily are given, and paradoxically the improved alertness induced by the drug may be increased by a reduction in dose to 200 mg twice daily.

In severe conditions with delusions and hallucinations, large doses up to 2.4 g daily may be necessary according to the response. Sulpiride has also been used at low dose levels in neurosis, depression and migraine.

Side-effects of sulpiride are similar to those of other neuroleptic drugs, and galactorrhoea may occur as a result of a rise in the serum prolactin level. Care is necessary in renal disease, and phaeochromocytoma is a contraindication.

Trifluperidol § (dose: 0.5–8 mg daily)

Brand name: Triperidol §

Trifluperidol is a butyrophenone with the actions, uses and side-effects of haloperidol but active in lower doses. It is used mainly in schizophrenia and mania, and is sometimes of value in Huntington's chorea. It is given in initial doses of 500 micrograms daily, increased at intervals of 3–4 days until an adequate response has been obtained up to a maximum dose of 6–8 mg daily. In children (6–12 years), an initial dose of 250 micrograms may be given, with a maximum dose of 2 mg daily.

ANXIOLYTIC TRANQUILLIZING AGENTS

The anxiolytic benzodiazepines (BZs), represented by diazepam, have also been termed minor tranquillizers. The term is a misleading one, as their mode of action differs from that of the chlorpromazine-like antipsychotic drugs, and they do not induce extrapyramidal symptoms. Their anxiolytic action appears to be mediated by a selective affinity for specific benzodiazepine (BZ) receptors in the cerebral cortex that are concerned with serotonin neurotransmission. They reduce emotional reactivity and associated somatic response without marked sedation. By their pharmacological nature, however, they reduce alertness, and patients should be warned that car-driving ability may be affected, an action that may be intensified if alcohol is also taken. The risks of dependence and the dangers of rapid withdrawal are referred to on page 33.

These benzodiazepines are of value in the short-term treatment of severe anxiety, but the lowest effective dose should be used, and therapy should be withdrawn slowly but without delay. Rapid withdrawal may evoke a rebound response, even after short-term treatment. The BZs have in general the same type of

Table 3.2 Butyrophenones and other powerful tranquillizers

Approved name	Brand name	Oral daily dose range	Dose by injection
benperidol	Anquil	0.25–1.5 mg	
clozapine	Clozaril	12.5–450 mg	
droperidol	Droleptan	15–100 mg	5–10 mg i.m. or i.v. 4–6 hourly
flupenthixol	Depixol	6–8 mg	
flupenthixol[a]	Depixol Depot		20–400 mg i.m. monthly
fluspirilene	Redeptin		2–20 mg i.m. weekly
haloperidol	Haldol, Serenace, Fortunan, Dozic	15–200 mg	2–10 mg i.m. 4–6 hourly
haloperidol decanoate	Haldol Decanoate		100–200 mg i.m. monthly
oxypertine	Integrin	80–100 mg	
pimozide	Orap	2–20 mg	
pipothiazine palmitate	Piportil Depot		50–200 mg i.m. monthly
risperidone	Risperdal	2–8 mg	
sulpiride	Dolmatil, Sulpitil	400 mg–2.4 g	
trifluperidol	Triperidol	6–8 mg	
zuclopenthixol	Clopixol	20–150 mg	200–400 mg i.m. monthly

[a] Flupenthixol is also used as an antidepressant.

action, but can be divided into the intermediate-acting and longer-acting drugs. The former include bromazepam, lorazepam and oxazepam, and have the advantage that accumulation of the drug is less likely, although there is a greater risk of withdrawal symptoms. The longer-acting BZs have a smoother initial action, and withdrawal usually causes less problems, but the risk of accumulation is greater, and the longer-acting BZs should be avoided in the elderly and in hepatic impairment. Table 3.3 indicates the range of benzodiazepine anxiolytics currently available. There is no specific treatment for overdose, and therapy should be symptomatic and supportive. The use of flumazenial in BZ overdose is under investigation (p. 35).

Table 3.3 Benzodiazepine anxiolytics

Approved name	Brand name	Average daily dose range
alprazolam	Xanax	750–1500 micrograms
bromazepam	Lexotan	3–18 mg
chlordiazepoxide	Librium	30–100 mg
clobazam	Frisium	20–30 mg
clorazepate	Tranxene	7.5–22.5 mg
diazepam	Atensine	5–30 mg
	Valium	
lorazepam[a]	Ativan	2.5–10 mg
medazepam	Nobrium	10–30 mg
oxazepam[a]		45–120 mg

[a] Intermediate-acting BZs.

Diazepam § (dose: 5–30 mg daily)

Brand names: Alupram §, Atensine §, Valium §

Diazepam is a benzodiazepine with anxiolytic, muscle relaxant and anticonvulsant properties. It is widely used in the treatment of anxiety and tension states, for the relief of anxiety complicating organic and psychosomatic illness, and for the short-term treatment of anxiety-associated insomnia. Diazepam is also given for premedication; and it is sometimes used in dentistry to reduce stress and apprehension. Diazepam has also been used for night terrors in children. It is also of value in the control of acute alcohol withdrawal symptoms. The use of diazepam in status asthmaticus is referred to on page 77.

In mild anxiety states, diazepam is given in doses of 2 mg three times a day, but in severe conditions doses up to 30 mg daily may be required. In insomnia complicated by anxiety, a dose of 5–15 mg at night may be effective. For the symptomatic treatment of acute alcohol withdrawal, large doses up to 20 mg, repeated 4-hourly, may be necessary.

Diazepam may also be given if required by suppository or rectal solution in doses of 5–15 mg. In severe conditions, and for the control of panic attacks, as well as in alcohol withdrawal, diazepam may be given by *slow* intravenous injection in doses of 5–10 mg, repeated after not less than 4 hours. Intramuscular injection should be avoided, as the response is unreliable, but intravenous injection requires care to avoid respiratory depression, hypotension and thrombophlebitis. (Diazemuls is an emulsified product for intravenous use that is better tolerated.)

Side-effects of diazepam include drowsiness, dizziness and ataxia, especially in the elderly, to whom half-doses should be given. It is not suitable for use with psychotic or depressed patients. The muscle relaxant and anticonvulsant properties of diazepam are referred to on pages 270 and 77.

Alprazolam § (dose: 750 micrograms–1.5 mg daily)

Brand name: Xanax §

Alprazolam is a benzodiazepine useful for the short-term treatment of anxiety, and of anxiety associated with depression. It is given in doses of 250–500 micrograms three times a day, with half-doses for elderly and debilitated patients. Higher doses may be required when depression is a complicating factor, but a total daily dose of 3 mg should not normally be exceeded.

Chlordiazepoxide § (dose: 50–100 mg daily)

Brand name: Librium §

Chlordiazepoxide has the anxiolytic action, uses and side-effects of diazepam. It is given in doses of 10 mg three times a day, increased if necessary up to 100 mg daily in the short-term treatment of severe anxiety states, with half-doses for elderly patients. It is also used as supplementary treatment in the control of the symptoms of acute alcohol withdrawal in doses of 25–100 mg, repeated at intervals of 2–4 hours according to need.

Lorazepam § (dose: 1–10 mg daily; 25 micrograms/kg by injection)

Brand names: Almazine §, Ativan §

Lorazepam has the actions, uses and side-effects of diazepam, but is effective in lower doses. In anxiety states it is given in doses of 1–4 mg or more three times a day, and as a dose of up to 5 mg at night for insomnia. In acute panic states lorazepam may be given by slow intravenous injection in doses of 25 micrograms/kg 6-hourly according to need. Larger doses of up to 50 micrograms/kg are sometimes given by injection for premedication. Lorazepam is also given intravenously in doses of 4 mg in status asthmaticus, but it may cause respiratory depression (p. 79).

Lorazepam is a relatively short-acting anxiolytic, and drowsiness as a side-effect may be less marked, but impairment of psychomotor performance may persist longer than with some related drugs.

OTHER ANXIOLYTIC DRUGS

Some other compounds, chemically unrelated to the benzodiazepines, have a similar anxiolytic action, and are useful when alternative therapy is required.

Buspirone § (dose: 15–45 mg daily)

Brand name: Buspar §

Buspirone is used for the short-term treatment of anxiety and anxiety associated with depression. It is thought to act on specific serotonin receptors, similar to but different from those acted on by the benzodiazepines as it lacks the muscle-relaxant properties of the BZs. Buspirone is given in doses up to 5 mg three times a day, gradually increased according to need, but the full response may not develop for 2 weeks, and patients should be warned accordingly. By the nature of its actions on specific receptors, patients on BZs cannot be switched directly to buspirone without the risk of a BZ withdrawal reaction. Buspirone should not be given with an MAOI, as the combination may cause a rise in blood pressure.

Side-effects include nausea, dizziness and headache.

Chlormezanone (Trancopal §), dose: 300–800 mg daily; hydroxyzine (Atarax §), dose: 200–400 mg daily; and meprobamate (Equanil §), dose: 1.2–1.6 g daily are other anxiolytic agents, but are used less extensively. The use of some beta-blockers such as propranolol in the control of tremor and apprehension is referred to on page 190.

ANTIDEPRESSANTS

Depression is a natural reaction to grief and disappointment and is normally self-limiting and relatively brief. However, depression may also occur without apparent cause, and the term depressive illness includes some common but not easily described psychiatric conditions. Depression that appears to come from within is referred to as endogenous depression, whereas reactive depression is often an excessive response to circumstances beyond the individual's immediate control. The terms neurotic and psychotic depression are also in use, and for further information on the types of depression specialist books should be consulted. The biochemical mechanism underlying depression is highly complex and still not clear, but it seems to be linked with a disturbance or abnormality in a central transmitter system. That disturbance may be due to an imbalance of or a deficiency in the brain of certain neurotransmitter substances such as dopamine, noradrenaline and serotonin (5HT), or to a dysfunction of the corresponding receptor sites. Treatment is aimed at the restoration of the balance of neuroregulating amines by drugs that block their normal physiological neuronal re-uptake in the brain, or those that bring about a similar effect by inhibiting their breakdown by enzymes such as amine oxidase. Attempts have been made to classify to some extent the wide range of antidepressant drugs in current use by their chemical structure, or by their mode of action, but some antidepressants may act at more than one receptor sites, their metabolites may not have quite the same action as the parent drug, and classification of antidepressants is correspondingly difficult. Here they will be dealt with basically in three groups, the tricyclic antidepressants, the monoamine oxidase inhibitors, and the serotonin re-uptake inhibitors, together with a few non-classified drugs.

TRICYCLIC ANTIDEPRESSANTS

These drugs form the largest group of antidepressant drugs in current use. The name refers to their three-ring chemical structure, although included in the group are a few with different but related ring formations. They all have the same basic action, but individual drugs may have supplementary effects that can determine individual preference although some 10–20% of patients may not improve with tricyclic drug therapy. Amitriptyline, for example, has certain sedative properties that are useful when depression is associated with agitation, anxiety and insomnia, whereas others, such as protripyline have a mild stimulant effect that is of value when the depression is linked with apathy and withdrawal. Response to treatment with tricyclic depressants is normally slow in onset over 2–4 weeks. Patients should be warned accordingly and encouraged to persist, as treatment for some months may be necessary to evoke a full response. Subsequent withdrawal of treatment should also be slow. The dose range in some cases is wide, and the aim of treatment is to obtain the optimum effective plasma level of the drug with a dose that will not evoke unacceptable side-effects. That optimum dose tends to vary from patient to patient, and careful adjustment of dose may be necessary initially to obtain an adequate response. Small doses should always be given initially to elderly patients, as the tricyclics have some hypotensive properties, and may cause dizziness by lowering the blood pressure. Caution is also necessary in epilepsy, as these drugs may lower the convulsive threshold and precipitate convulsions. For the same reason they may modify the action of antihypertensive drugs. They should never be given with a monoamine oxidase inhibitor (MAOI), or within 2 weeks of starting or stopping such treatment.

Side-effects. The side-effects mentioned here should be taken to refer in general to most tricyclic antidepressants, and will not be repeated again when dealing with individual drugs. Many are due to the anticholinergic properties of this group of drugs, so common side-effects include dryness of the mouth, blurred vision and urinary disturbances. Car-drivers should be warned that drowsiness may occur. Some degree of tolerance to these side-effects may develop with continued treatment. More serious side-effects are those on the cardiovascular system, as cardiac arrhythmias, heart block and sudden death have occurred during tricyclic antidepressant treatment. Severe haematological disturbances have occurred with mianserin.

The following notes refer to some individual drugs, and Table 3.4 indicates the range available.

Points about antidepressants

(a) Onset of action is slow (2–4 weeks).
(b) Encourage patients to persist with treatment.
(c) Maintain dose level for at least 1 month after improvement before lowering the dose.
(d) Drug withdrawal should be carried out slowly.
(e) Combined treatment with a MAOI is contraindicated and at least 2 weeks must elapse before commencing MAOI therapy after other treatment.
(f) Care is necessary in epilepsy, and in any machine-related activities.

Table 3.4   Tricyclic and similar antidepressants

Approved name	Brand name	Daily dose range
amitriptyline[a]	Domical	50–200 mg
	Lentizol	
	Tryptizol	
amoxapine	Asendas	100–300 mg
clomipramine	Anafranil	10–250 mg
desipramine	Pertofran	75–200 mg
dothiepin[a]	Prothiaden	75–150 mg
doxepin[a]	Sinequan	30–300 mg
imipramine	Tofranil	75–200 mg
iprindole	Prondol	45–180 mg
lofepramine	Gamanil	70–210 mg
maprotiline[a]	Ludiomil	25–150 mg
mianserin[a,b]	Bolvidon, Norval	30–90 mg
nortriptyline	Allegron	30–100 mg
	Aventyl	
protriptyline	Concordin	15–60 mg
trazodone	Molipaxin	150–300 mg
trimipramine	Surmontil	50–300 mg
viloxamine	Vivalan	300–400 mg

[a] These drugs have sedative properties that are of value when depression is
complicated by anxiety and insomnia.
[b] Mianserin is a tetracyclic compound.

Amitriptyline § (dose: 50–200 mg daily; 10–20 mg by intramuscular or intravenous injection)

Brand names: Domical §, Lentizol §, Tryptizol §

Amitriptyline is widely used in the treatment of depression, particularly when some sedative action is also required, as for agitated and anxious patients. It is given in initial doses of 25 mg three times a day, gradually increased up to a maximum dose of 200 mg daily, although maintenance doses of 100 mg daily are usually adequate. Half-doses should be given to elderly patients. If required the full daily dose can be given at night to avoid daytime sedation and at the same time to promote sleep. In severe conditions amitriptyline may be given by injection in doses up to 20 mg four times a day, followed by oral therapy as soon as possible. Following remission of symptoms, dosage should be reduced to a maintenance level, and therapy should be continued for at least 3 months to avoid a relapse, after which the drug should be gradually withdrawn.

By virtue of its anticholinergic action, amitriptyline is sometimes used in the treatment of nocturnal enuresis, and is given in doses of 10–20 mg at night for children aged 7–10 years, and 25–50 mg for children over 11 years. The use of tricyclic antidepressants in children is controversial, not least from the risk of accidental overdose. They are not recommended for children under 6 years of age.

Side-effects of amitriptyline are those of the tricyclic antidepressants generally referred to on page 64.

Amoxapine § (dose: 100–300 mg daily)

Brand name: Asendis §

One of the disadvantages of the tricyclic antidepressants is the slow onset of action, which may take 2 weeks or more to develop. Amoxapine is a derivative claimed to have a more rapid action, as an initial response may occur within 4–7 days. It is given in doses of 25 mg three to four times a day, with maintenance doses between 150 and 250 mg daily, with half-doses for elderly patients. Prolonged treatment is necessary to achieve a full response.

Amoxapine has the general properties and **side-effects** of the tricyclic antidepressants, and it may interact with other drugs, including antihypertensive agents and sympathomimetics.

Daytime drowsiness can be reduced by administration as a single dose at night. It may cause hormonal disturbances in female patients.

Clomipramine § (dose: 10–150 mg daily)

Brand name: Anafranil §

Clomipramine is a tricyclic antidepressant with the actions and uses of amitriptyline, but with reduced sedative properties. It is given in doses of 10 mg daily initially, subsequently increased according to need. Doses of 150 mg or more daily may be necessary. In severe depression, phobia and other severe conditions, clomipramine has been given by intramuscular injection or by intravenous infusion in daily doses of 100 mg (after a test dose of 25 mg).

Imipramine § (dose: 75–200 mg daily)

Brand names: Tofranil §, Praminil §

Imipramine was one of the first tricyclic antidepressants, and it has been widely used in the treatment of endogenous depression. It is given in doses of 25 mg three times a day initially and subsequently increased, although in some cases a single dose of 150 mg at night may be preferred, but the onset of action is slow, and may not be apparent for some 2–3 weeks. Extended treatment is necessary for the full remission of symptoms. Lower doses of 10 mg initially should be given to elderly patients. Withdrawal of the drug should be slow, but a course of treatment, including withdrawal, should not exceed 3 months.

Side-effects of imipramine are those of the tricyclic antidepressants in general (p. 64).

Imipramine has also been used for nocturnal enuresis in doses of 25 mg at night for children aged 8–12 years, and of 50 mg for older children. It is not recommended for younger children.

Desipramine § (dose: 75–200 mg daily)

Brand name: Pertofran §

Desipramine is the active metabolite of imipramine and it has the actions, uses and side-effects of the parent drug. It is used mainly in depressive illness uncomplicated by anxiety and agitation. Desipramine has a long half-life in the body, which permits administration by a single daily dose.

Mianserin § (dose: 30–90 mg)

Brand names: Bolvidon §, Norval §

Mianserin is a tetracyclic derivative with the actions, uses and side-effects of the tricyclic antidepressants. It is given initially in doses of 10 mg three times a day or as a single dose of 30 mg at night, slowly increased according to need. Mianserin is more likely to cause haematological disturbances than the tricyclic drugs, particularly in the elderly, and full blood counts are necessary during treatment, and the drug should be withdrawn if any signs of infection occur. An influenza-like syndrome may also develop and hepatic reactions as well as convulsions have also been reported.

Protriptyline § (dose: 15–60 mg daily)

Brand name: Concordin §

Most tricyclic antidepressants have a mild sedative effect, but protriptyline differs in having a stimulant action. It is correspondingly useful in the treatment of depression associated with apathy, and is given in doses of 5–10 mg three times a day. If insomnia is present, the third dose should be given before 4 p.m. Caution is necessary in the elderly, for whom a daily dose of 20 mg should not be exceeded, as in common with other antidepressants, protriptyline may cause hypotension and dizziness. Protriptyline is not suitable for the treatment of depression associated with anxiety as it may aggravate the symptoms.

Side-effects of protriptyline are in general similar to those of amitriptyline, but cardiovascular reactions are more common. Exposure to direct sunlight during treatment should be avoided, as a rash associated with photosensitization to protriptyline may occur.

Flupenthixol § (dose: 1–3 mg daily)

Brand name: Fluanxol §

Flupenthixol is a butyrophenone used in the treatment of schizophrenia (p. 59) but it also has some antidepressant and activating properties. It is sometimes used in the short-term treatment of depression, and it may relieve associated apathy and inertia, and may be effective when other depressants are unsatisfactory. It is not suitable for the treatment of severe depression. Flupenthixol is given as a single morning dose of 1 mg initially, increased after 7 days to 1 mg twice a day, with the second dose not later than 4 p.m. Half doses should be given to the elderly.

Flupenthixol has a more rapid action than most antidepressants, but if there is no response to treatment after 7 days, the drug should be withdrawn.

Side-effects include restlessness and insomnia, and care is necessary with excitable patients, and in confused states. Paradoxically, it may cause drowsiness initially in a few patients.

Viloxazine § (dose: 300–400 mg daily)

Brand name: Vivalan §

Viloxazine is also used in the treatment of depressive illness, and has the advantage of having less anticholinergic activity, and is less likely to cause sedation. It is given in doses of 200 mg in the morning, and 100 mg at midday, increased if necessary up to 400 mg daily. The last dose is best taken before 6 p.m.

Tryptophan §▼

Brand name: Optimax §▼

Tryptophan is an amino acid present in food, and is a precursor of serotonin. On the basis that depression may be linked with a deficiency of serotonin, tryptophan was used in severe depression, but the drug was withdrawn because of severe eosinophilia and myalgia, probably due to an impurity. It has now become available for the treatment of resistant depression under hospital supervision on a named-patient basis.

SELECTIVE SEROTONIN RE-UPTAKE INHIBITORS (SSRIs)

The tricyclic antidepressants inhibit the re-uptake of noradrenaline and serotonin at nerve terminals, and it is considered that drugs with a more selective action might have advantages, and have fewer anticholinergic (antimuscarinic) side-effects. Some selective inhibitors of serotonin re-uptake are now available, and they represent a distinct if not dramatic advance in the treatment of depression. They are less likely to cause sedation or cardiac disturbances, but are more likely to have gastrointestinal side-effects. Like the tricyclic antidepressants these serotonin re-uptake inhibitors are useful when depression is complicated by anxiety. By the nature of their action, these new drugs have some of the properties and side-effects of the tricyclic antidepressants, and similar care must be taken about car-driving and similar activities. They must not be used in combination with MAOIs, or within weeks of stopping or starting such therapy, or with any other drugs that might interfere with serotonin re-uptake. Such combined treatment may lead to a life-threatening syndrome of hyperthermia and convulsions. The following drugs are currently available:

Edwards J G 1992 Selective serotonin uptake inhibitors. British Medical Journal 304: 1644–1645

Fluoxetine § (dose: 20 mg daily)

Brand name: Prozac §

Fluoxetine differs to some extent from related drugs as it has a less sedative action. In depressive illness it is given in doses of 20 mg daily, but in the treatment of bulimia nervosa larger doses of 60 mg daily are needed. The use of fluoxetine requires care, as it has many side-effects, including dizziness, drowsiness, nausea and diarrhoea. It may also cause allergic reactions such as urticaria and anaphylaxis. The development of a rash requires withdrawal of the drug, as it may indicate the onset of a serious systemic reaction. Disturbances of the blood picture may also occur.

Anon 1990 Fluoxetine, another new antidepressive. Drug Therapy Bulletin 28: 33–34

Fluvoxamine § (dose: 100–300 mg daily)

Brand name: Faverin §

Fluvoxamine is used in depressive illness by initial doses of 100 mg daily, increased as required over 2 weeks or more up to a maximum of 300 mg daily. The tablets should be swallowed whole with water. Side-effects include agitation, insomnia, dizziness and tremor. Gastrointestinal disturbances are common. It is contraindicated in epilepsy, as it may lower the convulsive threshold and precipitate an attack, as may other SSRIs. The plasma levels of warfarin and propanolol may also rise.

Anon 1988 Fluvoxamine (Faverin) another antidepressive. Drug Therapy Bulletin 26: 11–12

Paroxetine §▼ (dose: 20–50 mg daily)

Brand name: Seroxat §▼

Paroxetine is an antidepressant of the fluoxetine type, and is given in all types of depressive illness, including depression accompanied by anxiety. It is given initially as a morning dose of 20 mg, and slowly increased up to 50 mg daily. The **side-effects** are similar to those of related drugs but extra-pyramidal symptoms have been reported more frequently.

Sertraline § (dose: 50–200 mg daily)

Brand name: Lustral §

Sertraline is used in the treatment of depressive illness as well as in prevention and recurrence, and is given initially in doses of 50 mg daily with food. The full response may not be noted for 2–4 weeks. When the response is incomplete, the doses may be slowly increased over some weeks, but a daily dose of 150 mg or more should not be continued for more than 8 weeks. **Side-effects** are nausea, diarrhoea and dryness of the mouth. The same precautions about combined therapy and car-driving should be observed with sertraline as with other serotonin up-take inhibitors.

Points about SSRIs

(a) Less sedative than the tricyclic antidepressants.
(b) Gastrointestinal side-effects are dose-related.
(c) Do not cause weight-gain.
(d) Caution necessary in epilepsy.
(e) A gap of 2–5 weeks must elapse between SSRI and MAOI therapy.
(f) As with tricyclics, care is necessary in car-driving and machine-related activities.

MONOAMINE OXIDASE INHIBITORS (MAOIs)

Monoamine oxidase is the enzyme that breaks down pressor substances like noradrenaline and serotonin. Suppression of that metabolic breakdown by monoamine inhibitors has a stimulant action by allowing the brain concentration of such pressor amines to rise. MAOIs have a general antidepressant action but they are now prescribed mainly for the treatment of depression resistant to other drugs. The onset of action is slow, and may take up to a month to reach a maximal level, but their main disadvantage is that of reacting with a wide range of other drugs, including pressor agents and potent analgesics. Combined treatment with a tricyclic antidepressant is hazardous.

The pressor action of tyramine, which is present in foods such as cheese, broad beans, pickled herrings and yeast extracts as well as wine and beer (including low alcohol beer) may also be potentiated to a dangerous extent. Ideally, supplementary treatment should not be given to patients receiving MAOI therapy, or within 14 days of withdrawal of such treatment, and all patients should carry the official MAOI warning card in case of accident. Nurses should also warn patients of the risks of self-medication, as some cough and cold remedies contain small doses of drugs with a pressor action, and that a throbbing headache with MAOI therapy is a warning of a potentially dangerous rise in blood pressure.

Table 3.5 Monoamine oxidase inhibitors

Approved name	Brand name	Initial daily dose
isocarboxazid §	Marplan §	30 mg
phenelzine §	Nardil §	45 mg
tranylcypromine §	Parnate §	20 mg

Moclobemide § (dose: 300–600 mg daily)

Brand name: Manerix §▼

Recently, an important advance has been made in MAOI therapy, as two forms of monoamine oxidase have been identified as MAO-A and MAO-B. The A-form binds preferentially with noradrenaline and serotonin, whereas both the A and B forms of the enzyme bind with dopamine and tyramine. A drug with a selective inhibitory action on the A-form would have clinical advantages over the older and non-selective MAOIs, and the first of that new type is moclobemide, sometimes referred to as an RIMA antidepressant (reversible inhibitor of monamine oxidase).

Moclobemide brings about a rapid inhibition of MAO-A activity within a few hours, but the effect fades after about 24 hours, as the drug is rapidly metabolized with restoration of enzyme activity, thus permitting single daily doses. Moclobemide is given in severe depression, but other therapy should be withdrawn for 2–3 weeks, after which the drug is given as an initial dose of 300 mg after food, subsequently increased according to response up to 150–600 mg daily for 2–3 weeks. It should not be given to agitated patients without prior sedation.

Side-effects include nausea, dizziness and sleep disturbances.

Points about MAOIs

(a) Potentiate the action of many pressor drugs.
(b) Throbbing headache may be a warning symptom of a rise in blood pressure.
(c) Combined treatment with other antidepressants contraindicated — tranylcypromine with clomipramine is dangerous.
(d) At least 2 weeks must elapse between MAOI therapy and other treatment.
(e) Warn patients not to eat cheese, broad beans, pickled herring, meat or yeast extracts.

Lithium carbonate § (dose: 0.25–1.6 g daily)

Brand names: Camcolit §, Liskonum §, Phasal §, Priadel §

Lithium carbonate is used in the prophylaxis and treatment of mania and recurrent depression, but the mode of action is unknown. It may be linked with changes in the pattern of electrolyte balance between intracellular and extracellular fluid, or with the balance between lithium and sodium ions. Lithium carbonate is given in doses of 250 mg daily initially, slowly increased according to regular laboratory reports to maintain a plasma level of 0.6–1.2 mmol lithium/litre, as the margin between the therapeutic and the toxic doses is narrow. The response is not immediate, and initial treatment is often combined with another antipsychotic drug.

For prophylaxis, extended treatment over 6–12 months may be required to obtain a full response, and continued for 3 years or more to maintain the remission. Such prolonged treatment may cause changes in renal function, and require a review of therapy. The same lithium product should be used throughout treatment, as the bio-availability of lithium from different products may vary widely, and a change of product requires reassessment of treatment. The anticonvulsant carbamazepine (p. 76) is sometimes used for patients not responding to lithium.

Side-effects of lithium therapy include gastrointestinal disturbances, tremor and polyuria, and it may also induce or exacerbate psoriasis, but toxic side-effects such as coarse tremor, drowsiness, lethargy and ataxia require immediate withdrawal of the drug. Toxicity may be increased by sodium loss induced by thiazide and other diuretics, and care is necessary in other conditions of sodium depletion, as plasma concentrations above 1.5 mmol lithium/litre may be fatal. **Lithium citrate** (Litarex) has similar actions and uses.

Points about lithium therapy

(a) Narrow therapeutic window between therapeutic and toxic dose.
(b) Lithium–plasma levels must be monitored.
(c) Adequate salt and fluid intake.
(d) Avoid diuretics.
(e) Warn patients that if a dose is missed, a compensatory double dose must not be taken.
(f) Prolonged treatment necessary.
(g) Withdraw treatment immediately if toxic symptoms occur.

ANTICONVULSANTS OR ANTI-EPILEPTICS
(Table 3.6)

Epilepsy, which is said to affect 1 in 200 people in Western countries, is a chronic condition characterized by seizures, popularly known as fits. The disease appears to be linked with dysfunction of certain neurotransmitter substances in the brain, and an imbalance between the central excitatory and inhibitory mechanisms. GABA, or gamma-aminobutyric acid, is a major inhibitory neurotransmitter, and deficiency leads to an excessive response to excitatory factors that may result in an epileptic seizure. These seizures have been classified as follows: (1) generalized tonic-clonic seizures or grand mal, with convulsions and loss of consciousness; (2) absence seizures or petit mal, characterized by transient loss of consciousness without convulsions, and (3) focal or Jacksonian epilepsy, similar in some ways to the clonic stage of grand mal.

Partial seizures, which are more difficult to control, include those with sensory, motor or autonomic symptoms, as well as the more complex temporal lobe or psycho-motor seizures. The atypical seizures of childhood may be associated with retardation or cerebral damage, and may respond poorly to treatment. Status epilepticus is a serious condition in which a series of convulsions may occur without an intervening recovery period.

The mode of action of anticonvulsant drugs is not yet clear. Some may act by mimicking the action of GABA, some by enhancing GABA-mediated inhibitory activity, and others by inhibiting the enzymatic breakdown of GABA. In any case, the successful treatment of epilepsy depends on the maintenance of an adequate plasma level of an effective anticonvulsant drug. Combined therapy with more than one drug may have disadvantages, as some drugs induce the production of liver enzymes which may both reduce the effective plasma levels and increase toxicity. In general, dosage must be individually adjusted to need and response, and patient compliance with treatment is essential, as prolonged medication is required. Any change of treatment from one drug to another must be carried out slowly, and withdrawal covered by overlapping doses, as convulsions may be precipitated by the rapid withdrawal of an anti-epileptic drug.

The use of anticonvulsants during pregnancy requires care, as they are potentially teratogenic, and there is an increased risk of neural tube defects with carbamazepine and valproate. The Committee of Safety of Medicines has advised that where appropriate, women should be informed of the risks and possible consequences, and if necessary offered specialist advice. In addition, during pregnancy the plasma levels of anticonvulsants should be monitored regularly, as the levels may fall, particularly during the later stages.

Table 3.6   Anticonvulsants

Approved name	Brand names
Those effective in petit mal:	
phenobarbitone	Luminal
methylphenobarbitone	Prominal
clonazepam	Rivotril
ethosuximide	Emeside, Zarontin
sodium valproate	Epilim
vigabatrin	Sabril
Those effective in grand mal and other types of seizure:	
phenobarbitone	Luminal
methylphenobarbitone	Prominal
carbamazepine	Tegretol
chlormethiazole[a]	Heminevrin
clonazepam[a]	Rivotril
diazepam[a]	Valium
gabapentin	Neurontin
lamotrigine	Lamictal
lorazepam[a]	Almazine, Ativan
phenytoin	Epanutin
primidone	Mysoline
sodium valproate	Epilim
vigabatrin	Sabril

[a]Indicates those drugs used in status epilepticus.

 Chadwick D 1988 The modern treatment of epilepsy. British Journal of Hospital Medicine 39: 104–110

Carbamazepine § (dose: 0.8–1.2 g daily)

Brand name: Tegretol §

Carbamazepine has an anticonvulsant action that is useful in most forms of epilepsy with the exception of petit mal. It is considered by some to be a first choice drug for the control of partial seizures.

Carbamazepine is given in doses of 200–400 mg daily initially, with food, rising slowly over 7–14 days to maintenance doses of 0.8–1.2 g daily, and control of seizures is usually achieved with a plasma level of the drug of 20–50 micromol/litre. Suppositories of carbamazepine (125 mg and 250 mg) are available for short-term treatment when oral administration is not possible, as post operatively, or when the patient is unconscious. Carbamazepine is also used occasionally in the treatment of trigeminal neuralgia, mania (p. 74) and diabetes insipidus (p. 365).

Side-effects, especially in the early stages of treatment, are drowsiness and dizziness, and gastrointestinal disturbances. Double vision may occur as higher plasma levels are reached with continued treatment. A generalized rash occurs in about 3% of patients receiving carbamazepine which may be severe enough to require withdrawal of the drug. Photosensitization and blood disorders have also been reported.

Clonazepam § (dose: 4–8 mg daily)

Brand name: Rivotril §

Clonazepam is chemically related to diazepam and has an anticonvulsant action that is of value in the control of all types of epilepsy. It is given in doses of 1 mg daily initially for a few days, usually at night as it has a sedative action, slowly increased over 2–4 weeks to a maintenance dose of 4–8 mg daily. Clonazepam is also effective in the control of status epilepticus, and is given in doses of 1 mg by slow intravenous injection, repeated as required. Its use requires care, as it may cause apnoea and hypotension requiring intensive treatment.

Side-effects of oral therapy include drowsiness, dizziness, fatigue and irritability. In children, clonazepam may cause respiratory side-effects by increasing bronchial and salivary secretion.

Diazepam § (dose: 10–20 mg intravenously)

Brand names: Diazemuls §, Valium §, Stesolid §

The anxiolytic drug diazepam has valuable anticonvulsant properties when given by intravenous injection, and is the drug of choice in the treatment of status epilepticus. It is given by slow intravenous injection in doses of 10–20 mg, repeated if necessary after 30–60 minutes, with subsequent doses by intravenous infusion after dilution with glucose 5% solution, up to a maximum of 3 mg/kg over 24 hours.

The injection solution frequently causes venous thrombosis, and an emulsified injection product (Diazemuls) is often preferred. Absorption after intramuscular injection is unreliable and when intravenous injection is not possible, diazepam may be given as a rectal solution in doses of 5–10 mg, repeated as required.

As with clonazepam, a **side-effect** of intravenous therapy is respiratory depression, and mechanical ventilation apparatus must be readily available.

Ethosuximide § (dose: 500 mg–2 g daily)

Brand names: Emeside §, Zarontin §

Ethosuximide is one of the preferred drugs for the treatment of petit mal (absence seizures). It is given in doses of 500 mg daily initially, slowly increased at weekly intervals up to a maximum of 2 g daily. An optimum response is associated with a plasma level of 300–700 micromol/litre. In mixed seizures, the incidence of grand mal may be increased by ethosuximide, requiring adjustment of other therapy.

Side-effects of ethosuximide are similar to those of related drugs, and include drowsiness, dizziness and gastrointestinal disturbances. Care is necessary in renal and hepatic impairment.

Chlormethiazole §

Brand name: Heminevrin §

Chlormethiazole is used mainly as an hypnotic (p. 36) but it also has some anticonvulsant properties that are useful in status epilepticus. It is then given by intravenous infusion of an 0.8% solution in doses of 40–120 mg/minute up to a total dose of 320–800 mg, continued if necessary with doses of 4–8 mg/minute.

The dose must be titrated against response, as the sleep induced by chormethiazole may otherwise easily pass into unconsciousness. It is used mainly when the epileptic state is continuous, or returns after treatment.

Side-effects of chlormethiazole include sneezing, conjunctival irritation, apnea and hypotension, and resuscitation facilities must be available. Local thrombophlebitis may occur at the injection site.

Gabapentin §▼ (dose: 300 mg–2.4 g daily)

Brand name: Neurontin §▼

Gabapentin is a new analogue of GABA, and has some useful anticonvulsant properties. The mode of action is not yet known, as it does not modify the brain level of GABA or inhibit GABA-transaminase activity, or bind to GABA receptors. At present it is used mainly as supplementary treatment in partial seizures not controlled by other drugs. It is given in a dose of 300 mg on the first day of treatment, 300 mg twice on the second day, 300 mg three times on the third day, after which the dose is increased according to need and response up to 1.2 g daily. Exceptionally, doses of up to 2.4 g daily may be required. Care is necessary in mixed seizures, some of which may be exacerbated, and reduced doses are advisable in renal impairment and the elderly.

Side-effects include drowsiness, dizziness, nausea, tremor and weight gain. Withdrawal of treatment should be carried out slowly with tapering-off doses over at least 1 week.

Lamotrigine §▼ (dose: 100–400 mg daily)

Brand name: Lamictal §▼

Lamotrigine is a new anticonvulsant discovered in a search for phenytoin-like compounds, but it is thought that it differs in action by inhibiting the release of an excitatory factor such as glutamate. It is used in resistant epilepsy as supplementary treat-ment with other anticonvulsants, and is given in doses of 50 mg twice a day initially for 14 days, with subsequent adjustment for maintenance doses of 100–200 mg twice a day. Half doses should be given when sodium valproate is being given. Withdrawal, if necessary, should be carried slowly over 2 weeks. Lamotrigine is not recommended for children or the elderly.

Side-effects include rash, fever, blurred vision and dizziness. Renal and hepatic impairment are contraindications, and such functions should be monitored in patients who develop side-effects.

Brodie M J 1992 Lamotrigine. Lancet 339: 1397–1400

Lorazepam § (dose: 4 mg by injection)

Brand names: Ativan §, Almazine §

Lorazepam is a benzodiazepine with the actions and uses of

diazepam that is occasionally used in status epilepticus. It is given by slow intravenous injection in a dose of 4 mg, repeated after 15 minutes if necessary. Apnoea and hypotension are **side-effects** that may be severe and require resuscitation.

Paraldehyde § (dose: 5–10 ml)

This old hypnotic drug (p. 36) is also of value in status epilepticus. It is given by deep intramuscular injection in doses of 5–10 ml, but not more than 5 ml at one site (with a glass syringe), or rectally in doses of 5 ml as a 10% solution in saline. In specialist centres it is sometimes given by slow intravenous injection in doses of 4–5 ml well diluted with saline, but great care is necessary, as intravenous paraldehyde may cause pulmonary oedema and haemorrhage.

Phenobarbitone § (dose: 60–180 mg daily; 50–200 mg by injection)

Phenobarbitone was once the standard drug for the treatment of epilepsy, and is still widely used. It has a general sedative as well as an anticonvulsant action, and is of value in all forms of epilepsy with the exception of absence seizures. Phenobarbitone is given in doses of 60–180 mg at night; the dose for children is on the weight basis of 8 mg/kg daily. In severe conditions, phenobarbitone may be given by intramuscular or intravenous injection in doses of 50–200 mg.

Side-effects include drowsiness and lethargy, although tolerance may develop, but the elderly may experience confusion and restlessness. In children, who sometimes require relatively high doses, phenobarbitone may have the paradoxical effect of causing hyperactivity. **Methylphenobarbitone** (Prominal) has similar actions and uses in doses of 100–600 mg daily.

Phenytoin sodium § (dose: 15–300 mg daily)

Brand name: Epanutin §

Phenytoin is used mainly in the control of grand mal and partial seizures, as it is of little value in petit mal. Following initial doses of 150–300 mg daily, maintenance doses range from 300–400 mg daily, although occasionally a dose of 600 mg may be required. Dosage must be adjusted in accordance with the drug plasma level to maintain a concentration of 40–80 micromol/litre as there are wide individual variations in the dose required to attain that level. Phenytoin should be taken after food to reduce gastric irritation.

In status epilepticus, phenytoin is given by slow intravenous injection in a loading dose of 15 mg/kg, followed by doses of 100 mg 6-hourly adjusted in accordance with the monitored plasma concentration. Such intravenous injections may cause hypotension and bradycardia, and facilities for resuscitation must be available.

Side-effects of phenytoin are numerous and include dizziness, headache, nausea and insomnia. Skin eruptions, acne and hirsutism may occur as well as overgrowth of the gums, and a megaloblastic anaemia may result from a disturbance of folate metabolism. Slurred speech may be a sign of overdose. The intravenous injection solution is alkaline and may cause local irritation.

Phenytoin binds easily to the plasma proteins, but can be displaced from such binding by a wide range of other drugs. Multiple therapy therefore requires care, as the plasma level of unbound drugs may rise sharply.

It is of interest that phenytoin has some antifolate properties that may play some part in its anticonvulsant activity, and in a search for more potent antifolate agents a drug of value in epilepsy was discovered (see lamotrigine on p. 79).

Primidone § (dose: 0.5–1.5 g daily)

Brand name: Mysoline §

Primidone has some chemical relationship to phenobarbitone, into which it is largely converted in the body. It is chiefly of value as alternative therapy in grand mal and psychomotor epilepsy when the response to other drugs is inadequate. Treatment is initiated with a dose of 125 mg daily at night, increased at intervals of 3 days to a daily dose of 0.5–1.5 g according to need. Children's doses are 10–15 mg/kg twice daily.

Primidone occasionally causes drowsiness, nausea, vertigo, fatigue, visual disturbances and skin eruptions, although these reactions may subside as treatment is continued.

Sodium valproate § (dose: 600 mg–2.5 g daily)

Brand names: Epilim §, Epilim Chrono §

Sodium valproate is effective in most types of epilepsy, but is less active against partial seizures. It appears to act by increasing the concentration in the brain of the inhibitory neurotransmitter GABA, possibly by reducing its enzymatic breakdown. It is given in doses of 200 mg three times a day initially, preferably after food, slowly increased as required at 3-day intervals up to a maximum of 2.5 g daily. In conditions where oral therapy is not possible, sodium valproate may be given by intravenous injection or infusion in doses of 400–800 mg, up to the same maximum daily dose of 2.5 g. Children's doses range from 20–40 mg/kg daily.

Epilim Chrono § is a product containing equal parts of sodium valproate and valproic acid. It is claimed that with the mixture there is less variation in the daily plasma levels of the anticonvulsant. Convulex § is a preparation of valproic acid.

Side-effects of sodium valproate are numerous, and include nausea, weight gain, and occasionally a transient loss of hair. Liver function may be impaired, sometimes severely, and the drug should be withdrawn immediately if vomiting, anorexia or jaundice occurs. In patients with a history of hepatic disease, regular monitoring of liver function should be carried out during the first months of treatment with sodium valproate. Blood platelet function and aggregation may also be disturbed. Care is necessary in pregnancy, as spina bifida has occasionally been associated with valproate therapy. As with phenytoin, interaction with a wide range of other drugs may occur, and multiple treatment requires care.

Vigabatrin § (dose: 2–4 g daily)

Brand name: Sabril §

Vigabatrin is a drug of promise in the treatment of epilepsy. It is an analogue of GABA, and has a highly specific and irreversible inhibitory action on GABA-transaminase, the enzyme concerned with breakdown of GABA. The administration of vigabatrin brings about an extended decline in the activity of GABA-transaminase that results in a rise in the brain level of GABA which is linked with the clinical response to the drug. Vigabatrin is well absorbed orally, it does not induce drug metabolising enzymes in the liver, and is excreted unchanged in the urine. Vigabatrin is used in the treatment of epilepsy not responding to other anticonvulsants, and is given as a supplement to such therapy, which should be continued. It is available as tablets and as sachets containing a sugar-free powder. The powder should be dissolved in water or other drink immediately before administration. Vigabatrin is given in doses of 2 g once or twice a day initially, subsequently adjusted as required, but doses above 4 g daily do not usually evoke an increased response. Reduced doses should be given to the elderly, and to patients with impaired renal function. Children may be given a starting dose of 40 mg/kg daily. Vigabatrin is well tolerated, but withdrawal, if necessary, should be by a gradual reduction of dose over 2 to 4 weeks. Abrupt withdrawal may lead to rebound seizures.

Side-effects of vigabatrin include drowsiness, fatigue, weight gain, dizziness and impairment of car-driving and related abilities. The sedative effects of the drug wane as treatment is prolonged. As with other anti-epileptic drugs, vigabatrin may cause an increase in seizure frequency in some patients, particularly those with myoclonic seizures. Vigabatrin does not become protein bound, so interactions with other drugs is less likely than with some other anti-epileptics.

 Anon 1990 Vigabatrin — a new anticonvulsant. Drug Therapy Bulletin 28: 95–96

Points about anti-epileptics

(a) They react variably and unpredictably with many other drugs.
(b) Plasma monitoring of drug level may be required, particularly in late pregnancy (as drug levels may fall).
(c) Mono-anticonvulsant therapy usually preferred.
(d) Change-over from one anti-epileptic to another must be made slowly and with care.
(e) Car-driving may be possible by patients who have had a seizure-free period of not less than 2 years.
(f) Care is necessary in pregnancy, as anti-epileptics are potentially teratogenic. Neural tube defects may occur with carbamazepine and valproate, and patients should be advised accordingly.

CENTRAL STIMULANTS

Many substances are known that have a stimulant effect on the central nervous system, but therapeutically they are of very limited value. There is no pharmacological basis for the use of stimulants in the treatment of depression, debility or fatigue, and they should not be so used. With amphetamines and related stimulants, the risks of misuse and dependence far outweigh any beneficial effects they might have.

Caffeine (dose: 250–500 mg)

Caffeine is the central stimulant constituent of tea and coffee. It acts mainly on the sensory cortex of the brain, increasing mental alertness and postponing drowsiness and fatigue.

Caffeine is present in a number of proprietary analgesic preparations available without prescription, but it adds little or nothing to the pain-relieving properties of such products.

Amphetamine sulphate*

Amphetamine has a marked stimulant effect on the cortex of the brain, causing a temporary increase in alertness, mediated by inhibiting the uptake and storage of noradrenaline and dopamine. The stimulant action of amphetamine has led to abuse, and it is now rarely prescribed.

Dexamphetamine sulphate* (dose: 10–60 mg daily)

Brand name: Dexedrine*

Dexamphetamine has the central stimulant properties of amphetamine, and is used mainly in the treatment of narcolepsy, an uncommon syndrome of recurrent periods of sleep with sudden loss of muscle tone. It is given in doses of 10 mg initially, slowly increased in divided doses up to 60 mg daily. Paradoxically, it has a central sedative action in some cases of brain damage, and it is used in the control of hyperkinesia in children. It is then given in initial doses of 5 mg daily, increased slowly according to need and response, up to 20 mg daily, although doses up to 40 mg daily have been given. Such use of dexamphetamine requires great care under expert supervision, as it may interfere with growth and development.

Side-effects of dexamphetamine include insomnia, restlessness and agitation, and with large doses personality changes with aggression may occur. Dexamphetamine has some appetite-depressant properties, and it has been used in the treatment of obesity. Dependence is a constant risk, and such use of dexamphetamine is no longer recommended. Phentermine §, (Duromine §, Ionamine §) and diethylpropion § (Apisate §, Tenuate Dospan §) have a similar action and carry similar risks of dependence. Fenfluramine § (Ponderax §) and dexfenfluramine § (Adifax▼) are other appetite depressants that differ in having mild sedative action. Although it is claimed that these alternative appetite depressants are less addictive, they should be regarded as short-term adjunctive agents in the treatment of severe obesity only. Treatment should be withdrawn slowly over at least a week to reduce the risk of a drug-withdrawal depression. They are contraindicated in epilepsy and any psychiatric illness.

Pulmonary hypertension may occur after fenfuramine, and treatment should not be continued for more than 3 months.

Pemoline § (dose: 20–40 mg daily)

Brand name: Volital §

Pemoline has a central stimulant action and was formerly used for lethargy in the elderly but it is now used only in the treatment of hyperkinesia in children. Its use requires care under supervision. In children over 6 years of age pemoline is given in doses of 10–20 mg morning and afternoon, but the response is variable.

Side-effects include insomnia, agitation and tachycardia. Hallucinations may sometimes occur with high doses.

4

Opioid (narcotic) analgesics and antagonists; non-narcotic analgesics; antimigraine drugs

The problem of pain has long puzzled both physicians and theologians, as pain, which has been described as a complex multidimensional experience, is very much more than a highly unpleasant sensation. Pain brings the patient to the doctor more quickly than any other symptom, and its relief has always been of considerable importance. The pain threshold varies in different individuals, and the perception of pain is subject to emotional and other influences; the so-called **gate theory** of the mechanism of pain has been put forward to explain certain aspects of pain perception.

It is considered that sensory stimuli pass from the periphery along small, unmyelinated fibres to the substantia gelatinosa, and are then transmitted to the higher centres of the brain to be perceived as pain. The theory suggests that the substantia gelantinosa (SG) acts as a gate that controls the passage of stimulatory impulses. It is normally closed against minor impulses, but an increased flow of impulses results in a widening of the gate to permit an increase in the number of impulses reaching the brain via the spinal transmitter cells (T). It is also thought that there may be other impulses from the brain to the SG along larger fibres that tend to have the effect of closing the gate against the increased transmission, and so reducing the perception of pain by a central action.

It has been postulated that substance P may be one of the neurotransmitters involved in the transmission of pain impulses from the SG to the T cells, and that its release and the transmission of pain impulses can be blocked by certain drugs. However the gate theory is but a partial explanation of a highly complex mechanism (Fig. 4.1) as there is evidence that certain natural substances, termed enkephalins and endorphins, are formed in the brain, and act upon specific receptor sites that are concerned with the perception of pain. They appear to function as endogenous analgesics.

NARCOTIC ANALGESICS

Opioid or narcotic analgesics are powerful drugs that both relieve pain and induce sleep. Non-narcotic analgesics relieve less severe pain but have little sedative action. Morphine, the main alkaloid of opium, is the oldest and one of the most widely used narcotic analgesics; aspirin and paracetamol are two of the common mild analgesics. Opioids reduce pain by binding to receptors that inhibit impulse transmission in the central synapses, and may stimulate pain-modulating factors. Not all pain is opioid sensitive, as muscle pain may be prostaglandin-mediated, and responds better to a prostaglandin synthetase inhibitor (p. 416).

When considering the use of analgesics, it may be that control of pain may be achieved and maintained with lower doses at optimum frequency more effectively than with larger doses given at longer intervals to suppress later break-through pain. It should be noted that the elderly are more susceptible to the side-effects

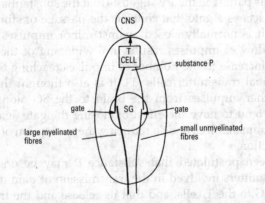

Figure 4.1   Diagram of gate control mechanism of pain perception.

of *any* opioid-containing analgesic preparation, and should be given correspondingly smaller doses.

Opium and Papaveretum*

Opium is the dried juice obtained from the seed-capsules of the opium poppy. It contains morphine, papaverine and codeine, and Papaveretum is a standardized preparation of those alkaloids. Omnopon* is a proprietary product of similar composition. Opium as such is rarely used in the UK; and papaveretum is used mainly as Papaveretum Injection and as Papaveretum and Hyoscine Injection. They are given by subcutaneous, intramuscular or intravenous injection for pre-operative medication and postoperative analgesia, but are now used less frequently as they may cause respiratory depression in the postoperative period. Papaveretum Injection is available in two strengths, 7.7 mg/ml and 15.4 mg/ml, equivalent to 5 mg and 10 mg of morphine. Papaverine and Hyoscine Injection contains 14.4 mg/ml together with hyoscine 400 micrograms/ml. Reduced doses ($\frac{1}{4}-\frac{1}{2}$) should be given intravenously.

Morphine* (dose: 10–20 mg)

Morphine is the oldest and most widely used narcotic analgesic, but its mode of action is complex and not yet clearly understood, as it both depresses and stimulates different areas of the CNS.

It is known that there are several opioid receptors for which morphine has an affinity, distinguished as the *mu, delta, kappa* and *sigma* receptors, and the various actions of morphine may be linked with different receptors. The affinity of morphine with the *mu* receptors is considered to bring about analgesia, the affinity for the *delta* receptors causes respiratory depression, whereas the *kappa* receptors appear to be linked with sedation and the *sigma* receptors with hallucinations. Morphine also stimulates the chemoreceptor trigger zone of the medulla, which causes the nausea and vomiting that are side-effects of the drug.

Whatever the mode of action, morphine remains a potent analgesic that is used for the relief of severe, acute pain in shock, biliary and renal colic, myocardial infarction, acute trauma, severe postoperative and cancer pain, acute pulmonary oedema and labour. It is of little value in trigeminal neuralgia. Morphine also brings about some mental detachment which reduces apprehension and anxiety, and may enhance the analgesia.

In acute pain, morphine is given in doses of 10 mg by intramuscular or subcutaneous injection, but in shock the former is preferred, as absorption from subcutaneous injection may be delayed because of the intense vasoconstriction that occurs after shock. If necessary, as in acute pulmonary oedema and myocardial infarction, morphine may be given by slow intravenous injection in doses of one-quarter to one half of those given intramuscularly. For pre-operative use, it is often given with atropine or hyoscine to reduce bronchial secretions. For the relief of chronic pain, morphine is given in oral doses of 5–20 mg 4-hourly, and in terminal illness the dose should be increased according to need, and doses of 100 mg or more may be required, if necessary together with an antiemetic to control any associated nausea. In such cases, the need to relieve pain outweighs the risks of possible dependence. In chronic and severe pain, the frequency of dose may be reduced by the use of long-acting products such as MST Continus and SRM-Rhotard.

Morphine may also be given as a 15 mg suppository. In severe, chronic intractable pain, morphine has been given by epidural and intrathecal injection. Another method of suppressing the severe pain of terminal malignancy that is under development is patient-controlled analgesia (PCA). This involves the use of an infusion pump that delivers a metered dose of the analgesic. The patient can control the frequency of the injection according to need, but not the delivered dose. The method offers an increased individual control of pain that in itself may improve the response to the analgesic. PCA has also been used to control the painful episodes of sickle-cell disease, even in young children.

 Grundy R, Howard R, Evans J 1993 Practical management of pain in sickling diseases. Archives of Disease in Childhood 69: 256–257

Oramorph is a solution of morphine (10 mg/5 ml) for oral use, and the so-called Brompton Cocktail or morphine elixir is a traditional mixture of varying quantities of morphine, cocaine, alcohol (often as gin) and chloroform water. Whether the inclusion of cocaine potentiates the analgesia or enhances mood is open to question.

Side-effects. Some of the side-effects of morphine are linked with its general action on the central nervous system. It depresses the respiratory centre, and care is necessary in patients with respiratory insufficiency, and in asthmatics, airway resistance may be increased by thickening of bronchial secretions and suppression of cough. Constipation may occur by a reduction in intestinal motility.

Morphine has a stimulant action on the chemoreceptor trigger zone of the medulla, causing nausea and vomiting, which can be reduced to some extent by combined treatment with small doses of chlorpromazine or a similar anti-emetic. Occasionally the pain of biliary colic is increased by morphine as it brings about a rise in intrabiliary pressure, and phenazocine is sometimes preferred. Care is necessary in patients with renal or hepatic impairment, and in those receiving antihypertensive therapy.

Children and the aged are particularly susceptible to morphine, and doses should be adjusted to need and response. The toxic dose varies, and in some patients even therapeutic doses may cause vomiting, restlessness and confusion. With larger doses, cyanosis may develop following respiratory depression, with coma and the pin-point pupils typical of opiate poisoning. The use of narcotic antagonists in the treatment of opiate poisoning is referred to on page 581.

Points about opioid analgesics

(a) Dose and timing are important, as analgesia may be more effective and controllable if given before severe pain develops.
(b) Subsequent doses should be given at suitable intervals to maintain analgesia before pain escapes from control.
(c) Nausea and vomiting are common side-effects, but may subside as opioid treatment is continued.
(d) In terminal analgesia, relief of pain is the primary aim, and outweighs any risks of drug-dependence.
(e) Pethidine should not be given to patients receiving MAOI treatment.
(f) Long-acting oral products should be swallowed whole, not chewed or crushed.
(g) Marked respiratory depression may indicate overdose; naloxone is specific treatment.

Drug dependence is a problem with all narcotic analgesics, and arises from the euphoric side-effects of those drugs. For that reason extended treatment should be avoided, except in terminal illness, where the risks of tolerance and drug addiction are much less important than the need to relieve pain.

Diamorphine* (dose: 5–10 mg)

Diamorphine, also known as heroin, is prepared from morphine and has a similar but more powerful analgesic action. It is of great value when increasing doses are required for severe pain in the terminal stages of carcinoma, as its greater solubility permits the use of smaller volumes of injection solution. In chronic pain, diamorphine is given orally or by injection in doses of 5–10 mg which should be repeated according to need, and increased as required. Similar doses can be given for the short-term treatment of acute pain, but intravenous doses should be reduced to one quarter to one half of the intramuscular dose. Diamorphine is also given by subcutaneous infusion in the control of the pain of terminal disease.

It is also a powerful cough centre depressant, and is sometimes given as a linctus (3 mg/5 ml) in the severe and intractable cough of terminal disease.

Side-effects of diamorphine, including constipation, are essentially similar to those of morphine. It is very liable to cause addiction, and diamorphine should be used only when less dangerous drugs are ineffective.

Alfentanil*   (dose: 500 micrograms intravenously initially)

Brand name: Rapifen*

Alfentanil is a potent narcotic analgesic, similar to fentanyl, but mainly used in operative procedures when a rapid onset and short duration of action is required. When used with thiopentone anaesthesia, it permits a reduction in dose of thiopentone, and a more rapid recovery that is useful in out-patient surgery and in poor-risk patients. Doses of 500 micrograms are given initially, followed by doses of 250 micrograms at intervals of 4–5 minutes according to need. In case of assisted ventilation, an initial dose of 50–100 micrograms/kg is given by intravenous infusion, with supplementary doses of 0.5–1 micrograms/kg/minute as required. Alfentanil may occasionally cause severe respiratory depression which may extend over the postoperative period. It can be reversed by **naloxone** or **doxapram** (p. 443).

Buprenorphine* (dose: 200–400 micrograms by injection, 200 micrograms sublingually)

Brand name: Temgesic*

Buprenorphine is a powerful analgesic with a long action that may extend for 8–12 hours, but is less likely to cause dependence. It is given by subcutaneous or intramuscular injection in doses of 200–400 micrograms 6–8 hourly. It is also given orally as sublingual tablets of 200 micrograms. Paradoxically, it also has some of the properties of an opioid antagonist, and may cause withdrawal symptoms in opioid-dependent patients.

Buprenorphine may cause drowsiness, vomiting and dizziness, and although it has a relatively wide margin of safety, some respiratory depression may occur. The action, which may be prolonged in hepatic disease, is only partly reversed by naloxone.

Dextromoramide* (dose: 5–20 mg)

Brand name: Palfium*

Dextromoramide is a powerful narcotic analgesic that is used mainly in the severe pain of terminal disease. It is less sedating than morphine, but the duration of action is shorter, and may not extend over 3 hours. Dextromoramide is given orally in doses of 5–20 mg, or 10 mg by suppository.

Dihydrocodeine § (dose: 30 mg orally, 50 mg by injection)

Brand name: DF-118 §

A derivative of codeine with increased analgesic potency. It is valuable in the treatment of a variety of moderate to severe painful conditions where the use of more powerful narcotic analgesics is not justified. It also has some cough suppressant properties. Dihydrocodeine is given orally after food in doses of 30 mg up to 4-hourly as necessary, or in doses of 50 mg by intramuscular or deep subcutaneous injection. The injection, but not the oral form, is subject to CD regulation. DHC Continus § is a long-acting oral product containing 60 mg of dihydrocodeine, given twice daily.

Side-effects are similar to those of morphine, but less severe, and dependence is also less likely to occur.

Co-dydramol § (Paramol §) is a mixed product containing dihydrocodeine 10 mg and paracetamol 500 mg.

Dipipanone* (dose: 40–120 mg daily)

Dipipanone is a synthetic narcotic analgesic that is less potent and less sedating than morphine, and less liable to cause respiratory depression.

It is used as the mixed product **Diconal***, which contains dipipanone 10 mg and cyclizine 30 mg. Cyclizine is added to reduce the **side-effects** of nausea and vomiting, but the mixed product is not suitable for extended use.

Fentanyl* (dose: 50–200 micrograms by intravenous injection)

Brand name: Sublimase*

Fentanyl is a morphine-like analgesic but of considerably higher potency. It is used mainly as an analgesic during thiopentone anaesthesia, as it permits a reduction in the dose of anaesthetics, and the combination is of value in poor-risk patients. Fentanyl is given by intravenous injection in doses of 50–200 micrograms initially, with subsequent doses of 50 micrograms as required, but if assisted ventilation is used, initial doses of 300–500 micrograms are given.

Fentanyl is also used in association with **droperidol** and **phenoperidine (Thalamonal)*** to promote anaesthesia in children and the aged, and for neuroleptoanalgesia during certain diagnostic procedures.

The **main side-effects** are respiratory depression, nausea and vomiting, but bradycardia and transient hypotension may also occur. Care is necessary in respiratory and liver disease, and in myasthenia gravis.

Meptazinol* (dose: 800 mg–1.6 g daily orally; 100–150 mg by injection)

Brand name: Meptid*

Meptazinol is a potent synthetic analgesic with reduced sedative effects, and appears to have a selective action on the *mu*-receptors thought to mediate the action of the opiate analgesics. It is used in the short-term treatment of postoperative and obstetric pain, in renal colic and other conditions of moderate to severe pain in oral doses of 200 mg four to eight times a day. Meptazinol is also given by intramuscular injection in doses of 75–150 mg 2–4 hourly according to need, and in acute pain it is given by slow intravenous injection in doses of 50–100 mg.

Meptazinol is relatively free from opiate side-effects, and is less likely to cause respiratory depression, but nausea and dizziness may occur.

Methadone* (dose: 5–20 mg by injection)

Brand name: Physeptone*

Methadone is a powerful synthetic analgesic resembling morphine in general activity, but with less sedative or euphoric potency, and with an action lasting up to 8 hours. It is given orally or by subcutaneous or intramuscular injection in doses of 5–10 mg three or four times a day according to need, and is useful when adequate analgesia without sedation is required. For extended use, twice daily dosage should not be exceeded in order to avoid accumulation and subsequent overdose.

Methadone also has cough centre depressant properties, and is useful for the control of useless cough in malignant lung conditions. Methadone *linctus* contains 2 mg/5 ml, and is for adult use only. Methadone is also used in the withdrawal and replacement treatment of drug addiction and dependence as **methadone mixture**, which contains 5 mg/5 ml.

Nalbuphine* (dose: 10–20 mg by injection)

Brand name: Nubain*

Nalbuphine is a synthetic, rapidly acting morphine-like analgesic with reduced side-effects and a lower abuse potential. It is given in moderate to severe pain in doses of 10–20 mg by intramuscular, subcutaneous or intravenous injection at intervals of 3–6 hours according to need.

Nalbuphine is also used to control the pain of myocardial infarction as a dose of 10–20 mg by slow intravenous injection, repeated after 30 minutes if required. When used as a supplementary drug in anaesthesia, it is given in doses of 250–500 micrograms/kg at 30-minute intervals.

Side-effects include respiratory depression and sedation, but nausea and vomiting are less common. Care is necessary in renal and hepatic disease, and in pre-existing respiratory depression.

Pentazocine* (dose: 25–100 mg orally; 30–60 mg by injection)

Brand name: Fortral*

Pentazocine has the general analgesic properties of morphine, but is less likely to cause addiction. Its action is less potent and less prolonged, and after oral administration much of a dose is lost by first-pass liver metabolism. Pentazocine is given orally in doses of 50–100 mg after food, up to a maximum of 600 mg daily, or by injection (subcutaneous, intramuscular or intravenous), according to the severity of the pain, up to 360 mg daily. Pentazocine may also be used as 50 mg suppositories up to four times a day. It may be of value in biliary colic, as it appears to be less likely to cause an increase in biliary pressure than some related analgesics. Care is necessary with patients already receiving an opioid analgesic, as pentazocine, like buprenorphine, may paradoxically increase the pain and bring about withdrawal symptoms.

Side-effects of pentazocine include nausea, dizziness, lightheadedness and hallucinations. As transient hypertension may occur, pentazocine should be avoided in hypertensive states and after myocardial infarction. Convulsions have followed large intravenous doses.

Pethidine* (dose: 50–100 mg orally; 25–100 mg by intramuscular injection; 25–50 mg intravenously)

Pethidine is an old synthetic drug with some of the properties of both morphine and atropine, and has analgesic, and antispasmodic actions. Although less potent than morphine, and with a shorter action, it is widely used for the relief of moderate to severe pain, including postoperative pain, in labour, and as a supplementary drug in general anaesthesia. It is not suitable for the treatment of severe and constant pain, as in terminal illness.

Pethidine is given mainly by intramuscular injection in doses of 25–100 mg, repeated 4-hourly as required, or subcutaneously. It may also be given by slow intravenous injection in doses of 25–50 mg, (10–25 mg as an adjunct to anaesthesia) but vasodilatation and hypotension may occur. Pethidine may also be given orally in doses of 50–150 mg, but the response is less rapid and less intense. It is also used by injection as an obstetric analgesic, although labour may be prolonged, and some neonatal respiratory depression may occur, but to a lesser extent than with other narcotic analgesics.

Side-effects of pethidine are those of the narcotic analgesics generally, but some stimulation of the CNS may occur, and convulsions have been reported after high doses. It is less likely to cause constipation, and has no antitussive properties. The prolonged use of pethidine should be avoided, as addiction may result.

Phenazocine* (dose: 5–20 mg)

Brand name: Narphen*

Phenazocine is a synthetic analgesic with the general properties of morphine, but with an increased potency, and effective in lower doses. It is used for the relief of severe painful conditions, including pancreatitis, and in renal colic as it is less likely to increase the biliary pressure. Phenazocine is given orally in doses of 5 mg, repeated 4–6 hourly as required, but single doses up to 20 mg may sometimes be necessary. It may be given sublingually when nausea and vomiting complicate oral treatment.

Side-effects include nausea and vomiting, but phenazocine is less sedating than morphine, and is less likely to cause constipation. Dependence remains a risk with extended use.

Phenoperidine* (dose: 0.5–5 mg by injection)

Brand name: Operidine*

Phenoperidine is an analgesic of the pethidine type, but it is used mainly as a supplementary drug in general anaesthesia. In patients with spontaneous respiration, it is given intravenously as an initial dose of 1 mg, followed by supportive doses of 500 micrograms at intervals of 40–60 minutes according to need. With assisted respiration, doses of 2–5 mg may be given initially, with subsequent doses of 1 mg as needed. Phenoperidine may cause some respiratory depression, which may be controlled and terminated by naloxone (p. 99).

In conjunction with **droperidol** or **fentanyl**, phenoperidine produces a state of mental detachment and analgesia referred to as neuroleptanalgesia. This indifference to the environment is of particular value where certain procedures, such as pneumo-encephalography, have to be carried out where analgesia is essential but cooperation from the patient is also required. Phenoperidine is also useful as an analgesic during the treatment of severe burns.

Tramadol § (dose: 50–100 mg)

Brand name: Zydol §

Tramadol is a centrally-acting analgesic, but the mode of action is not yet clear, as it has a low affinity for opioid receptors. Tramadol is used in the short-term or intermittent management of moderate to severe pain, and is given in oral doses of 50–100 mg 4–6 hourly. Doses of more than 400 mg daily are seldom required. In severe pain, tramadol may be given in similar doses by intramuscular or intravenous injection. The dosage intervals should be extended in renal and hepatic impairment. Tramadol has a low dependence potential, and cannot suppress morphine-withdrawal symptoms, but prolonged use should be avoided. **Side-effects** include drowsiness, dizziness and fatigue.

NARCOTIC ANTAGONISTS

Lofexidine §▼(dose: 0.4–2.4 mg daily)

Brand name: Britlofex §▼

It is thought that the symptoms of opiate withdrawal may finally be due to an excessive rebound release of noradrenaline in the brain. It is known that clonidine (p. 210) has an inhibitory action on such noradrenaline release, but its value in opiate withdrawal is limited because of its antihypertensive properties. Lofexidine is a related drug with a more selective action on brain noradrenergic activity. It is used in the rapid control of opiate withdrawal symptoms, and may prove useful as transitional treatment before naltrexone therapy is commenced. Lofexidine is given in initial doses of 200 micrograms twice a day, slowly increased according to need and response up to a maximum if required of 2.4 mg daily. At the end of treatment the dose should be tapered off over 2–4 days. **Side-effects** are drowsiness and dryness of mucous membranes. Lofexidine has certain mild hypotensive properties, and should be used with caution in marked bradycardia.

Naloxone § (dose: 1.5–3 micrograms/kg by injection)

Brand name: Narcan §

Naloxone is a short-acting specific antagonist of the opioid analgesics, and is used in the treatment of narcotic-induced postoperative respiratory depression and of narcotic overdose. In such respiratory depression, naloxone is given by intravenous injection as an initial dose of 1.5–3 micrograms/kg (or 100–200 micrograms), followed by 100 microgram doses at intervals of 2 minutes as required. For neonates, doses of 10 micrograms/kg, or a single dose of 200 micrograms may be given. It should be noted that naloxone reverses the analgesic action of the opioids as well as their depressant action on respiration, so dosage in the postoperative period must be controlled to avoid the return of pain.

In suspected narcotic overdose or poisoning, naloxone is given intravenously in doses of 0.8–2 mg, repeated at 2-minute intervals according to response, up to a total dose of 10 mg. Alternatively, a dose of 2 mg, after dilution, may be given by continuous intravenous infusion. The absence of a response indicates that the respiratory depression is not due to narcotic overdose.

Naltrexone § (dose: 25–50 mg daily)

Brand name: Nalorex §

Naltrexone is a powerful, long-acting narcotic antagonist that binds selectively with the opioid receptors (p. 89). It is used only to maintain recovery from opioid drug addiction, and prevents re-addiction only while the drug is being taken, so prolonged maintenance therapy is required. It is given in doses of 25 mg initially, later increased to 50 mg daily. Naltrexone must not be given to patients who are still opioid-dependant, as relapse and an acute withdrawal syndrome may be precipitated within minutes. Its use requires care under specialist supervision. Caution is necessary in hepatic and renal dysfunction, as naltrexone is metabolized in the liver and excreted in the urine.

Some less powerful narcotic analgesics

Codeine § (dose: 60–180 mg daily orally; 30 mg by injection)

Codeine is one of the alkaloids present with morphine in opium. It is much less powerful than morphine, and its analgesic value is limited, but it is given in doses of 30–60 mg up to a maximum of 180 mg daily in mild to moderate pain. An increase in dose does not increase the analgesic response. It is occasionally given by injection in doses up to 30 mg.

Side-effects include constipation, nausea and sedation. It is contraindicated in respiratory depression.

Co-codamol is a mixed product containing codeine 8 mg and paracetamol 500 mg; **Co-codaprin** contains codeine 8 mg with aspirin 400 mg, and a number of proprietary mild analgesic products are formulated on a similar basis. The analgesic value of the small doses of codeine in these preparations is open to question. The use of codeine as a cough centre depressant is referred to on page 444.

Dextropropoxyphene § (dose: 65 mg)

Brand name: Doloxene §

Dextropropoxyphene is an analgesic resembling codeine, but less likely to cause constipation. It is used in the relief of mild to moderate pain in doses of 65 mg three or four times a day, often in association with paracetamol as **co-proxamol** (Distalgesic §), which contains dextropropoxyphene 32.5 mg with paracetamol 325 mg.

Co-proxamol is used in a wide range of chronic and recurring painful conditions, but the maximum dose of eight tablets daily should not be exceeded. Overdose, especially if taken with alcohol, may cause opioid-induced respiratory depression and collapse requiring prompt treatment with naloxone. Subsequently, severe paracetamol hepatotoxicity may develop (see p. 581).

MILD ANALGESICS

Several mild analgesics are available for the relief of the many minor painful and rheumatic conditions that do not call for treatment with more powerful drugs. The more specific antirheumatic drugs, dealt with in Chapter 15, also have useful mild analgesic properties.

Points about mild analgesics

(a) Ask patients about any aspirin hypersensitivity.
(b) Take with food or milk to reduce the risks of gastric irritation.
(c) Aspirin-soluble and similar products should be dissolved in water to promote rapid absorption.
(d) In general, alcohol should be avoided, as car-driving and similar abilities may be affected.
(e) Aspirin should not be given to children under 12 years of age.

Aspirin, acetylsalicylic acid (dose: 2–4 g daily)

Although introduced in 1899, aspirin remains one of the most valuable and widely used of the mild analgesics. It acts mainly by inhibiting the biosynthesis of prostaglandins (p. 420) and is the principal constituent of a variety of popular pain-relieving preparations, often with paracetamol and other drugs.

Aspirin relieves the pain of headache, toothache, neuritis, myalgia and a variety of other conditions requiring mild analgesic therapy. It is given in doses of 300–600 mg five to six times a day, up to a maximum as an analgesic of 4 g daily. In larger doses up to 8 g daily it is given for the treatment of acute and chronic inflammatory conditions such as rheumatoid arthritis.

Aspirin has some antiplatelet activity (see p. 311) and may potentiate the effects of warfarin.

Side-effects. Aspirin is in general well tolerated, but it can cause nausea, indigestion, and gastric irritation with blood loss, and may be the cause of an unsuspected iron-deficiency anaemia when aspirin is taken for prolonged periods.

Idiosyncrasy to aspirin is not uncommon, and in susceptible patients even small doses may precipitate hypersensitivity reactions such as paroxysmal bronchospasm, which may be severe or even fatal.

Some of the gastric side-effects can be reduced by taking the drug after meals, or in association with an alkali, and Dispersible Aspirin Tablets and similar proprietary products are formulated on that basis and contain calcium carbonate.

In high doses, aspirin may cause dizziness, confusion, tinnitus, deafness and hypothrombinaemia. Toxic doses may cause respiratory failure and cardiovascular collapse.

Aspirin may be a causative factor in Reye's syndrome. That syndrome, an acute encephalopathy and fatty degeneration of the liver, is a rare but potentially fatal illness in children. It is now recommended that aspirin should not be given to children under 12 years of age for minor or febrile illness, but be reserved for conditions such as juvenile rheumatoid arthritis (Still's disease).

> Waldman R J et al 1982 Aspirin as a risk factor in Reye's syndrome. Journal of the American Medical Association 247: 3089–3094

Benorylate (dose: 4–8 g daily)

Brand name: Benoral

Benorylate is a chemical compound of aspirin and paracetamol and has the anti-inflammatory and analgesic properties of the parent substances but with reduced side-effects. Dose 1.5–2 g three times a day. It should not be given to a patient with a known hypersensitivity to aspirin, or to children under 12 years of age.

Diflunisal § (dose: 500 mg–1 g daily)

Brand name: Dolobid §

Diflunisal is chemically related to aspirin, and has a similar pattern of activity, but is less likely to cause gastrointestinal side-effects. It has both analgesic and anti-inflammatory properties and is used in post-traumatic and postoperative pain, in some chronic painful conditions, and in osteoarthritis. Diflunisal is given in initial doses of 500 mg twice daily, preferably after food, later reduced to 250 mg twice daily.

Side-effects are similar to those of aspirin, and diflunisal should not be given to aspirin-sensitive patients, or those with a history of peptic ulcer. **Salsalate** § (Disalcid §) is a compound with a basically similar action, and given in doses of 0.5–1 g three of four times a day, after food.

Ibuprofen (dose: 1.2–2.4 g daily)

Brand names: Brufen, Fenbid, Motrin

Ibuprofen is an analgesic anti-inflammatory drug of the NSAID type (p. 416) used in the treatment of mild to moderate musculoskeletal pain, including the pain of dysmenorrhoea and in mild rheumatoid conditions. It is given in doses of 400–800 mg three times a day, after food. It is also given in doses of 20 mg/kg daily in the treatment of pain and febrile conditions in children.

Side-effects are usually mild, but are basically those common to related drugs and bronchospasm may occur in sensitive patients. **Fenoprofen** (Progesic; Fenopron), dose, 200–400 mg three times a day, has similar actions and uses. Codafen Continus contains ibuprofen 300 mg with codeine phosphate 20 mg.

Ketorolac §▼ (dose: 40 mg daily)

Brand name: Toradol §▼

Ketorolac is a NSAID (p. 416) with increased analgesic potency, and is used in the short-term treatment of acute postoperative pain. It is given in doses of 10 mg 4- to 6-hourly up to a maximum of 40 mg daily for up to 7 days. Ketorolac may also be given by deep intragluteal or slow intravenous injection in doses of 10–30 mg at intervals of 4–6 hours, but in the initial postoperative period 2 hourly administration may be required. A transfer to oral therapy should be made as soon as possible, but on the day of transfer the total dose given should not normally exceed 90 mg. In elderly patients, lower doses at longer intervals should be given. Ketotolac is a peripherally acting analgesic and does not interfere with opiate-binding receptors, and may be used together with opiate analgesics for the control of severe pain. It has no sedative or anxiolytic action. Ketorolac is contraindicated in patients sensitive to aspirin or any other NSAID, in active or latent ulcer, or in patients with asthma or coagulation disorders. Ketorolac has many side-effects, and for details the manufacturer's literature should be consulted.

Mefenamic acid § (dose: 1.5 g daily)

Brand name: Ponstan §

Mefenamic acid has analgesic and mild anti-inflammatory properties, and is useful in mild to moderate pain of varied origin, including simple menorrhagia, and in rheumatic states, including Still's disease. The adult dose is 500 mg three times a day after food; children's doses for short-term treatment are 25 mg/kg daily in divided doses.

   Side-effects include diarrhoea, which is an indication for withdrawal, as is haemolytic anaemia, hypersensitivity and bronchospasm, rash and jaundice. Blood tests are necessary during prolonged treatment. Overdose may cause convulsions.

Nefopam § (dose: 90–270 mg daily orally; 20 mg by injection)

Brand name: Acupam §

Nefopam is an analgesic with aspirin-like properties, although its mode of action differs, as it has no effect on prostaglandin synthesis. It is used in the relief of moderate and chronic pain in doses of 30–60 mg three times a day up to a maximum of 270 mg daily or more according to need. It is also given in doses of 20 mg up to 6-hourly by intramuscular injection, but some local pain at the injection site may occur. Nefopam has some anticholinergic properties, and may cause dryness of the mouth and urinary retention. Other side-effects include nausea, dizziness, tachycardia and confusion. It may give a pink colour to the urine. It is contraindicated in convulsive disorders and myocardial infarction.

Paracetamol (dose: 1–4 g daily)

Brand names: Panadol, Calpol

Paracetamol is a very widely used mild analgesic, and is also present in a range of mixed products available under brand names. It has the great advantage over aspirin of being much less likely to cause any gastric irritation but it has no anti-inflammatory action. Paracetamol is given in doses of 0.5–1 g four to six times a day, up to a maximum dose of 4 g daily. In suitable doses, it is useful in febrile conditions in children. In post-immunization pyrexia in infants, paracetamol is given in a dose of 60 mg, followed if necessary by a second dose, administered as Paracetamol Paediatric Elixir (Oral Solution) via an oral syringe. Not more than two doses should be given without medical advice. (Co-codamol is a mixed product containing, unless otherwise prescribed, 8 mg of codeine and 500 mg of paracetamol.)

Paracetamol has few **side-effects**, but excessive and prolonged use may cause liver damage. In acute paracetamol poisoning *early* treatment is essential, as a severe and potentially fatal hepatonecrosis may develop (p. 581).

Sodium salicylate (dose: 5–10 g daily)

Sodium salicylate has the general properties of salicylates as referred to under aspirin, but is more irritant and is now rarely prescribed.

TREATMENT OF MIGRAINE AND CLUSTER HEADACHE

Migraine is a complex of symptoms, consisting essentially of periodic recurrent pulsating headache, frequently unilateral at first, and accompanied by gastric disturbance. The attack is often heralded and followed by visual disturbances and photophobia. Cluster headache, sometimes referred to as migrainous neuralgia, is characterized by short-lived but intense attacks of unilateral head pain, that may recur at intervals at the same time of day for some weeks.

The mechanism of migraine attacks is by no means clear, but the migraine headache is considered to be due to a vascular dilatation and rigidity of the cranial blood vessels. No neuro-logical cause for migraine has been found, and there is probably a constitutional tendency that is triggered off by a variety of apparently unrelated factors which may include vasoactive amines present in chocolate, cheese and other foods, and oral contraceptives are known to precipitate and exacerbate migraine attacks.

Treatment is largely based on ergotamine, but sumatriptan is a newer alternative. For prophylaxis the use of serotonin antagonists may be helpful. Mild analgesic products such as Migraleve, Migravess and Paramax, have but a limited place.

Ergotamine tartrate § (dose: 1–2 mg orally)

Brand name: Lingraine §

Ergotamine is one of the alkaloids of ergot (p. 449) but it is used only for the relief of migraine, as it has a powerful constrictor action on the cranial arteries. The best response is obtained if the drug is taken in adequate dose before an attack has fully developed. It relieves the headache, but may aggravate nausea and vomiting, and combined treatment with an anti-emetic may be required.

The optimum oral dose of ergotamine is best determined by experience, and the initial dose of 2 mg should be taken at the first sign of an attack, preferably sublingually and repeated after 30 minutes. Not more than 6 mg should be taken in any single day, or more than 12 mg in 1 week. Ergotamine may also be given by oral inhalation for a more rapid effect, and the Medihaler-Ergotamine delivers a dose of 360 micrograms, which may be repeated after 5 minutes, but not more than six doses should be taken in 24 hours, or 15 during 1 week. Alternatively, when nausea prevents oral therapy, ergotamine may be given as a 2 mg suppository.

Ergotamine in high doses has a powerful peripheral vasoconstrictor action, and it should be withdrawn immediately if any tingling or numbness in the extremities is noted, as gangrene due to vasoconstriction has occurred. For that reason ergotamine is not used prophylactically.

Side-effects of ergotamine include nausea, vomiting and abdominal pain. Cafergot and Migril are mixed products containing caffeine, which may be better tolerated.

Clonidine § (dose: 100–150 micrograms daily)

Brand name: Dixarit §

Clonidine is used in doses of 50–75 micrograms twice daily in the prophylaxis of migraine and other recurring vascular headaches. It appears to act by reducing the sensitivity of the cranial vessels to circulating amines, but it is of no value in the treatment of an established attack.

Side-effects include dizziness, dryness of the mouth, nausea and occasional rash. It should be noted that the dose and brand name differ from the clonidine product used in hypertension (p. 210).

Methysergide § (dose: 2–6 mg daily)

Brand name: Deseril §

Serotonin may play some part in the migraine syndrome, and the action of ergotamine may be due in part to its anti-serotonin properties. Methysergide has a similar but more powerful action, and it also potentiates the vasoconstrictor action of noradrenaline. It is used under hospital supervision for the long-term prophylaxis of very severe recurrent migraine and cluster headache in doses of 1–2 mg three times a day.

Treatment should not be continued for more than 6 months without a break. Care is necessary in patients with cardiovascular disease and liver or renal damage. Retroperitoneal fibrosis and fibrosis of the heart valves have occasionally followed the prolonged use of methysergide, and the drug is best reserved for those patients not responding to other therapy. Methysergide is also of value in other conditions associated with serotonin release, such as carcinoid disease, where it may give prompt relief of the associated severe diarrhoea. It is then given in doses of 12–15 mg daily under hospital supervision.

Pizotifen § (dose: 0.5–6 mg daily)

Brand name: Sanomigran §

Pizotifen is a serotonin and histamine antagonist similar to **cyproheptadine** and is effective in the *prophylaxis* of migraine and cluster headache. It is given in doses of 1.5 mg at night, or in doses of 500 micrograms or more three times a day, up to a maximum of 6 mg daily, but a single dose should not exceed 3 mg.

Pizotifen may cause drowsiness, weight gain and nausea, but other **side-effects** are linked with its mild anticholinergic properties, and it should not be used in closed angle glaucoma or urinary retention.

Sumatriptan §▼ (dose: 100 mg)

Brand name: Imigran §▼

Sumatriptan is a serotonin-like (5-HT$_1$) receptor agonist, with a selective vasoconstrictor action. It is given for the relief of acute migraine as a single dose of 100 mg as soon as an attack occurs, which can be repeated if the attack returns after an initial response up to a total of 300 mg in 24 hours. If no initial relief is obtained, a second dose should not be given. In severe migraine, and in cluster headache, sumatriptan can be given by subcutaneous injection in a dose of 6 mg, repeated after not less than 1 hour if the attack recurs. Not more than two doses in 24 hours. **Side-effects** include fatigue and dizziness. Chest pain has occurred after injections of sumatriptan. It should not be given intravenously, as angina and coronary vasospasm may be precipitated. It should not be given together with other drugs, or until ergotamine therapy has been withdrawn for at least 24 hours.

Goadsby P J 1991 Oral sumatriptan in acute migraine. Lancet 338: 782–783

Points about migraine treatment

(a) Early treatment advisable before the attack develops.
(b) Mild analgesics helpful, but should be taken with a hot drink to promote absorption.
(c) Ergotamine is more specific in action, side-effects may limit effective dose.
(d) Treatment should not be repeated for at least 4 days or more than twice a month.
(e) Ergotamine should not be given for prophylaxis.
(f) Sumatriptan is a new drug of value in acute migraine, but not more than two doses in 24 hours; and ergotamine treatment should have been withdrawn at least 24 hours previously.

Other antimigraine drugs

Other drugs that have a secondary action that may be useful in the prophylaxis of migraine are **beta-blockers** such as propranolol, metoprolol, nadolol and timolol; **tricyclic antidepressants** represented by amitriptyline, and **calcium channel blocking agents** such as nifedipine and verapamil.

The feverfew plant has long had a reputation of being useful as a prophylactic against migraine, but it is not a prescribed product.

5

Antibiotics and other anti-infective chemotherapeutic agents

CHEMOTHERAPY

Chemotherapy was originally defined as the treatment of infective diseases by drugs, but the term now includes the drug treatment of malignancy. In this chapter antimicrobial chemotherapeutic agents are reviewed.

Although bacteria can be killed by antiseptics, in the past it was considered that an antibacterial substance would be too toxic for systemic use in the control of infections. The problem was first solved when the unusual antibacterial properties of the sulphonamides were discovered in 1936, and the realization of their value in pneumonia and puerperal sepsis resulted in a dramatic widening of medical thought on the treatment of bacterial disease. Although the sulphonamides have been largely replaced by the less toxic antibiotics, they still have a limited place in the treatment of urinary infections and chronic bronchitis, and for historical reasons they will be considered here before the antibiotics.

SULPHONAMIDES

The sulphonamides have an indirect antibacterial action, as they have the ability to inhibit the uptake of para-aminobenzoic acid by certain bacteria, which require that acid for the subsequent formation of folic acid. Folic acid is essential for bacterial development. The sulphonamides interrupt folic acid synthesis and so inhibit further bacterial growth. They are therefore bacteriostatic and not bactericidal in action. (Those bacteria that do not need folic acid for their development are obviously resistant to the action of the sulphonamides.)

The sulphonamides are active against a wide range of Gram-positive and Gram-negative bacteria, but acquired resistance is now common in many pathogenic organisms. Attempts have been made to extend the action of the sulphonamides by the combined use of trimethoprim, which interrupts bacterial metabolism at another point, and some resistant infections may respond to such combined therapy.

Common **side-effects** are nausea, vomiting and malaise, but more serious adverse effects include allergic reactions, cyanosis and agranulocytosis, requiring withdrawal of treatment. Crystalluria may occur, but can be largely prevented by an adequate fluid intake. The Stevens–Johnson syndrome, a form of erythema multiforme with widespread lesions of the skin and mucous membranes, is more likely to occur with the long-acting sulphonamides and may be fatal.

Points about sulphonamides

(a) High fluid intake is necessary to avoid crystalluria.
(b) Best avoided in the elderly and other patients with a folate deficiency.
(c) Trimethoprim now often preferred for most infections.

Sulphadimidine § (dose: 1.5–4 g daily)

Sulphadimidine is used mainly in the treatment of infections of the urinary tract. It is given as a loading dose of 2 g, followed by doses of 0.5–1 g every 6–8 hours, with an adequate fluid intake. It is also used in the prophylaxis of meningococcal meningitis in doses of 2 g daily for 5 days.

Sulphadiazine § (dose: 4–6 g daily)

Sulphadiazine is the preferred sulphonamide for the treatment of sulphonamide-sensitive meningococcal meningitis. In severe conditions it is given by intravenous infusion in doses of 1–1.5 g 4-hourly for 2 days, followed by oral doses of 1 g every 4–6 hours. It may also be given by deep intramuscular injection, but the solution is irritant, and great care is necessary to ensure that it does not damage the subcutaneous tissues.

Sulfametopyrazine § (dose: 2 g weekly)

Brand name: Kelfizine W §

Sulfametopyrazine is a long-acting sulphonamide as it binds extensively with plasma proteins. It is used mainly in the treatment of urinary tract infections and in the control of chronic bronchitis in a dose of 2 g weekly. A disadvantage is that if side-effects occur, they will be slow in subsiding after the withdrawal of the drug, and the Stevens–Johnson syndrome is more likely to occur with sulfametopyrazine than with more rapidly eliminated sulphonamides.

Sulphamethoxazole §

Sulphamethoxazole has the general properties of the sulphonamides, but is now used mainly as a constituent of **co-trimoxazole.**

Co-trimoxazole § (dose: 1.92 g daily)

Brand names: Bactrim §, Septrin §

Co-trimoxazole is a mixture of sulphamethoxazole and trimethoprim. The antibacterial range of trimethoprim is similar to that of the sulphonamides, but it interrupts the folic–folinic acid metabolic process at a different point. The mixture thus permits a two-pronged antibacterial attack which increases the activity. Co-trimoxazole is widely used in the treatment of urinary infections, the exacerbations of chronic bronchitis, in some bone and joint infections, in typhoid fever and salmonellosis.

Co-trimoxazole is the drug of choice in the treatment of

pneumonia caused by *Pneumocystis carinii* in immunocompromised and AIDS patients.

In the prophylaxis of recurrent urinary infections, co-trimoxazole is given in doses of 480 mg daily, but the therapeutic dose in severe infection is 960 mg 12-hourly, together with adequate fluids. For extended treatment, and in patients with reduced renal efficiency, doses of 480 mg twice a day are preferred. In very severe infections, co-trimoxazole is given by intramuscular injection or intravenous infusion in doses of 960 mg twice daily. In gonorrhoea, 1.92 g is given 12-hourly for 2 days, or as two doses of 2.4 g separated by an 8-hour interval. High doses of 120 mg/kg daily are used in *Pneumocystis carinii* infections.

Side-effects of co-trimoxazole are similar to those of the sulphonamides, but the trimethoprim component may cause a depression of haemopoiesis. Care is necessary in renal impairment, and it is no longer recommended for patients over 65 as a folate deficiency may be present. Blood counts are advisable during prolonged treatment, and the drug should be withdrawn immediately if a rash occurs. It is contraindicated in severe liver damage or marked renal insufficiency, and in pregnancy.

Trimethoprim § (dose: 400 mg daily)

Brand names: Ipral §, Monotrim §, Trimopan §

Trimethoprim is an antibacterial agent with a wide range of activity similar to that of the sulphonamides. Although it is often used in combination as co-trimoxazole, trimethoprim is also widely used alone in the treatment of respiratory and urinary tract infections, including acute bronchitis, and is given in doses of 200 mg twice a day. In severe infections, it may be given by intravenous injection or infusion in doses of 150–250 mg 12-hourly. In chronic infections, and for prophylaxis, trimethoprim is given in doses of 100 mg at night. It is also suitable for administration to children in doses adjusted to age (25 mg twice daily for a child of 1–5 years).

Side-effects are gastrointestinal disturbances, rash and pruritus, and some depression of haemopoiesis may occur. Blood counts are necessary during prolonged treatment. Severe renal insufficiency is a contraindication.

ANTIBIOTICS

Antibiotics can be broadly defined as antibacterial substances produced by fungal and other organisms. They owe their use to the chance observation by Professor Fleming in 1928 that the growth of some cultures of staphyloccoci had been inhibited by the growth of a contaminant mould.

It was found that a substance formed by the mould could prevent the growth of certain bacteria, and the active compound was eventually extracted and termed penicillin, a name derived from the name of the contaminant mould. Penicillin came into therapeutic use in 1941, and since that time many other antibiotics have become available. Table 5.1 indicates the *main* type of activity of some principal antibiotics. They have no antiviral properties.

Mode of action

The antibiotics have a bactericidal action by interfering with the development of bacterial cell walls and cross linkages. The walls

Table 5.1   Main type of activity of some principal antibiotics

Against Gram-positive organisms	Against Gram-negative organisms	Against Gram-positive and Gram-negative organisms	Antitubercular antibiotics
Penicillins	Amikacin	Amoxycillin	Capreomycin
Clindamycin	Aztreonam	Ampicillin	Cycloserine
Cloxacillin	Colistin	Azlocillin	Rifampicin
Erythromycin	Gentamicin	Bacampicillin	Streptomycin
Flucloxacillin	Kanamycin	Carbenicillin	
Sodium fusidate	Netilmicin	Carfecillin	
Vancomycin	Pivmecillinam	Cephalosporins[a]	
	Polymyxin	Chloramphenicol	
	Spectinomycin	Ciclacillin	
	Ticarcillin	Imipenem	
	Tobramycin	Mezlocillin	
		Neomycin	
		Piperacillin	
		Pivampicillin	
		Tetracyclines[b]	

[a]See Table 5.4 on page 130.
[b]See Table 5.5 on page 136.

have a lattice-like structure containing the polymer peptidoglycan, and are strengthened by cross linkages of peptide chains
to resist the osmotic pressure of the cell. Penicillins, and similar
antibiotics, which must first enter the cell, inhibit further cell wall
synthesis by linking with certain penicillin-binding proteins
(PBPs) concerned with peptidoglycan production. As a result, the
cell wall becomes weakened as growth and repair are inhibited
and it eventually bursts under the internal pressure, with lysis of
the cell. That explains why antibiotics are mainly active against
rapidly growing bacteria, as mature or quiescent organisms are
less susceptible to cell wall breakdown. Gram-negative organisms
have cell walls of a more complex structure containing a higher
proportion of lipids that prevent the entry of many penicillins,
and so are more resistant to antibiotic attack.

The aminoglycosides act by inhibiting the synthesis of proteins
by the cell ribosomes, or by the formation of non-functioning
proteins, whereas the tetracyclines inhibit the attachment of
aminoacids to extending peptide chains, and inhibit protein
synthesis by another mechanism.

Ideally, antibiotics should be used after the infecting organisms
have been identified, and their sensitivity determined, but that is
not always possible, and an empirical choice of drug based on
experience is often necessary.

Bacterial resistance

Although the antibacterial range of some antibiotics may be wide,
the *degree* of activity may vary as bacteria can differ markedly in
their sensitivity, especially to penicillin, even among those
groups of organisms that are normally susceptible. These changes
may be linked with an ability of the organism to tolerate the
antibiotic, as initially, the most sensitive organisms will be eliminated, and less sensitive bacteria will tend to survive, or require
increased doses of the antibiotic to ensure bacterial kill.
Resistance is also linked with the fact that some bacteria possess
enzymes, referred to as penicillinases, that can inactivate antibiotics before they can enter bacterial cells. Resistance to one antibiotic is often associated with resistance to related antibiotics, as
cross-resistance between penicillin and cephalosporins is well
known. One of the most important penicillinases is beta-lactamase,
which inactivates penicillin by breaking the beta-lactam ring

of the penicillin structure. Some semi-synthetic penicillins, such as cloxacillin, are not inactivated by beta-lactamase, and so are active against penicillin-resistant organisms. Others are active against normally non-susceptible organisms, such as the ubiquitous and highly resistant *Pseudomonas aeruginosa*.

Resistance may also be acquired by the transfer of genetic material when bacteria are in contact. In that way, a gene carrying resistance may be transferred to another organism, a process known as transduction, and is thought to be the method by which many strains of *Staphylococcus aureus* have acquired resistance.

Resistance has often occurred through the over-use of antibiotics for trivial infections, or the use of wide-ranging antibiotics before the identity and sensitivity of the invading organisms have been confirmed. Fortunately there is now a tendency to avoid the indiscriminate use of antibiotics in hospitals by devising an antibiotic policy, and so restrict the use of specific antibiotics for the treatment of infections where they are most likely to be effective.

Antibiotic-associated colitis

Diarrhoea is a common side-effect of antibiotic therapy, and may be due to a disturbance of the normal balanced bacterial flora of the intestinal tract. It may be mild and self-limiting, but a much more serious condition is pseudomembranous colitis, now known as antibiotic-associated colitis (AAC), which may occur occasionally with virtually all antibiotics, but most frequently with clindamycin. It is due to the overgrowth of *Clostridium difficile*, the release of diarrhoea-causing toxins and the superficial necrosis of the bowel mucosa. It occurs most frequently in elderly and debilitated patients, especially after abdominal surgery. Treatment is with metronidazole (p. 150) or vancomycin (p. 144).

Sensitivity reactions

Some degree of sensitivity to antibiotics, particularly the penicillins, is relatively common, and nurses should always enquire about such sensitivity before giving an antibiotic. Most sensitivity reactions are allergic in character, and may be immediate or delayed. Immediate reactions may be itching, flushing and sneezing, but breathing difficulties indicate the possibility of an anaphylactic reaction requiring urgent treatment with adrenaline. Later reactions include urticaria, and delayed reactions are characterized by bullous eruptions and dermatitis.

Points about antibiotic therapy

(a) Antibiotics are antibacterial, not antiviral agents: whenever possible, the nature of infective organism and its sensitivity to antibiotics should be determined before treatment is commenced.

(b) Other factors governing choice of antibiotic include previous treatment and hypersensitivity, hepatic and renal efficiency, whether patient is immunocompromised or pregnant.

(c) Route of administration and duration of treatment depends on severity of infection: a simple urinary tract infection may respond to short-term therapy; bone infections require prolonged treatment; serious and life-threatening infections require intravenous high-dose therapy.

THE PENICILLINS

Penicillin once referred to what is now known as benzylpenicillin or penicillin G, but many semisynthetic penicillin derivatives with varying patterns of activity are in use. Table 5.2 indicates the wide range of penicillins now available.

Points about penicillins

(a) Bactericidal, not bacteriostatic.

(b) Renal excretion can be delayed by probenecid.

(c) Hypersensitivity to one penicillin includes all others and may extend to the cephalosporins.

(d) Oral therapy may cause diarrhoea, and is not suitable for severe infections as absorption is variable.

(e) Most staphylococci are resistant to ampicillin.

(f) Penicillinase-resistant and broad-spectrum penicillins are not effective against *Pseudomondas aeruginosa*.

(g) With high doses or renal impairment, accumulation of electrolytes (sodium/potassium) may occur.

Benzylpenicillin §, penicillin G §

Brand name: Crystapen §

Penicillin is highly active against many Gram-positive bacteria, but it is also active against a few Gram-negative and other organ-

Table 5.2 Types of penicillins

Approved name	Brand name	Administration
Standard penicillins		
benzylpenicillin	Crystapen	i.m; i.v.
phenoxymethyl penicillin		oral
procaine penicillin	Bicillin	i.m.
Broad-spectrum penicillins		
amoxycillin	Amoxil	oral; i.m; i.v; ivf.
ampicillin	Penbritin	oral; i.m; i.v; ivf.
ampicillin with cloxacillin	Amplicox	oral; i.m; i.v; ivf.
bacampicillin	Ambaxin	oral
co-amoxiclav (amoxycillin with clavulanic acid)	Augmentin	oral; i.m; i.v; ivf.
co-fluampicil (ampicillin with flucloxacillin)	Magnapen	i.m; i.v; ivf.
pivampicillin	Pondocillin	oral
Penicillinase-resistant penicillins		
cloxacillin	Orbenin	oral; i.m; i.v; ivf.
flucloxacillin	Floxapen	oral; i.m; i.v; ivf.
temocillin	Temopen	i.m; i.v; ivf.
Penicillins active against *Pseudomonas aeruginosa*		
azlocillin	Securopen	i.v; ivf.
carbenicillin	Pyopen	i.m; i.v; ivf.
piperacillin (with tazobactam)	Pipril	i.m; i.v; ivf.
	Tazocin	i.v; ivf.
ticarcillin (with clavulanic acid)	Ticar	i.m; i.v; ivf.
	Timentin	ivf.

ivf = intravenous infusion.

isms. It is effective in a wide range of infections, including those in Table 5.3.

Benzyl penicillin is not very effective orally, as it is rapidly broken down by gastric acid, and is best given by intramuscular injection. The initial dose of 600–1200 mg is followed by maintenance doses of 600 mg two to four times a day, and when the organism is susceptible to penicillin, the response to treatment is usually prompt.

In bacterial endocarditis much larger doses are necessary. In that disease the valves of the heart are infected by *Streptococcus viridans* (although other organisms may also be involved) and become inflamed. In these inflamed tissues large numbers of bacteria are present, and to achieve an adequate cardiac tissue level of penicillin, daily doses of 7.2 g are given by slow intra-

Table 5.3   Infections for which benzylpenicillin is effective

Organism	Disease
β-haemolytic *Streptococcus*	Septicaemia, tonsillitis
Staphylococcus	Septicaemia, osteomyelitis
Pneumococcus	Pneumonia
Meningococcus	Meningococcal meningitis
Streptococcus viridans	Infective endocarditis
Clostridium tetani	Tetanus
Clostridium welchii	Gas gangrene
Corynebacterium diphtheriae	Diphtheria
Treponema pallidum	Syphilis
Actinomyces	Actinomycosis
Neisseria gonorrhoeae	Gonorrhoea

venous infusion together with gentamicin. Prolonged therapy is necessary to avoid relapse.

Penicillin has been used prophylactically against bacterial endocarditis in patients with heart valve lesions as with such patients a dental extraction may lead to bacteraemia, but oral amoxycillin is now preferred.

In meningitis, penicillin penetrates through the normally resistant blood–brain barrier and is given in doses of 2.4 g by slow intravenous injection or infusion every 4–6 hours.

Procaine-penicillin is a long-acting form, given by intramuscular injection, from which penicillin is slowly released over 24 hours. It is used mainly in the treatment of primary syphilis as Bicillin, which contains procaine-penicillin and benzyl penicillin.

Side-effects. Although benzylpenicillin and its modifications are virtually non-toxic, allergic reactions and hypersensitivity may occur and are referred to on page 11.

Phenoxymethylpenicillin § (Penicillin V) § (dose: 1–2 g daily)

Benzylpenicillin is not very active orally except in patients with hypoacidity or achlorhydria, but phenoxymethylpenicillin is an acid-stable derivative suitable for oral use. It is used mainly in streptococcal tonsillitis and respiratory infections in children, in doses varying from 62.5 to 250 mg every 6 hours. It is also useful for maintenance therapy after a satisfactory response to penicillin by injection. It is also given prophylactically against re-infection after recovery from streptococcal rheumatic fever in doses of 250 mg twice a day. Phenoxymethylpenicillin is not suitable in any severe condition in which high plasma levels of the antibiotic are required, as absorption is variable.

PENICILLINASE-RESISTANT PENICILLINS

Cloxacillin § (dose: 2 g daily orally)

Brand name: Orbenin §

Although staphylococci were originally largely susceptible to penicillin, the extensive use of the drug has been accompanied by the emergence of resistant strains, and now most staphylococci are resistant to penicillin. Some semisynthetic penicillins such as cloxacillin are largely immune to enzymatic breakdown, and are of great value in the treatment of infections caused by penicillinase-producing staphylococci generally.

Cloxacillin is acid stable, and is active orally as well as by injection. The standard oral dose in staphylococcal infections is 500 mg every 6 hours, 30 minutes to 1 hour before food to secure maximum absorption. In severe infections, it may be given by intramuscular or slow intravenous injection or infusion in doses of 250–500 mg 6-hourly.

Side-effects are those of penicillin generally.

Flucloxacillin § (dose: 1 g daily orally)

Brand names: Floxapen §, Stafoxil §

Flucloxacillin is a beta-lactamase-resistant penicillin very similar to cloxacillin, but is absorbed much better after oral administration, and is effective in doses of 250 mg 6-hourly, preferably well before food. In severe conditions it may be given by i.m. or i.v. injection in doses of 250–500 mg or more every 6 hours. Flucloxacillin is used in many conditions associated with penicillin-resistant *Staphylococcus aureus*, including osteomyelitis, endocarditis and pneumonia. Co-fluampicil (Magnapen) is a mixture of flucloxacillin and ampicillin.

Temocillin § (dose: 2–4 g daily by injection)

Brand name: Temopen §

Temocillin is a penicillin derivative active against many beta-lactamase-producing Gram-negative bacteria, including most enterobacteria. It has little action against Gram-positive cocci or *Pseudomonas aeruginosa*. Temocillin is used mainly in urinary and respiratory tract infections, and in septicaemia associated with susceptible Gram-negative organisms. It is given in doses of 1–2 g every 12 hours by intramuscular or intravenous injection or infusion. As the former may be painful, the antibiotic can be dissolved in 1% lignocaine solution if required. The dose should be adjusted in cases of severe renal impairment. In simple infections of the urinary tract it is given as a single daily dose of 1 g.

Temocillin is well tolerated, and **side-effects** are uncommon, but if a rash or other indications of sensitivity develop, the drug should be withdrawn.

PENICILLINS ACTIVE AGAINST PSEUDOMONAS AERUGINOSA

Benzylpenicillin and related penicillins are inactive against *Pseudomonas aeruginosa*, but some semisynthetic derivatives have a largely specific action against that ubiquitous and normally resistant organism. The first to be introduced was carbenicillin, but more powerful antibiotics such as ticarcillin which are not inactivated by penicillinases, are now available.

Carbenicillin § (dose: 5–20 g daily by injection)

Brand name: Pyopen §

Carbenicillin has a largely specific action against *Ps. aeruginosa*, but the degree of activity is not great, so large doses are required.

In severe systemic infections due to *Ps. aeruginosa* or some strains of *Proteus*, carbenicillin is given by intravenous infusion in doses of 5 g or more every 4–6 hours. It is essential to maintain a high blood level of the drug, as it is rapidly excreted. In urinary tract infections, doses of 2 g are given 6-hourly by intramuscular injection. The activity of carbenicillin is increased by gentamicin, but the two antibiotics should be injected separately at different times.

The large doses of carbenicillin that are necessary may cause electrolyte disturbances and hypokalaemia. Lower doses should be given in cases of renal dysfunction.

Azlocillin § (dose: 6–15 g daily intravenously)

Brand name: Securopen §

Azlocillin is a broad spectrum antibiotic markedly effective against *Pseudomonas aeruginosa* and *Proteus spp.* It is also active against some anaerobic organisms, including *Bacteroides* and *Clostridium.* In pseudomonal infections of the respiratory and urinary tracts, and in septicaemia, azlocillin is given by intravenous injection in doses of 2 g 8-hourly; in serious infections doses of 5 g 8-hourly by intravenous infusion may be necessary. In renal impairment, the dosage interval should be extended. Azlocillin may be given in conjunction with an aminoglycoside such as gentamicin in pseudomonal septicaemia, but the drugs must be given separately.

Piperacillin § (dose: 100–300 mg/kg daily by injection)

Brand name: Pipril §

Piperacillin is a derivative of ampicillin that resembles carbenicillin in its antipseudomonal pattern of activity, but it is more potent, and active against a wider range of organisms. It is used mainly in severe infections due to *Pseudomonas* and associated organisms, including bacterial septicaemia and endocarditis, and is given in divided doses of 100–150 mg/kg daily by intramuscular or slow intravenous injection or infusion, increased in very severe or life-threatening infections up to 16 g or more daily.

In pseudomonal septicaemia piperacillin is given with an aminoglycoside antibiotic, as such combined treatment is synergistic, but the antibiotics should be injected separately. It may also be given with metronidazole in mixed aerobic/anaerobic infections. Piperacillin has also been given by intramuscular injection in doses of 2 g every 12 hours in the extended treatment of uncomplicated urinary tract infections, and a single dose of 2 g has been used in gonorrhoea. In cases of renal impairment the interval between doses should be extended.

The antibacterial potency of piperacillin can be extended to organisms normally resistant to the antibiotic by combined administration with tazobactam as Tazocin ▼. Tazobactam is a potent inhibitor of beta-lactamase, and combined use extends the antibacterial spectrum to include many beta-lactamase-producing bacteria that are normally resistant to piperacillin and other beta-lactam antibiotics. Tazocin is indicated in a wide range of infections, including mixed infections with both aerobic and anaerobic organisms and is given in doses of 2.25–4.5 g 8-hourly by intravenous injection or slow infusion.

Ticarcillin § (dose: 15–20 g daily by injection)

Brand name: Ticar §

Ticarcillin resembles azlocillin in its general properties, and is used mainly in infections due to *Pseudomonas* and *Proteus spp.* Combined treatment with gentamicin or a related aminoglycoside has a synergistic effect, but the two antibiotics should be given separately.

The dose of ticarcillin is 15–20 g daily in divided doses, which may be given by intramuscular or slow intravenous injection or by intravenous infusion. In cases of renal impairment, reduced doses of 2 g every 8–12 hours should be given. In the treatment of acute, uncomplicated urinary tract infections, doses of 3–4 g daily by intramuscular injection may be given, but as such injections may be painful, the antibiotic can be dissolved in 0.5% lignocaine.

Side-effects are few, but skin and mucous membrane haemorrhages have occasionally been reported.

Timentin § contains ticarcillin and clavulanic acid. The mixture is active against penicillase-producing bacteria that are otherwise resistant to ticarcillin and is given by intravenous infusion in doses of 3.2 g three or four times a day.

Cholestatic jaundice is a late-onset side-effect thought to be associated with clavulanic acid.

BROAD-SPECTRUM PENICILLINS AND OTHER ANTIBIOTICS

The broad-spectrum semisynthetic penicillins not only have the general action of penicillin, but a range of activity that includes many Gram-negative pathogens, with the exception of *Pseudomonas*. They are not resistant to the penicillinases. Ampicillin is a typical member of the group but some of its derivatives may be better absorbed, and give higher plasma levels.

Ampicillin § (dose: 1–4 g daily)

Brand names: Amfipen §, Penbritin §

Ampicillin is widely used in the treatment of respiratory infections such as chronic bronchitis, which is often associated with *Streptococcus pneumoniae* and *Haemophilus influenzae* as well as in ear, nose, throat and urinary infections, including gonorrhoea.

The oral dose of ampicillin is 250 mg–1 g every 6 hours, but in severe infections it is given in doses of 500 mg 4–6-hourly by intramuscular or intravenous injection. Pain after intramuscular injection can be avoided by reconstituting the antibiotic with 0.5% lignocaine solution. In gonorrhoea, a single 2 g oral dose with 1 g of probenecid may be adequate.

Ampicillin should always be given *before* meals as absorption is incomplete, and is further decreased by the presence of food in the intestine. It is inactivated by penicillinases, and most staphylococci are now resistant to ampicillin, as are many strains of *Escherichia coli.*

Diarrhoea is a common **side-effect**, and a reaction of the urticarial type is usually indicative of a penicillin allergy. A macropapular rash is common in patients with infectious mononucleosis or chronic lymphatic leukaemia, but is not usually a penicillin-allergy reaction.

Co-fluampicil (Magnapen) is a mixture of ampicillin and flucloxacillin.

Amoxycillin § (dose: 750 mg–1.5 g daily)

Brand names: Almodan §, Amoxil §

Amoxycillin is a derivative of ampicillin, and has the action and uses of the parent drug, but it is more active when given orally, and higher plasma levels are obtained from smaller doses. The standard dose is 250 mg 8-hourly, but double doses may be given in severe infections, or a dose of 500 mg may be given by intramuscular injection, or up to 1 g by intravenous infusion every 6–8 hours. Amoxycillin is of value in bronchial and purulent respiratory infections, in which doses of up to 3 g 12-hourly are given. It is also used in the treatment of typhoid fever, and prophylactically in bacterial endocarditis and dentistry.

Side-effects are similar to those of ampicillin, but diarrhoea is less common.

Co-amoxiclav (Augmentin) is a mixture of amoxycillin and clavulanic acid. That acid, which has no intrinsic antibacterial properties, is an effective inhibitor of penicillinases, and the mixture extends the action of amoxycillin to include otherwise resistant strains of *Staphylococcus aureus*, *Escherichia coli*, *Haemophilus influenzae*, and *Bacteroides*. The dose is one or two tablets 8-hourly.

Care is necessary with co-amoxiclav in hepatic impairment, and cholestatic jaundice has occurred up to 6 weeks after co-amoxiclav treatment.

Other broad-spectrum ampicillin-like antibiotics are **bacampicillin** § (Ambaxin), dose 800 mg–2.4 g daily, and **pivampicillin** § (Pondocillin), dose 1–2 g daily.

MACROLIDE AND LINCOSAMIDE ANTIBIOTICS

This group of antibacterial agents is considered here because the oldest and still used member, erythromycin, has a range of activity similar to that of benzylpenicillin. They have a much more complex chemical structure than the penicillins, and have a bacteriostatic action by affecting bacterial ribosomes and so inhibiting bacterial protein synthesis. The lincosamide antibiotics, represented by clindamycin, have a similar action, but are of limited therapeutic value.

Points about macrolide antibiotics

  (a) Penicillin-like range of activity, so useful in penicillin sensitivity and against some penicillin-resistant staphylococci.
  (b) Tissue concentrations higher with azithromycin and clarithromycin with reduced gastrointestinal disturbances.
  (c) Combined treatment with astemizole or terfenadine should be avoided.

Erythromycin § (dose: 1–2 g daily)

Brand names: Erythrocin §, Erycen §, Erythroped §, Ilosone §

Erythromycin has a penicillin-like range of activity with the advantage of being active orally, and is suitable for use in penicillin-sensitive patients. It is active against many Gram-positive cocci, and as it is taken up by the phagocytes, it is of value in many respiratory infections including *Mycoplasma pneumoniae* and Legionaire's disease, which is due to *Legionella pneumophilia*. Those organisms multiply intracellularly, so are more exposed to attack by macrolide antibiotics which enter the phagocytes. Erythromycin is used mainly for short-term therapy, and is given in doses of 250–500 mg four times a day, but in severe infections it may be given by intravenous infusion in doses of 2–4 g daily.

Side-effects of erythromycin include nausea and vomiting and diarrhoea may occur after large doses. Care is necessary with patients receiving warfarin, as the action of the anticoagulant may be potentiated.

Azithromycin § (dose: 500 mg daily)

Brand name: Zithromax §

Azithromycin is chemically related to erythromycin but it is more acid stable. It is well absorbed after oral administration, giving high tissue levels which decline slowly, and so permit single daily doses. It is effective in many soft tissue infections, bronchitis and atypical pneumonia. Such pneumonia, caused by *Mycoplasma* and similar organisms, is becoming more common, and resistant to many antibiotics. The invading organisms migrate to the phagocytes, and azithromycin appears to be concentrated in the phagocytes to a greater degree than erythromycin. It is given in single daily doses of 500 mg for 3 days, 1 hour before or after food. Gastrointestinal disturbances are the main side-effect. It is contraindicated in hepatic disease.

Clarithromycin § (dose: 500 mg daily)

Brand name: Klaricid §

Clarithromycin is a derivative of erythromycin with similar actions and uses. It is acid stable, and so has a greater degree of bioavailability. Clarithromycin is given in doses of 250 mg twice a day for 7 days, doubled in severe infections, with treatment continued if necessary for 14 days. It may also be given by intravenous infusion in divided doses of 1 g daily for 5–7 days. Headache, rash and gastrointestinal disturbances are side-effects. Care is necessary in renal and hepatic impairment.

Clindamycin § (dose: 600–1200 mg daily)

Brand name: Dalacin C §

Clindamycin is a lincosamide antibiotic that is taken up selectively and concentrated in bone, and is used in the control of staphylococcal bone and joint infections. It is also active against some intestinal anaerobic pathogens, and is used in abdominal sepsis.

Clindamycin is given orally in doses of 150–300 mg (with water) four times a day, and in severe infections by intramuscular injection or intravenous infusion in divided doses of 600 mg–2.4 g daily.

A serious and potentially fatal **side-effect** of clindamycin is the occasional development of a severe pseudomembranous colitis, particularly in elderly patients after abdominal surgery. It may occur with almost any other antibiotic, and is now referred to as antibiotic-associated colitis (AAC) (p. 117). If any diarrhoea occurs, the drug should be withdrawn at once (see vancomycin and metronidazole).

CEPHALOSPORINS AND ASSOCIATED ANTIBIOTICS

The cephalosporins are a group of semi-synthetic antibiotics with some chemical relationships to the penicillins. In general they have a wide range of activity against both Gram-positive and Gram-negative infections, and have an antibacterial action by an interference with cell-wall and cross-link synthesis.

These antibiotics are widely used in a variety of systemic infections not responding to the penicillins, or when alternative therapy is required, and as they are excreted largely unchanged in the urine, they are also used in the treatment of various urinary infections not responding to other treatment.

Some members of the group are largely inactivated by beta-lactamase, and so are not effective against many staphylococcal infections, although others such as cefuroxime and cephamandole, are less susceptible to such inactivation.

Side-effects. A wide range of side-effects have been reported with the cephalosporins, some of which occur mainly with the higher doses. Allergic reactions are the most common and include rash, pruritus, urticaria, arthralgia and fever. Cross-sensitivity may occur in 10% of patients sensitive to penicillin. Gastrointestinal disturbances and disturbances of liver enzyme activity may occur, and an interference with blood clotting factors has also been noted. The cephalosporins are excreted mainly in the urine, and may cause renal disturbance in elderly patients. Powerful diuretics such as frusemide, when given in high doses, may increase the risk of renal damage and the dose of cephalosporin may require adjustment.

Points about cephalosporins

(a) Wide-range bactericidal antibiotics.
(b) Some are less susceptible to inactivation by beta-lactamases.
(c) Cefsulodin and ceftazidime are exceptional in being active against *Pseudomonas*.
(d) Ceftriaxone has a long action that permits single daily doses.
(e) Cefoxitin is active against intestinal organisms.
(f) Main side-effect is hypersensitivity, and 10% of penicillin-sensitive patients are also cephalosporin-sensitive.
(g) Exclude such sensitivity before cephalosporin therapy.

Table 5.4 indicates the range of available products, but clinically there is often little difference between many members of the group, although **cefsulodin** and **ceftazidime** are exceptional in having a more specific action against *Pseudomonas aeruginosa*. Extended treatment with wide-range cephalosporins carries the risk of superinfection with resistant organisms.

Cefaclor § (dose: 750 mg–4 g daily)

Brand name: Distaclor §

Cefaclor is an orally active cephalosporin effective against a wide range of Gram-positive and Gram-negative bacteria, but less active against *Haemophilus influenzae*. It is often useful in urinary tract infections not responding to other treatment. It is given in doses of 250 mg 8-hourly, with double doses in severe infections.

Table 5.4 Cephalosporins

Approved name	Brand name	Route of administration	Daily dose	Notes
cefaclor	Distaclor	oral	750 mg–4 g	Typical cephalosporin
cefadroxil	Baxan	oral	1–2 g	Twice daily dose
cefixime	Suprax	oral	200–400 mg	Single daily dose
cefodizime	Timecef	i.m., i.v., ivf	2 g	More active against some Gram-negative organisms
cefotaxime	Claforan	i.m., i.v., ivf	2–12 g	More active against some Gram-negative organisms
cefoxitin	Mefoxin	i.m., i.v., ivf	3–12 g	More active against intestinal bacteria
cefpodoxime	Orelox	oral	200–400 mg	Resistant respiratory tract infections
cefsulodin	Monaspor	i.m., i.v., ivf	1–4 g	Used in pseudomonal infections
ceftazidime	Fortum	i.m., i.v., ivf	1–6 g	Active against Gram-negative organisms
ceftriaxone	Rocephin	i.m., i.v., ivf	1–4 g	Single daily dose
ceftizoxime	Cefizox	i.m., i.v., ivf	2–8 g	Active against Gram-negative organism
cefuroxime	Zinacef	i.m., i.v., ivf	2–6 g	Active against *Haemophilus Influenzae* and *Neisseria gonorrhoeae*
	Zinnat	oral	0.5–1g	
cephalexin	Ceporex	oral	2–6 g	Not for severe infection
	Keflex	oral		
cephamandole	Kefadol	i.m., i.v., ivf	2–12 g	Active against *Haemophilus influenzae* and *Neisseria*
cephazolin	Kefzol	i.m., i.v., ivf	2–4 g	Now used less frequently
cephradine	Velosef	oral	1–2 g	Now used less frequently
		i.m., i.v., ivf	2–4 g	

i.m. = intramuscular; i.v. = intravenous; ivf = intravenous infusion.

Cefaclor may cause skin reactions in some patients, particularly in children.

Cefadroxil § (dose: 1–2 g daily)

Brand name: Baxan §

Cefadroxil has a longer duration of action than some other oral cephalosporins, and is effective in doses of 500 mg–1 g twice daily. It is used mainly in soft tissue, skin and urinary tract infections. It has little action against *Haemophilus influenzae*.

Cefixime § (dose: 200–400 mg daily)

Brand name: Suprax §

Cefixime is a long-acting and powerful cephalosporin given in doses of 200–400 mg as a single daily dose. At present it is used only in acute infections.

Cefoxitin § (dose: 3–8 g daily by injection)

Brand name: Mefoxin §

Cefoxitin is a cephamycin antibiotic, closely related chemically to the cephalosporins, and having similar actions and uses against a wide range of infections. It is largely resistant to enzymatic breakdown by beta-lactamases, with an increased activity against Gram-negative organisms, and is of value in surgery for the prevention and treatment of intra-abdominal infections associated with *Bacteroides fragilis* and similar organisms, as well as in mixed infections.

Cefoxitin is given in doses of 1–2 g either by intramuscular or slow intravenous injection at intervals of 6–8 hours, but in severe infections, doses up to 12 g daily may be required. Lower doses are given in renal impairment. The intramuscular injection, which should be made deeply into a large muscle, can be painful, and if necessary the drug may be dissolved in 0.5 or 1% lignocaine solution.

Side-effects are hypersensitivity and occasional gastrointestinal disturbances, but diarrhoea may indicate the development of pseudomembranous colitis.

Cefpodoxime §▼ (dose: 200–400 mg daily)

Brand name: Orelox §▼

Cefpodoxime is mainly indicated in the treatment of chronic and recurrent respiratory tract infections, and those resistant to other antibiotics, as it is more active than some other oral cephalosporins. It is given in doses of 100–200 mg twice a day with meals, although in sinusitis, double doses are recommended. The side-effects of cefpodoxime are similar to those of the cephalosporins generally.

Ceftriaxone §▼ (dose: 1–4 g daily by injection)

Brand name: Rocephin §▼

Ceftriaxone is a representative of the so-called 'third generation' cephalosporins with increased activity against Gram-negative organisms, and is of value in serious infections such as septicaemia, pneumonia and meningitis. It is given by deep intramuscular injection or by intravenous injection/infusion as a single daily dose of 1 g, increased if necessary to 2–4 g daily. The intramuscular injection site should be varied. For presurgical prophylaxis a single dose of 1 g may be given. A single dose of 250 mg is used in gonorrhoea. It is excreted mainly via the bile with the possible formation of biliary deposits of the calcium salt. The side-effects of ceftriaxone are those of the cephalosporins generally.

Cefuroxime § (dose: 2.25–6 g daily by injection; 500 mg daily orally)

Brand names: Zinacef §, Zinnat §

Cefuroxime is a cephalosporin that is active against both Gram-positive and Gram-negative organisms, including *Staphylococcus aureus*, *Haemophilus influenzae* and *Neisseria gonorrhoeae*, and with an increased resistance to enzymatic breakdown by beta-lactamases. It is used in a wide range of respiratory and urinary tract infections, in bone infections such as osteomyelitis, and in obstetric and gynaecological infections.

Cefuroxime is given by intravenous or intramuscular injection in doses of 750 mg 8-hourly, with double doses by intravenous injection in severe infections. High doses of 3 g intravenously at intervals of 12 hours are given in meningitis. In mixed infections, combined treatment with an aminoglycoside antibiotic may be indicated. In gonorrhoea, in cases where penicillin is unsuitable, a single intramuscular dose of 1.5 g may be given. Reduced doses are necessary in severe renal impairment. Cefuroxime is also used in conjunction with metronidazole for prophylaxis in colonic surgery.

Cefuroxime axetil (Zinnat) is an oral pro-drug form which is hydrolyzed after absorption to release the free antibiotic in the circulation. It is given in doses of 250 mg twice a day, doubled in severe infections, but in urinary infections doses of 125 mg twice a day are given. A single dose of 1 g is used in gonorrhoea.

Cephalexin § (dose: 1.5–6 g daily)

Brand names: Ceporex §, Keflex §

Cephalexin is a well-absorbed, orally effective antibiotic with a wide range of activity against both Gram-positive and Gram-negative organisms. It is largely excreted in the urine, and is used in acute and chronic infections of the urinary tract, in respiratory infections, including bronchitis, and in ear, nose and throat infections.

Cephalexin is given in doses of 500 mg three times a day, but in severe or deep-seated infections, doses up to 1.5 g four times a day may be given. Doses should be reduced in renal impairment.

Side-effects include nausea and diarrhoea. False-positive reactions for glucose in the urine may occur when using copper-based test solutions.

Aztreonam § (dose: 3–8 g daily by injection)

Brand name: Azactam §

Aztreonam is described as a monobactam antibiotic, and has a range of activity limited to Gram-negative organisms. It is useful as an alternative to the aminoglycoside antibiotics and certain newer cephalosporins in infections caused by *Pseudomonas aeruginosa*, *Haemophilus influenzae* and *Neisseria gonorrhoea*, as it is resistant to breakdown by beta-lactamases produced by those organisms. It is given by intramuscular or intravenous injection in doses of 1–2 g 6–8-hourly according to the severity of the infection, with doses of 0.5–1 g twice daily for urinary infections. A single intramuscular dose of 1 g is given in gonorrhoea.

Side-effects include nausea, diarrhoea, urticaria, rash, hepatitis and blood disorders. Care is necessary in renal and hepatic impairment. Aztreonam is not suitable for use in pregnancy or breast-feeding.

> Brogden R N, Heel R C 1986 Aztreonam: a review of its properties and therapeutic use. Drugs 31: 96–130

Imipenem § (dose: 2–4 g daily by intravenous infusion)

Brand name: Primaxin §

Imipenem is a beta-lactam antibiotic that acts by inhibiting cell wall synthesis. It is active against virtually all clinically significant pathogens, including Gram-positive and Gram-negative aerobes and anaerobes, and those resistant to other antibiotics. Imipenem is very stable against attack by beta-lactamases, but it is partly inactivated by the renal enzyme dehydropeptidase, with the formation of toxic metabolites, and so it is always given with an equal dose of cilastatin, a specific inhibitor of that enzyme.

Imipenem is used in the control of both single and mixed infections, and is given by intravenous infusion in divided doses of 1–2 g daily, increased if necessary to a maximum dose of 4 g daily. For pre-operative prophylaxis two doses of 1 g are given. Reduced doses are necessary in renal impairment. Care is necessary in known sensitivity to related antibiotics.

Side-effects of imipenem are those of the beta-lactam antibiotics generally, and include gastrointestinal and blood disorders, allergic reactions and confusion. A drug-related diarrhoea may be indicative of a pseudomembranous colitis.

TETRACYCLINES

The mode of action of the tetracyclines differs from that of penicillin, as they interfere with bacterial protein synthesis, and so are bacteriostatic and not bactericidal in action. They have a wide range of activity against most Gram-positive and Gram-negative organisms, with the exception of *Pseudomonas aeruginosa* and most strains of *Proteus*, and are active orally as well as by injection.

They have been very widely used, but drug resistance to the tetracyclines is now common and their importance has declined.

The main therapeutic applications of the tetracyclines include the control of the exacerbations of chronic bronchitis, as they are active against *Haemophilus influenzae*; the treatment of rickettsia, Q-fever and chlamydial infections represented by trachoma, mycoplasma[1] infections, brucellosis and cholera. They are sometimes useful in infections not responding to other antibiotics, and small doses are used in the long-term treatment of severe acne.

All the tetracyclines have the disadvantage of being taken up and deposited in teeth and growing bones, and are contraindicated in pregnancy, and should never be given to children under 12 years of age. The tetracyclines are generally well tolerated, and allergic reactions are uncommon, but absorption after oral administration is hindered by antacids, including milk, and by preparations of aluminium, calcium, iron and magnesium. Doxycycline and minocycline are the exceptions, as their absorption is less affected. They are also the only tetracyclines that are not contraindicated in renal failure.

Table 5.5 indicates the ranges of tetracyclines available, and tetracycline is discussed as a representative member of the group, with short references to doxycycline and minocycline.

Tetracycline § (dose: 1–2 g daily)

Brand names: Achromycin §, Sustamycin §, Tetrabid §, Tetrachel §

Tetracycline is given orally in doses of 250–500 mg four times a day, but in severe infections it may be given by intramuscular injection in doses of 100 mg 4–8-hourly, or by intravenous infusion in doses not exceeding 500 mg 6-hourly. Oral therapy

---

[1]Mycoplasma are small organisms that differ from viruses in their ability to live and multiply outside a living cell, and differ from bacteria in the absence of a cell wall. *Mycoplasma pneumoniae* infections are difficult to diagnose, and are resistant to penicillin. The organism is susceptible to the tetracyclines, although the clinical response may be disappointing.

Table 5.5 Tetracyclines

Approved name	Brand name	Average oral dose
chlortetracycline	Aureomycin	250–500 mg 6-hourly
clomocycline	Megaclor	170–340 mg 6-hourly
demeclocycline	Ledermycin	150 mg 6-hourly
doxycycline	Vibramycin, Nordox	200 mg initially, then 100 mg daily
lymecycline	Tetralysal	400 mg twice daily
minocycline	Minocin	200 mg initially, then 100 mg twice a day
oxytetracycline	Berkmycen, Imperacin, Terramycin	250–500 mg 6-hourly
tetracycline	Achromycin Sustamycin Tetrachel	250–500 mg 6-hourly

should be given as soon as possible, and continued for at least 48 hours after the symptoms of infection have subsided. It is contraindicated in pregnancy, renal failure, and for children under the age of 12.

Side-effects of tetracycline include nausea, which may be reduced by taking the antibiotic with food, and diarrhoea, but allergic reactions are uncommon. A more serious side-effect is a 'super infection' or staphylococcal enteritis, due to the overgrowth of a tetracycline-resistant organism. Fungal overgrowth with *Candida* may also occur in the same way.

Doxycycline § (dose: 100 mg daily)

Brand names: Vibramycin §, Nordox §

Doxycycline has the general action of the tetracyclines and it has also been used in the treatment of prostatitis associated with *Proteus*, and as an adjunct to amoebicides in the control of acute intestinal amoebiasis. It has the advantage of being effective in low doses, and treatment is commenced with a dose of 200 mg, followed by maintenance doses of 100 mg daily. In the long-term treatment of acne, doses of 50 mg daily are given.

Unlike most tetracyclines, the absorption of doxycycline is not influenced by food, and it may be used with care in patients with renal disease. Some oesophageal ulceration has occurred with doxycyline, and to reduce that risk, it is now recommended that a dose should be given at least 1 hour before bedtime, with a full glass of water, and with the patient in a sitting or standing position.

Minocycline § (dose: 200 mg daily)

Brand name: Minocin §

Minocycline is of value in many tetracycline-sensitive infections, and the standard dose is 200 mg initially, followed by doses of 100 mg twice a day. In gonorrhoea, single doses of 300 mg are given to adult males, but females require longer treatment. It is also useful in non-gonococcal urethritis and prostatitis. In the prophylactic treatment of meningococcal carriers, minocycline is given in doses of 100 mg twice a day for 5 days. In acne, a dose of 50 mg twice a day is given for at least 6 weeks. Absorption is not influenced to any extent by food.

Minocycline may be given to patients with renal impairment, but reduced doses should be used in cases of severe renal insufficiency.

Side-effects are those of tetracycline.

Points about tetracyclines

(a) Broad-spectrum antibiotics, value now largely limited by bacterial resistance.
(b) Used mainly in infections caused by chlamydia, rickettsia and mycoplasma.
(c) Tetracyclines bind with calcium, and are deposited in teeth, so should not be given to children under 12 years of age, or used in pregnancy.
(d) Absorption of most tetracyclines is decreased by milk and antacids (except doxocycline and monocycline).
(e) Most tetracyclines may increase renal failure if present, with the same exceptions.

AMINOGLYCOSIDES

The aminoglycosides, of which streptomycin was the first to be discovered, are a group of potent antibiotics which differ from the penicillins and cephalosporins in several respects. They act partly by binding to ribosomes and inhibiting the synthesis of normal proteins, and partly by the production of non-functioning proteins. The aminoglycosides have a wide range of action, and as they are not absorbed orally, for systemic use they must be given by injection. Their use requires care, as they are potentially nephrotoxic and ototoxic, particularly in the elderly, and monitoring of drug serum levels during treatment is advisable, as any renal dysfunction may reduce excretion and increase toxicity. Treatment should not normally be for longer than 7 days.

Care is necessary if potentially ototoxic diuretics such as frusemide are also given. Aminoglycosides should be avoided during pregnancy, as they cross the placenta, and may damage the eighth cranial nerve of the fetus. But within those limits they are drugs of exceptional value, as they are active in many infections caused by Gram-negative organisms where other antibiotics may be less effective.

Gentamicin will be considered as a representative member of this valuable group of aminoglycoside antibiotics. The use of streptomycin in tuberculosis is referred to on page 156.

Points about aminoglycosides

(a) Wide-range bactericidal antibiotics.
(b) Not absorbed orally.
(c) Side-effects are dose-related, and treatment should not exceed 7 days.
(d) Excreted renally; dose should be decreased and dose-interval extended in renal impairment.
(e) Main side-effects are ototoxicity and nephrotoxicity, and may be exacerbated by some potent diuretics.
(f) Plasma levels of aminoglycosides should be monitored.

Gentamicin § (dose: 2.5–5 mg/kg daily by injection)

Brand names: Cidomycin §, Genticin §

Gentamicin is active against a wide range of Gram-negative and Gram-positive organisms, including *Pseudomonas aeruginosa*, and is a valuable drug in septicaemia, meningitis, endocarditis and many other severe systemic infections. In bacterial endocarditis caused by *Streptococcus viridans* or *Strep. faecalis*, combined treatment with penicillin is necessary. It is also effective in the control of biliary and urinary infections, but it is of less value against haemolytic streptococcal infections and is inactive against anaerobes.

The standard dose of gentamicin is 2–5 mg/kg daily, given in divided doses at 8-hourly intervals by intramuscular injection, slow intravenous injection or intravenous infusion. In severe infections, the dose may be doubled and later adjusted according to the serum level findings, as determined 1 hour after injection and again just before the next injection is due. Dosage should be adjusted so that the post-dose level is not greater than 10 mg/l, and the pre-dose level should not fall below 2 mg/l. In severe mixed infections, it can be used in association with penicillin or metronidazole, but as gentamicin should not be mixed with penicillins or cephalosporins, the injections should be at different sites to avoid inactivation.

Treatment should not normally exceed 7 days, as longer therapy may lead to renal impairment and ototoxicity. Lower doses at longer intervals are essential in renal impairment. In bacterial meningitis, gentamicin has been given by intrathecal injection of 1 mg, increased to 5 mg daily supported by intramuscular therapy, under laboratory control. The use of gentamicin in ocular infections is referred to on page 524.

Early signs of *toxicity* include headache, dizziness, rash and fever. Vestibular damage and nephrotoxicity are later symptoms of toxicity. Gentamicin should not be used in pregnancy.

Amikacin § (dose: 1 g daily by injection)

Brand name: Amikin §

Amikacin is a semi-synthetic aminoglycoside with the actions and uses of gentamicin, and although less potent it is more resistant to enzyme inactivation. Amikacin is effective in many infections caused by Gram-negative organisms, including *Pseudomonas aeruginosa*, as well as some staphylococcal infections, but it is mainly used in severe infections resistant to gentamicin.

Amikacin is given by intramuscular or slow intravenous injection in divided doses of 15 mg/kg daily (average adult dose 500 mg twice daily) up to a maximum total dose of 15 g. Intramuscular doses of 250 mg twice daily may be effective in urinary infections, other than those due to *Pseudomonas*, and the urine should be kept alkaline to increase the antibacterial action.

Side-effects, precautions and contraindications are those of the aminoglycosides generally.

Kanamycin § (dose: 0.5–1 g daily by injection)

Brand name: Kannasyn §

Kanamycin is a wide-range aminoglycoside antibiotic, and has been used in the systemic treatment of severe infections due to Gram-negative organisms, and in some resistant staphylococcal infections. It is not effective against *Pseudomonas aeruginosa*. Kanamycin is now used less frequently, as gentamicin is the preferred antibiotic, but it remains of value in severe infections resistant to gentamicin, and as an occasional alternative drug in the treatment of tuberculosis (p. 152). A standard dose is 500 mg twice a day by intramuscular injection for about 6 days, although it has been given by intravenous infusion in doses of 15–30 mg/kg daily.

Kanamycin, like other drugs in the aminoglycoside group, has nephrotoxic and ototoxic **side-effects**, requiring adjustment of dose, or in severe cases withdrawal of treatment.

Netilmicin § (dose: 300 mg daily by injection)

Brand name: Netilin §

Netilmicin is a semi-synthetic aminoglycoside with the general action and uses of gentamicin but is less active against *Pseudomonas aeruginosa*. It is active against some infections resistant to gentamicin and related antibiotics, and is used mainly in severe septicaemia and urinary tract infections not responding to the other aminoglycosides. It is given in doses of 4–6 mg/kg daily, but an average adult dose is 100 mg 8-hourly, or 150 mg 12-hourly, by intramuscular injection or intravenous infusion. In very severe infections, netilmicin may be given in doses of 7.5 mg/kg daily in three divided doses, for 48 hours or so, and subsequently reduced to the 6 mg/kg-daily level. In urinary infections, netilmicin is given in single daily doses of 150 mg for 5 days.

Peak serum concentrations of netilmicin should not exceed 12 micrograms/ml.

If combined treatment with an antipseudomonal penicillin is given the injections should be made at different sites to avoid inactivation.

Netilmicin has the advantage of having a reduced toxic effect on the eighth cranial nerve, so hearing and vestibular disturbance may be less than with related drugs and it may be of particular value in the elderly. The dose must be reduced in cases of renal impairment, and the combined use of powerful diuretics, which may also have an ototoxic effect, should be avoided.

Neomycin § (dose: 6 g daily)

Brand names: Mycifradin §, Nivemycin §

Neomycin is an aminoglycoside antibiotic with a wide range of activity, but it is too toxic for systemic use. It is not absorbed orally and is sometimes given in doses of 1 g 4-hourly for intestinal infections, and for pre-operative preparation for bowel surgery. It is also widely used locally in eye, ear and skin infections (0.5%).

Some skin sensitization may follow extended local application and ototoxicity has occurred following absorption from extensively damaged skin areas.

Tobramycin § (dose: 200–350 mg daily)

Brand name: Nebcin §

Tobramycin has the action and uses of gentamicin, and is given by intramuscular injection or intravenous infusion in doses of 3–5 mg/kg daily in divided doses. Peak plasma concentrations 1 hour after injection should not exceed 10 mg/l, or fall below 2 mg/l before the next dose is given.

UNCLASSIFIED ANTIBIOTICS

In this section a few unrelated antibiotics are referred to which either have a limited value, or are sometimes useful in special circumstances.

Chloramphenicol § (dose: 50 mg/kg daily)

Brand names: Chloromycetin §, Kemecetine §

Chloramphenicol acts by interfering with protein synthesis in bacterial cells, and is highly effective against *Haemophilus influenzae* and many other organisms. It was introduced as a wide-range orally active antibiotic, but is now considered too toxic for routine use. It remains of value in life-threatening infections due to *H. influenzae* and in typhoid fever and other conditions not responding to conventional therapy. The standard dose orally or by intravenous injection is 50 mg/kg daily in divided doses, which may be doubled in septicaemia and meningitis. The main toxic effect of chloramphenicol is a severe depression of bone marrow activity leading to aplastic anaemia; blood counts should be carried out before and during treatment, with careful monitoring of the plasma levels of the drug. Other side-effects are nausea, vomiting and diarrhoea.

Care is necessary when chloramphenicol is given to neonates, as they may exhibit the 'grey syndrome' of vomiting, respiratory depression, cyanosis and collapse. The condition is associated with a reduced ability of the infant to metabolize and excrete chloramphenicol.

The local use of chloramphenicol in bacterial conjunctivitis is referred to on page 524.

Colistin §

Brand name: Colomycin §

Colistin is a polymyxin antibiotic that has been used by injection in Gram-negative infections in doses of 2 mega units 8-hourly, but has now been replaced by gentamicin. It is used occasionally for pre-operative preparation for bowel surgery in oral doses of 2–3 mega units three times a day. It has also been used by inhalation of a nebulized solution in doses of one mega unit 12-hourly.

Polymyxin B §

Polymyxin B is related to colistin, and is present with other antibiotics in Polybactrin Spray for topical use.

Sodium fusidate § (dose: 1.5 g daily)

Brand name: Fucidin §

Sodium fusidate is unusual amongst antibacterial agents in possessing a steroid structure. It is highly effective against penicillinase-producing staphylococci, but the organisms may soon develop a resistance to the drug, and in practice it is used together with erythromycin or another antibiotic to prevent the emergence of such resistance.

Sodium fusidate is used mainly in staphylococcal osteomyelitis, as it penetrates well into bone. It is given orally in doses of 500 mg three times a day. In severe infections it can be given by intravenous infusion in doses of 1.5 g over 24 hours. It is usually well tolerated, although some gastrointestinal disturbances may occur. As it is excreted largely in the bile, there is no need to adjust the dose in renal insufficiency.

A reversible jaundice may follow intravenous administration, especially after high doses, and in such cases oral therapy should be commenced as soon as possible, and liver function tests should be carried out.

Sodium fusidate is also used topically as a 2% ointment, cream or gel in the control of staphylococcal skin infections.

Spectinomycin §

Brand name: Trobicin §

Spectinomycin is an antibiotic that is used solely in the treatment of gonorrhoea when penicillin is ineffective or otherwise contraindicated. It is given by deep intramuscular injection as a single dose of 2 g, doubled in severe infections.

Side-effects are nausea, chills, dizziness and urticaria. It is not recommended for use during pregnancy.

Teicoplanin § (dose: 200–400 mg by injection)

Brand name: Targocid §

Teicoplanin is an antibiotic with a wide range of activity against aerobic and anaerobic Gram-positive organisms, including resistant staphylococci. It acts by interfering with the biosynthesis of peptidoglycan, which forms the lattice-like structure of the bacterial cell wall. Teicoplanin is used in the treatment of serious staphylococcal infections in patients who have failed to respond to other antibiotics, or where such antibiotics are contraindicated.

Teicoplanin is given by intramuscular or intravenous injection as a loading dose of 400 mg, followed by single doses of 200 mg daily. In very severe infections, three doses of 400 mg are given at intervals of 12 hours, maintained by single daily doses of 400 mg. In severe burns, and in endocarditis due to *Staphylococcus aureus*, intravenous maintenance doses up to 12 mg/kg have been given. Dosage must be adjusted in renal impairment. Gastrointestinal **side-effects**, dizziness and anaphylactic reactions may occur with teicoplanin, and blood counts with liver and kidney function tests should be carried out, as it is potentially nephrotoxic.

Vancomycin §

Brand name: Vancocin §

Vancomycin is chemically related to teicoplanin, and has a similar pattern of antibacterial activity. It is used for the treatment of severe staphylococcal or streptococcal infections which have not responded to other antibiotics, including staphylococcal endocarditis, osteomyelitis, and antibiotic-associated colitis (p. 117). Vancomycin is not suitable for intramuscular injection, and is given intravenously in doses of 500 mg 6-hourly according to need, with monitoring of the plasma concentrations, which should not exceed a peak of 30 mg/l 1 hour after injection. In staphylococcal endocarditis treatment for 3 weeks or longer may be required.

Vancomycin is the drug of choice for the treatment of the pseudomembranous colitis that may follow the use of clindamycin and other antibiotics, and is then given orally in doses of 125–250 mg four times a day for 7–10 days.

Care is necessary with injections as vancomycin is irritant to the tissues, and other **side-effects** include nausea, chills, fever, urticaria and rash. Blood counts and renal function tests are advisable. Tinnitus may be an indication of ototoxicity, especially in the elderly, and deafness may be progressive even if treatment is withdrawn.

Fekety R et al 1984 Treatment of antibiotic-associated colitis with vancomycin. Journal of Antimicrobial Chemotherapy 14: (suppl D) 97–102

OTHER ANTIBACTERIAL AGENTS

It is convenient to refer here to some other antibacterial drugs unrelated to the antibiotics, many of which are useful in the treatment of urinary infections.

A high urinary output plays an important part in controlling urinary infections, and before potent urinary antiseptics became available, potassium citrate was widely used to promote diuresis, and to make the urine alkaline, as in some infections the urine becomes very acid.

Urine is virtually a culture medium for some organisms that gain access to the urinary system, and infection may be confined to the lower urinary tract, and cause dysuria and cystitis, or reach the pelvis and parenchyma of the kidney and cause pyelonephritis. In lower urinary tract infections a drug is required that is chiefly concentrated and excreted in the urine, but in infections of the kidney, a drug that will also penetrate into the kidney tissues is necessary.

Most of the organisms associated with urinary infections are Gram-negative, such as *Escherichia coli*, *Proteus spp.*, but *Streptococcus faecalis* is Gram-positive. Such infections often respond to a suitable antibiotic or a sulphonamide but a few unrelated substances also have a place in the treatment of urinary infections. The following drugs are in current use, some of which are described chemically as 4-quinolones.

QUINOLONE ANTIBACTERIALS

Bactericidal agents of the 4-quinolone group act by inhibiting the enzyme DNA gyrase. That enzyme controls the supercoiling of the long strands of DNA within bacterial cells, and the inhibition of the enzyme by a quinolone brings about irreversible chromosome damage.

The quinolones have many side-effects, and they may cause convulsions in patients with or without a history of epilepsy, and that risk may increase if a NSAID is also taken. Treatment should be stopped if any neurological disturbances or hypersensitivy reactions occur after the first dose. Most members of the group are used in the treatment of infections of the urinary tract, but ciprofloxacin has a wider therapeutic range.

Table 5.6 4-Quinolones

Approved name	Brand name	Dose
acrosoxacin	Eradacin	300 mg as a single dose
cinoxacin	Cinobac	500 mg twice a day
ciprofloxacin	Ciproxin	250–750 mg twice a day
nalidixic acid	Mictral	1 g four times a day
	Negram	
	Uriben	
norfloxacin	Utinor	400 mg twice a day
ofloxacin	Tarivid	200–400 mg daily

 Hooper D C, Wolfson J S 1991 Fluoquinolone antibacterial agents. New England Journal of Medicine 324: 384–394

Ciprofloxacin § (dose: 500 mg–1.5 g daily)

Brand name: Ciproxin §

Ciprofloxacin is highly active against Gram-negative organisms, including *Pseudomonas* and *Proteus*, and it is also active against streptococci and other Gram-positive bacteria.

Ciprofloxacin is of value in many systemic infections resistant to other antibacterial agents, in respiratory and urinary tract infections, and in bone and joint infections. In mixed infections, it may be used in association with aminoglycoside or beta-lactam antibiotics, as cross-resistance is uncommon. It is given orally in doses of 250–750 mg twice a day in the treatment of most infections, but in gonorrhoea a single dose of 250 mg may be adequate. In severe infections, ciprofloxacin may be given by intravenous infusion in doses of 200 mg twice a day, reduced to 100 mg twice a day in urinary infections, and to a single 100 mg daily dose in gonorrhoea. An adequate fluid intake is necessary during ciprofloxacin therapy to avoid crystalluria.

Ciprofloxacin is also given for surgical prophylaxis as a single dose of 750 mg 60–90 minutes before operation.

Care is necessary in epilepsy, as ciprofloxacin may lower the convulsive threshold. It is not recommended for use in children or adolescents as there is a possible risk of damage to weight-bearing joints. Ciprofloxacin, in common with most other

4-quinolones, may increase the plasma levels of theophylline, and enhance the effects of warfarin.

Side-effects are nausea, diarrhoea, dizziness, rash, pruritus, confusion, visual disturbances and blood disorders. Some local irritation may occur at an injection site.

Points about quinolone antibacterials

(a) Ciprofloxacin has the widest range of activity, being effective against Gram-positive and Gram-negative pathogens.
(b) To be used with caution in epileptic patients, and may cause convulsions in other patients.
(c) Action may increase if NSAIDs are also taken.
(d) Treatment with any quinolone should be withdrawn if neurological or other disturbances occur after the first dose.

Acrosoxacin § (dose: 300 mg)

Brand name: Eradacin §

Acrosoxacin is used only for the treatment of gonorrhoea in patients allergic to penicillin, or when the infecting organism is resistant to other treatment. It is given as a single dose of 300 mg, before food.

Side-effects include dizziness and gastrointestinal disturbances.

Cinoxacin § (dose: 1 g daily)

Brand name: Cinobac §

Cinoxacin is effective in both upper and lower urinary tract infections, and it is also useful as a prophylactic agent in reducing the frequency of recurrent infections.

Cinoxacin is well absorbed orally, and is given in doses of 500 mg twice a day for 7–14 days in acute infections, and in prophylaxis, a single nightly dose of 500 mg is used. It is not suitable for use in cases of severe renal impairment.

In general cinoxacin is well tolerated, but **side-effects** include gastrointestinal disturbances and abdominal cramps. *Hypersensitivity* reactions such as rash, itching and urticaria have occurred and anaphylactoid reactions have been reported.

Nalidixic acid § (dose: 2–4 g daily)

Brand name: Negram §

Nalidixic acid has a similar range of antibacterial activity to that of cinoxacin, and is used mainly for treatment of urinary tract infections. The standard dose is 1 g 6-hourly for 7 days, but if longer treatment is required, half doses should be given.

   Side-effects include nausea and vomiting, as well as urticaria and other manifestations. Visual disturbances may also occur, but are transient, but patients should avoid strong sunlight as phototoxicity is a possible side-effect. Care is necessary in renal impairment. Nalidixic acid is not suitable for young children, or in epileptics, as it may precipitate convulsions.

Norfloxacin § (dose: 800 mg daily)

Brand name: Utinor §

Norfloxacin is an antibacterial agent of the quinolone group, active against many Gram-negative urinary pathogens, and effective in the treatment of acute and chronic infections of the urinary tract. In uncomplicated infections it is given in doses of 400 mg a day, but in more severe infections doses of 400 mg twice a day are required. In chronic infections, doses of 400 mg twice a day may be given for up to 12 weeks, although if a response occurs earlier, the dose may be reduced to 400 mg daily. That lower dose should also be given in cases of renal impairment. In general, single daily doses should be taken in the morning.

   Side-effects include nausea, dizziness, abdominal pains and diarrhoea. Photosensitivity and dermatitis have also been reported. Norfloxacin may displace warfarin from serum albumin binding sites, and a rise in plasma levels of theophylline and cyclosporin may occur, and adjustments may be necessary with patients receiving those drugs.

Ofloxacin § (dose: 200–800 mg daily)

Brand name: Tarivid §

Ofloxacin is a fluorinated quinoline with actions and uses similar to those of ciprofloxacin. It is used mainly in urinary and lower respiratory tract infections, and is given as a single dose of up to

400 mg, preferably in the morning with water (larger doses should be taken as two divided doses), for 5–10 days, except in gonorrhoea, where a single dose may be adequate. Absorption may be reduced if iron or antacid preparations are taken within 2 hours of a dose of ofloxacin. In severe infections oflaxacin may be given by intravenous infusion in doses varying from 200 mg to 800 mg daily according to the seriousness of the infection.

Side-effects include hypersensitivity reactions, dizziness and other disturbances of the central nervous system. Exposure to strong sunlight should be avoided. Dosage should be reduced in impairment of renal function based on the creatinine clearance rate.

URINARY ANTIBACTERIAL DRUGS

Fosfomycin §▼ (dose: 3 g)

Brand name: Monuril §▼

Fosfomycin is a phosphonic acid antibiotic active against a range of Gram-positive and Gram-negative organisms that includes *Staphylococcus aureus* and some enterobacteria. It is used in lower urinary tract infections, and as a prophylactic in urethral instrumentation, and is given as a single nightly dose of 3 g after the bladder has been emptied. In urethral investigations it is given as one dose 3 hours beforehand, followed by a second dose of 3 g 24 hours later. It is not recommended in patients over 75 years of age, or when marked renal impairment is present, as the necessary urinary concentration may not be obtained. **Side-effects** include heartburn, nausea, diarrhoea and rash.

Nitrofurantoin § (dose: 200–600 mg daily)

Brand names: Furadantin §, Macrodantin §, Macrobid §

Nitrofurantoin is a wide-spectrum antibacterial agent that is well absorbed orally, but it is excreted so rapidly in high concentration in the urine that it is of value only in urinary tract infections and after prostatectomy. It is given in doses of 100 mg four times a day with food for 7 days. The urine should be kept acid, as nitrofurantoin is inactive in an alkaline urine. As the tissue concentration of the drug is low, it is not suitable in acute pyelonephritis.

Nitrofurantoin is sometimes used in doses of 50–100 mg at night as a suppressive drug in the long-term treatment of urinary infections. It should not be given to infants, or to patients with glucose-6-phosphate dehydrogenase deficiency, as in such patients it may cause haemolytic anaemia.

Side-effects are nausea, vomiting, rash, urticaria and pruritus. Peripheral neuropathy may occur and any tingling is an indication for withdrawal of the drug. Pulmonary infiltration has occasionally been reported, and lung and liver function tests are necessary during long-term treatment. Marked renal impairment is a contraindication.

Metronidazole § (dose: 1.2 g daily)

Brand names: Flagyl §, Metrolyl §, Zadstat §

Most pathogenic organisms can be divided into two groups, those that can develop in the presence or absence of oxygen (aerobes), and the anaerobes, which develop only in the absence of oxygen. Certain anaerobes such as *Bacteroides fragilis* are the cause of some colonic infections, and metronidazole has a selective action against anaerobic organisms by interfering with DNA activity.

In anaerobic infections, which are usually treated for 7 days, metronidazole is given as an initial dose of 800 mg, followed by doses of 400 mg 8-hourly. Alternatively, suppositories of 500 mg may be used three times a day. In severe infections metronidazole is given by intravenous infusion in doses of 500 mg at 8-hourly intervals. In less severe infections such as acute ulcerative gingivitis and in dental infections, doses of 200 mg are given 8-hourly for 3–7 days. Metronidazole is also of value in pre-surgical prophylaxis when given in doses of 400 mg 8-hourly 24 hours before surgery, supported by postoperative intravenous infusion or rectal use in doses of 500 mg 8-hourly until oral treatment can be given. In antibiotic-associated colitis (AAC) (p. 117) it is given in doses of 400 mg three times a day.

Metronidazole has no action against aerobic organisms, so in mixed infections with coliform or other organisms, combined treatment with gentamicin has been used. Metronidazole is in general well tolerated, but nausea, drowsiness and dizziness may occur. It has been used during pregnancy, but some adjustment of dose may be required.

Transient convulsions have followed high dose treatment, and peripheral neuropathy has been reported after prolonged therapy. Nurses should note that metronidazole tablets may cause gastric disturbances, and should be taken with or after food. Metronidazole mixture on the other hand, which contains a modified form of the drug, should be given at least 1 hour *before* food. A disulfiram-like reaction may occur if alcohol is taken (p. 9).

Metronidazole also has applications in the oral treatment of infected leg ulcers and pressure sores. It is also used locally as a 0.8% gel (Metrotop) in the control of malodorous fungating tumours associated with anaerobic bacteria by application to the cleaned area once or twice a day. Metronidazole gel (Elyzol) is used locally for chronic periodontal disease. The use of metronidazole in amoebiasis is referred to on page 474, in trichmoniasis on page 456, and in acne rosacea on page 535.

Bartlett J G 1982 Anti-anaerobic antibacterial agents. Lancet ii: 478–481

Tinidazole § (Fasigyn) has similar action, uses and side-effects to those of metronidazole, with the advantage of a longer plasma half-life. Dose 2 g initially, followed by 500 mg twice a day.

Noxythiolin §

Brand name: Noxyflex §

Noxythiolin is a wide-range antibacterial agent used in bladder infections by the instillation of a 2.5% solution. The instillation solution may cause pain, and it is usual to add a local anaesthetic such as amethocaine (10 mg).

Hexamine (dose: 600 mg–2 g)

Hexamine is an old drug that has been used in the treatment of recurrent urinary infections. It is a formaldehyde compound, and in an acid urine it slowly breaks down to release small amounts of formaldehyde, to which the antibacterial action is due. It survives as hexamine hippurate (Hiprex).

Dimethyl sulphoxide

Dimethyl sulphoxide is used mainly as a solvent, but a 50% solution is available as **Rimso 50**. This product is intended for the symptomatic relief of interstitial cystitis (Hunner's ulcer) and is used by the instillation in the bladder of 50 ml of the product.

Urinary pH

As hexamine is active only in acid urine, it is convenient here to note the influence of urinary pH on the activity of some drugs. The symbol pH refers to the *degree* of acidity or alkalinity of an aqueous solution and the neutral point is pH 7. All acid solutions have a lower pH, and the *degree* of acidity increases as the pH figure becomes lower. Similarly, all alkaline solutions have a pH greater than 7. An acid pH of the urine increases the activity of nitrofurantoin and the tetracyclines, and an alkaline pH may increase the activity of sulphonamides, prevent the formation of uric acid crystals and relieve the discomfort of dysuria.

The urine may be made acid by large doses of ascorbic acid, methionine or ammonium chloride, but it should be noted that where the urine is alkaline by the infection of *Proteus*, an organism that can break down urea and liberate ammonia in the urine, acidifying agents are of little value. On the other hand, the urine may be made alkaline by large doses of sodium bicarbonate. Potassium citrate is no longer recommended as an alkalizing agent, because of the danger of hyperkalaemia if any renal failure is present.

ANTITUBERCULAR DRUGS

Tuberculosis is caused by the parasitic bacillus *Mycobacterium tuberculosis*, and may become established in the body before symptoms or other evidence of the disease are detected.

Following the introduction of streptomycin, the first antibiotic to be introduced after penicillin, it was thought that tuberculosis would soon be brought under complete control. In fact, drug resistant *M. tuberculosis* has now become a major problem and the WHO recently declared tuberculosis a 'global emergency'. Treatment of tuberculosis requires multi-drug therapy and when possible antitubercular therapy is given in two stages, an initial stage of triple-drug treatment, and a secondary stage using two drugs. Drug resistance occurs rapidly in tuberculosis if any drug is used alone, and the initial phase of treatment is designed to bring the condition under control as rapidly as possible, and to reduce the risks of drug resistance.

The secondary phase of treatment is initiated after tests have shown which drugs are most active against the strains of organisms of the individual patient, and must be continued for many months. Initial therapy is commenced with any three of the following drugs: isoniazid, rifampicin, pyrazinamide, streptomycin or ethambutol.

Points about antitubercular drugs

(a) Initial or first-phase treatment with three drugs, usually with isoniazid, rifampicin and pyrazinamide.
(b) Continuation phase with two, usually isoniazid and rifampicin.
(c) Compliance with treatment is essential; some patients must be supervized.
(d) Peripheral neuropathy is a side-effect of isoniazid and ethambutol; advise patients to report any numbness or tingling in the extremities or visual disturbances.

Isoniazid § (dose: 300 mg daily)

Isoniazid is a highly selective antibacterial drug, as although it is active against *Mycobacterium tuberculosis* it has virtually no action against other organisms. It is widely used with other drugs in the primary treatment of pulmonary tuberculosis, as following oral administration, isoniazid is rapidly absorbed and penetrates easily into the body tissues and fluids, including the cerebrospinal fluid, and also into caseous areas.

Isoniazid is given in doses of 300 mg daily, orally or by intramuscular injection, but with the slow inactivators (see p. 154), doses of 1 g twice weekly may be given. In tuberculous meningitis, supplementary doses of 25–50 mg have been given by intrathecal injection.

Isoniazid is well tolerated and **side-effects** are not usually serious. Skin reactions may occur, and convulsions, psychotic reactions and liver damage have also been reported. Peripheral neuropathy is an occasional hazard with higher doses and pyridoxine in doses of 50–100 mg daily should be given as a prophylactic, as isoniazid may interfere with normal pyridoxine metabolism.

This effect on pyridoxine occurs mainly with the 'slow inactivators'. Isoniazid is inactivated by acetylation in the liver, but the speed of inactivation varies. Patients can be divided into slow-acetylators and rapid-acetylators and a gene factor is involved. As the steady state plasma level of isoniazid is lower with the rapid inactivators, frequent, regular and adequate dosing is necessary to maintain the anti-tubercular action, whereas slow acetylators are more likely to develop peripheral neuropathy.

Rifampicin § (dose: 450–600 mg daily)

Brand names: Rifadin §, Rimactane §

Rifampicin is one of the rifamycin group of antibiotics and it has a wide range of antibacterial activity. It is highly effective against *Mycobacterium tuberculosis* and *Mycobacterium leprae* (leprosy). It penetrates well into the tissues, and reaches intracellular organisms. It is of low toxicity and well tolerated. Rifampicin is a first-line antitubercular drug, and is given as a single daily dose of 450–600 mg, preferably on an empty stomach to obtain maximum absorption.

Side-effects are of varying severity, including nausea, diarrhoea and rash, and it may evoke an influenza-like reaction with chills, fever, and respiratory stress which in some cases may extend to shock and collapse. Thrombocytopenic purpura may also occur.

Rifampicin is mainly excreted in high levels in the bile, but much is re-absorbed by the enterohepatic circulation system and care may be necessary in liver impairment. Jaundice may require a change of treatment. Rifampicin may give a red colour to the urine and sputum, but the colouration is of no significance, and may even be useful as a test of compliance with therapy. It may also stain contact lenses.

Combined therapy with other antitubercular drugs, particularly ethambutol or isoniazid, remains essential, and **Rifinah** and **Rimactazid** represent products containing both rifampicin and isoniazid. **Rifater** contains rifampicin, isoniazid and pyrazinamide. Rifampicin is also used with dapsone in the initial treatment of leprosy (p. 476). (Rifampicin has a secondary use in the prophylactic treatment of meningococcal meningitis in doses of 600 mg twice daily for 2 days.)

It should be noted that rifampicin stimulates the hepatic metabolism of many drugs, and adjustment of dose of other therapeutic agents such as warfarin may be required. It also reduces the effectiveness of oral contraceptives and is contraindicated in pregnancy.

Rifabutin §▼ (dose: 300–600 mg daily)

Brand name: Mycobutin §▼

Rifabutin is a semi-synthetic derivative of rifampicin, and has a similar range of activity, and in pulmonary tuberculosis it is given as part of combined therapy in doses of 150–450 mg daily for at least 6 months. It is also of value in the prophylaxis and treatment of non-tuberculous mycobacterial disease such as that caused by *Mycobacterium avium-intracellulare* complex (MAC). That organism is the cause of severe opportunistic infections in AIDS patients, and is resistant to many antibacterial agents. Rifabutin is effective against most strains of MAC, and in prophylaxis it is given in doses of 300 mg daily as monotherapy. For treatment, it is given in doses of 450–600 mg daily as part of a multi-drug regimen for 6 months after negative cultures have been obtained. The side-effects of rifabutin are similar in general to those of rifampicin, including the effects on co-administrated drugs mediated by hepatic enzymes such as cytochrome 450 (p. 6). Care is necessary in hepatic insufficiency.

Ethambutol § (dose: 15–25 mg/kg daily)

Brand name: Myambutol §

Ethambutol is sometimes used as part of the primary treatment of tuberculosis, as it is active mainly against young and dividing cells. Its main use is in the early stages of treatment to prevent the emergence of resistance to other drugs. It is given as a single daily dose of 15 mg/kg, although in some cases the higher dose of 25 mg/kg may be necessary.

Although generally well tolerated, it is considered less suitable for children or the elderly.

Side-effects include peripheral neuritis. It may also cause a retrobulbar neuritis with loss of visual acuity and a green–red colour blindness. These ocular toxic effects are more likely in patients with some renal dysfunction who are receiving high doses and usually disappear slowly with a change of treatment. Patients should be warned to report any such visual disturbances without delay. **Mynah 250** is a mixed product containing 250 mg of ethambutol and 100 mg of isoniazid.

Streptomycin § (dose: 1 g daily by injection)

Streptomycin, one of first antibiotics to be introduced after penicillin, was once widely used in the treatment of tuberculosis, but ototoxicity limits its use. It survives as part of multiple therapy for use in resistant tuberculosis, and is given in doses of 1 g daily by intramuscular injection. Permanent deafness has followed the prolonged use of the drug because of its toxic effects on the eighth cranial nerve. Other reactions include paraesthesia of the lips, and hypersensitivity reactions may occur. Care is necessary in renal insufficiency and liver dysfunction. Great care should be taken when handling streptomycin, as skin sensitization with dermatitis may occur, and protective gloves should be worn. Hypersensitivity may also occur by the inhalation of streptomycin, which may happen if a poor technique is used during the preparation of an injection of streptomycin.

Continuation or secondary phase

Once sensitivity tests have been carried out, treatment should be continued for 9–12 months with a two-drug regimen. Normally, one of these two should be isoniazid, together with rifampicin.

SUPPLEMENTARY ANTITUBERCULAR DRUGS

These drugs are used mainly as alternative therapy in cases of intolerance to conventional drugs, or where resistance requires a change of therapy.

Capreomycin § (dose: 1 g daily by injection)

Brand name: Capastat §

Capreomycin is an antibiotic used in tuberculosis resistant to first-line drugs. It is given in doses of 1 g daily by deep intramuscular injection, which may cause pain and induration.

Side-effects include urticaria, renal damage, tinnitus and vertigo. It should not be used with streptomycin or other ototoxic drugs.

Pyrazinamide § (dose: 20–30 mg/kg daily)

Brand name: Zinamide §

Pyrazinamide is an antitubercular drug, active against the intracellular dividing forms of the tubercle bacillus. It is of value in tuberculous meningitis as it penetrates well into the CSF. Pyrazinamide is given in divided doses of 20–30 mg / kg daily or 2 g three times a week. As it is most effective during the early stages of treatment, it should not be given for longer than 2 months.

The main disadvantage of pyrazinamide is its *hepatotoxicity*, which can be serious and lead to liver failure, and liver function should be checked during treatment. Care is also necessary in renal impairment and diabetes. Other side-effects are nausea, arthralgia and urticaria.

Cycloserine § (dose: 500 mg–1 g daily)

Cycloserine is used occasionally in tuberculosis resistant to conventional first-line drugs in doses of 250–500 mg twice a day. It diffuses well into the tissues, but it is slowly excreted, and it may cause **side-effects** such as drowsiness, twitching, and convulsive seizures, indicative of central nervous system involvement. Epilepsy and psychotic states are contraindications.

ANTIVIRAL DRUGS

Viruses are simple organisms that can develop only in living cells, and so can be regarded as obligate intracellular parasites.

They consist of little more than a nucleic acid core and protein capsid which may be surrounded by a lipoprotein envelope. In most cases the nucleic acid core is DNA, from which RNA is subsequently formed, but in some viruses, termed retroviruses, RNA forms the genetic core, and one of these retroviruses is of particular interest as being the cause of the acquired immune deficiency syndrome (AIDS).

Viruses replicate by entering a cell and interrupt the normal cell metabolism by using the cell's nuclear apparatus for the development of new viral particles and so causing viral disease (Fig. 5.1).

When a virus for example enters the mucosal cells of the nasopharynx, the damaged cell metabolism leads to death of the infected cells, and the shedding of the dead cells gives rise to catarrh and other cold symptoms. The dead cells are soon replaced by new and non-infected cells, and the viral infection is correspondingly short-lived. In other viral infections, antibodies may be formed to attack the invading virus, and such an immune reaction inhibits viral development, and the viral attack may be self-limiting. In others, the virus may become dormant, and may be reactivated long afterwards. The re-appearance of cold sores is an example of such reactivation, and persistent viruses with long incubation periods may be the cause of Alzheimer's and other degenerative diseases. The search for antiviral drugs is hampered

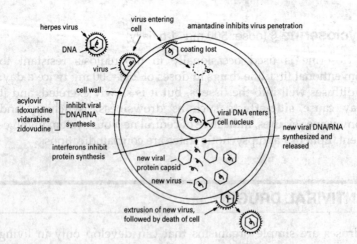

Figure 5.1 Diagram of virus replication.

because of the many changes in the nature of the virus protein coat that occur, and a receptor site common to many viruses that would be a vulnerable point of attack has yet to be distinguished. Antiviral drugs have little if any action on latent viruses.

Points about antiviral agents

(a) Mainly virustatic, not virucidal in action.
(b) Early treatment necessary.
(c) Some are inactivated by gastric acid and should be given fasting or between meals.
(d) Some of those given by injection are skin irritants—avoid direct skin contact.

Although the tetracyclines have a limited value in some viral diseases, such as trachoma, and amantadine is used in the prophylaxis of A2 viral influenza, few specific antiviral drugs are yet available, but the following are of considerable interest, and further advances can be expected.

Acyclovir §

Brand name: Zovirax §

Acyclovir, also known as acycloguanosine, is an antiviral drug of great value, as it has a wide range of activity against different types of herpes virus. Acyclovir as such is inactive, but when it enters a virus-infected cell, it is activated by a viral enzyme to form acyclovir phosphate, which blocks the replication of viral DNA, with little effect on normal cell activity. (It is therefore unlikely to be of any value in eradicating latent herpes infections.)

Acyclovir is given orally in doses of 200 mg five times a day in the early treatment of herpes virus infections of the skin and mucous membranes, but it is effective only when given in the early stages of infection. It also reduces the acute pain, and the risk of post-herpetic neuralgia. Similar doses can be given in the prophylaxis of immunocompromised patients.

In systemic herpes infection early treatment is also essential, and acyclovir is given by intravenous infusion in doses of 5 mg/kg 8-hourly, increased to 10 mg/kg in immunocompromised patients with varicella zoster infections.

Acyclovir has many **side-effects**, including rash, gastro-intestinal and neurological disturbances. Care must be taken to avoid extravasation, as severe local inflammation may occur. Caution is necessary in renal impairment, as the drug is excreted by the kidneys, and monitoring of renal function is advisable. For the treatment of herpes simplex conjunctivitis, acyclovir is used as a 3% ointment to be applied to the infected eye five times a day.

Amantadine § (dose: 200 mg daily)

Brand name: Symmetrel §

Amantadine, used in the treatment of parkinsonism, also has some antiviral properties, and is used in the prophylaxis of influenza A infections, and in the treatment of *Herpes zoster*. It is given as a prophylactic in doses of 100 mg 12-hourly for 7–10 days, but it has recently been recommended that the prophylactic dose should be reduced to 100 mg daily, particularly in the elderly. In shingles a 14-day course of treatment is given, extended if post-herpetic pain persists.

Side-effects include dizziness, gastrointestinal disturbances and insomnia. Skin discolouration has been reported occasionally. Amantadine should not be given to patients with a history of epilepsy or duodenal ulceration.

Didanosine §▼ (dose: 250–400 mg daily)

Brand name: Videx §▼

Didanosine is an antiviral agent chemically related to zidovudine (p. 163) and is used similarly in the symptomatic treatment of human immunodeficiency virus (HIV) infections. Its action is virostatic, not virucidal, so while it inhibits the spread of the virus, it does not eradicate an established infection. Didanosine is used mainly in the treatment of HIV infections no longer responding to zidovudine and is given orally in doses of 200 mg twice a day (250 mg daily for patients weighing less than 60 kg). It is rapidly broken down by gastric acid, and absorption is reduced in the presence of food. Didanosine should therefore be given at least 30 minutes before a meal, or in the fasting state. Didanosine tablets contain antacids to reduce gastric acid hydrolysis, and must be chewed, crushed, or dispered in water for administration. **Side-effects** include diarrhoea (occasionally severe), nausea, vomiting, fever, peripheral neuropathy and hyperuricaemia. Pancreatitis is a complication of HIV infection, and should be excluded before starting didanosine treatment.

Famciclovir §▼ (dose: 750 mg daily)

Brand name: Famvir §▼

Famciclovir has the general action of acyclovir, and is used similarly in the treatment of herpes zoster (shingles). Like acyclovir, it is phosphorylated in the herpes virus-infected cells, but persists longer, and is effective in doses of 250 mg three times a day. The usual course of treatment is 7 days. Reduced doses may be required in renal impairment.

Ganciclovir § (dose: 5–10 mg/kg daily by injection)

Brand name: Cymevene §

Ganciclovir is chemically related to acyclovir, but is more active and effective against a wide range of human herpes viruses, including cytomegalovirus (CMV). CMV is a major pathogen in immunocompromised patients and is a common cause of death in AIDS. It also causes a progressive retinitis that may be sight-threatening. Ganciclovir is indicated in the treatment of life- and sight-threatening CMV infections in immunocompromised patients, and in drug-induced immunosuppression associated with organ transplants. It is given by intravenous infusion in doses of 5 mg/kg every 12 hours for 14–21 days, followed by maintenance doses of 5 mg/kg daily for 5 days a week. Solutions of ganciclovir are very alkaline, so the administration of the drug requires care. Protective glasses and gloves should be worn when preparing the injection solution.

Ganciclovir has many **side-effects**, and neutropenia may be severe, so regular blood counts are essential. Zidovudine and other drugs affecting bone marrow function should not be used with ganciclovir.

Foscarnet § (Foscavir §) is an antiviral agent for the treatment of CMV retinitis in AIDS patients when ganciclovir is contraindicated or unsuitable. It is given as an initial dose of 20 mg/kg by intravenous infusion, followed by maintenance doses of 20–200 mg/kg daily, according to need.

Side-effects include nausea and hypocalcaemia, but adequate fluid intake is essential, as foscarnet may cause renal impairment leading to acute renal failure. Monitoring of the serum creatinine levels should be carried out every second day.

Idoxuridine §

Idoxuridine acts as a blocking agent in the development of the herpes virus, as it interferes with the uptake of thymidine during the formation of viral DNA. It is used mainly in ophthalmology for the treatment of keratitis due to *Herpes simplex*. Even severe dendritic ulcers respond to the local application of idoxuridine as a 0.5% ointment every 4 hours. Treatment should not be continued for more than 3 days after healing of the ulcer, as corneal damage may occur.

Idoxuridine is also used as 5% solution in dimethylsulphoxide (**Herpid; Iduridin; Virudox**) for the local treatment of herpes simplex infections. A stronger solution (40%) is used for *severe* cutaneous herpes zoster infections. If used early and regularly for 4 days, the lesions are soon checked, and there is less post-herpetic neuralgia. The 40% solution is *not* suitable for the treatment of herpes labialis. Idoxuridine has also been used occasionally by intravenous infusion in severe conditions such as herpes encephalitis, but its toxicity limits its value.

Inosine pranobex § (dose: 4 g daily)

Brand name: Imunovir §

The relationship between the biosynthesis of viral and normal cell DNA is so close that most antiviral drugs are toxic to some extent to the host cells, and a balance must be struck between the therapeutic and toxic doses. Clinically acceptable antiviral drugs are few, but a different approach would be the use of a drug that could stimulate the immune system of the body, and have an indirect but wide-ranging antiviral action.

Inosine pranobex, also known as isoprinosine, has some of the required antiviral properties and appears to act by increasing the proliferation of T and B cells (p. 557) which is depressed during viral infections.

Inosine pranobex is used in the treatment of mucocutaneous herpes simplex infections, and is given orally in doses of 1 g four times a day for 7–14 days. It is well tolerated but care is necessary in gout and renal impairment, as it increases uric acid levels.

Interferon

The interferons (alpha, beta and gamma) are glycoproteins produced in mammalian cells after infection by viruses, and are part of the natural defence system of the body. They not only inhibit viral growth in infected cells, but also protect surrounding cells from attack. Although they have potential value as antiviral agents, at present they are used mainly for their antitumour activity (p. 298).

Tribavarin §

Brand name: Virazid §

Tribavarin is a synthetic antiviral agent effective against many influenzal viruses, but indicated in the treatment of young children with severe respiratory syncytial virus (RSV) infections. The virus infects most children up to 3 years of age, and the infection is usually mild, but severe infections require hospital treatment by nebulization of a 2% solution of tribavarin for 12–18 hours daily for at least 3 days, if necessary with assisted ventilation.

Zidovudine § (dose: 1.2–1.8 g daily)

Brand name: Retrovir §

Zidovudine, also known as azidothymidine or AZT, is an antiviral agent used in the suppressive treatment of acquired deficiency syndrome (AIDS) and the control of secondary conditions referred to as AIDS-related complex. The disease is due to a retrovirus (human T-cell lymphotropic virus) or HIV, which has an affinity for T-cells that play an essential part in the defence of the body against infection. The synthesis of viral RNA requires thymidine, and zudovidine, which has a chemical relationship with thymidine, functions as a 'false thymidine, and blocks the formation of viral RNA, and so inhibits further viral development.

Zidovudine is used in the treatment of the more severe manifestations of AIDS, and is given orally in doses of 200–300 mg 4-hourly day and night, and continued as long as necessary, as extended treatment is usually required. Lower doses of 500 mg daily are given in the treatment of asymptomatic patients. It may also be given by intravenous infusion in doses of 2.5 mg/kg every 4 hours in patients unable to cope with oral therapy, but such infusion treatment should not be given for more than 2 weeks. Its action is virustatic and suppressive, and it is not capable of eliminating an established infection.

Side-effects are numerous and anaemia, neutropenia and leucopenia are common and severe, and may be increased if paracetamol is taken. Regular blood counts are essential. Other side-effects are nausea, rash, anorexia, fever, insomnia and myalgia. The value of zidovudine in other viral infections has yet to be assessed.

SYSTEMIC ANTIFUNGAL AGENTS

Fungal diseases, both local and intestinal, are common, but systemic fungal infections have become more frequent and important as a consequence of the lowering of host resistance following the increasing use of immunosuppressive drugs and the spread of AIDS. The antifungal agents in current use include some antibiotics as well as synthetic drugs.

Of importance is the group referred to as the imidazoles, represented by econazole, ketoconazole and miconazole. Fluoconazole and itraconazole have a related triazole structure. They are fungistatic rather than fungicidal in action. The imidazoles act by influencing fungal membrane permeability, so the transport of amino acids and subsequent protein synthesis is impaired.

The triazoles appear to have a more specific effect on the fungal cytochrome P450 enzyme system, and inhibit the biosynthesis of ergosterol. As a result, ergosterol intermediates accumulate in the fungal cells, which leads to subsequent degeneration and breakdown of the fungal cell structure. These antifungal agents are used mainly for superficial fungal infections such as candidiasis, others are used for systemic infections, and some have both types of activity. A few old drugs such as salicylic acid are still in use for the local treatment of some fungal infections of the skin. Care is necessary when triazoles are given with other drugs that influence metabolism, and combined use with astemizole or terfenadine should be avoided (risk of cardiac arrhythmias).

Amphotericin § (dose: 250 micrograms/kg daily by injection; 400–800 mg daily orally)

Brand names: AmBisome §, Amphocil §, Fungilin §, Fungizone §

Amphotericin is an antibiotic with no antibacterial action, but it is highly effective against many yeast-like and filamentous fungi, and is one of the few antifungal antibiotics that can be given by injection. It is of value in the treatment of deep fungal infections such as cryptococcosis, histoplasmosis and systemic candidiasis, and is given in doses of 250 micrograms/kg daily by slow intravenous injection, often preceded by a test dose of 1 mg. The injection solution should be freshly prepared, and protected from light during administration. The dose is slowly increased up to 1 mg/kg daily, but treatment for some months may be required, with frequent change of the injection site, as amphotericin is an irritant, and may cause local pain and thrombophlebitis.

The dose of amphotericin is normally limited by the nephrotoxic effects of the drug and the development of renal insufficiency. The risk of toxicity has recently been reduced with the introduction of two new presentations of amphotericin for intravenous infusion, AmBisome and Amphocil. AmBisome is a liposome-encapsulated preparation of amphotericin, from which the drug is slowly released; Amphocil is a complex of amphotericin with sodium cholesteryl sulphate. When the complex is reconstituted for intravenous infusion, it forms a colloidal dispersion (not a solution). With both products the toxicity of amphotericin has been markedly reduced, permitting daily doses of 1 mg/kg to be given initially, increasing as required to 3–4 mg/kg daily. The side-effects of conventional forms of amphotericin when given intravenously have been largely eliminated.

Amphotericin is not absorbed orally, and so is correspondingly useful in oral and intestinal candidiasis. It is given in doses of 100–200 mg 6-hourly. An ointment and cream of amphotericin 3% is used for cutaneous infections due to *Candida* and other yeast-like fungi.

Side-effects of standard therapy are numerous and may be dose-limiting, and include nausea, malaise, chills and rash, as well as blood and neurological disorders. Disturbances of liver function require immediate withdrawal. Amphotericin is also nephrotoxic, and renal function tests are necessary during amphotericin therapy. If treatment is withdrawn for more than 7 days, dosage should be recommenced at the low initial level.

Fluconazole § (dose: 50 mg daily)

Brand name: Diflucan §

Fluconazole has a triazole structure, and has a selective action on the fungal cytochrome P450 enzyme system; it inhibits fungal development by interrupting the biosynthesis of ergosterol. In mucosal candidiasis it is given in doses of 50 mg daily for 7–14 days, but in vaginal candidiasis fluconazole is given as a single dose of 150 mg. For fungal infections of the skin such as tinea, similar doses are given but continued for 2–4 weeks or more.

Fluconazole is also given prophylactically in immunocompromised patients in doses of 50–100 mg daily. It is also given by intravenous infusion in systemic fungal infections such as cryptococcosis, cryptococcal meningitis and systemic candidiasis. In such infections, fluconazole is given as an initial intravenous dose of 400 mg, followed by doses of 200 mg daily. Duration of treatment depends on response, and may have to be continued for 6–8 weeks. Dosage must be modified in renal impairment. Combined treatment with astemizole or terfenadine should be avoided (risk of cardiac arrhythmias).

Side-effects include nausea and abdominal discomfort.

Flucytosine § (dose: 100–200 mg/kg daily)

Brand name: Alcobon §

Flucytosine is a synthetic antifungal agent that is active against yeast-like fungi by interfering with nucleic acid synthesis. It is well absorbed and widely distributed, and is used in the treatment of systemic infections with *Cryptococcus, Candida, Torulopsis* and other fungi. Flucytosine is given orally in doses of 50 mg/kg four times a day, but in severe conditions it may be given by intravenous infusion in doses of 100–200 mg/kg daily, for up to 7 days, when oral therapy can be given.

It is usually well tolerated, but nausea, diarrhoea, rash and blood disturbances may occur, so blood counts should be taken. Resistance to flucytosine is common, and may develop during treatment, and sensitivity tests may be required before and during the use of the drug. Flucytosine is excreted in the urine, and lower doses are necessary in renal impairment.

Griseofulvin § (dose: 0.5–1 g daily)

Brand names: Fulcin §, Grisovin §

Griseofulvin is an antibiotic that has no antibacterial properties but is effective in ringworm and other fungal infections of the keratin-containing tissues, i.e. hair, skin and nails. Griseofulvin appears to be taken up selectively by such tissues, and prevents further penetration by the fungus. The new tissues formed are therefore free from infection, but response to treatment is correspondingly slow, and complete elimination of the fungus awaits the natural shedding of infected hair or nails. It is not effective in systemic infections, and is of no value for local application. Griseofulvin is given orally in doses of 125–250 mg four times a day for some months.

In general it is well tolerated, but headache, allergic reactions and gastrointestinal disturbances may occur. Care is necessary in liver damage.

Itraconazole § (dose: 100–200 mg daily)

Brand name: Sporanox §

Itraconazole becomes bound to the keratinocytes in the basal layer of the epidermis, and has a sustained antifungal action that is terminated by the natural shedding of the skin. In tinea infections, it is given in doses of 100 mg daily for 15–30 days, but in pityriasis versicolor a 7-day course of 200 mg daily is usually adequate. Itraconazole is also used for the 1-day treatment of vulvo-vaginal candidiasis as two doses of 100 mg. The side-effects include headache, nausea and abdominal pain. It is metabolized in the liver, and care is necessary in hepatic disease. Combined use with astemizole or terfenadine should be avoided.

Points about systemic antifungal agents

(a) When used for oral infections, any dentures should first be removed.
(b) In dermatophyte infections of the hair, as much infected hair as possible should be removed.
(c) Special care with ketoconazole — risk of severe hepatotoxicity — limit treatment to 14 days.
(d) Combined use of azoles and astemizole and terfenadine should be avoided — risk of cardiac arrhythmias.
(e) Should not be used for superficial infections.

Ketoconazole § (dose: 200–400 mg daily)

Brand name: Nizoral §

Ketoconazole is one of the imidazole group of antifungal agents. It is well absorbed orally, and effective in systemic and resistant mycoses, as well as in vaginal candidiasis. It has also been used in the prophylactic treatment of immunocompromised patients.

The standard dose is 200 mg daily with food, increased if necessary to 400 mg in deep-seated and systemic infection.

Side-effects include nausea and pruritus, but jaundice and fatal liver damage have followed ketoconazole therapy, and careful monitoring is essential during treatment. It should not be given for superficial fungal infections. If treatment is continued for more than 14 days, liver function tests should be carried out regularly. Hepatic impairment is a contraindication. Combined use with astemizole or terfenadine should be avoided.

Miconazole § (dose: 1–2 g daily)

Brand name: Daktarin §

Miconazole is a systemic antifungal agent with antibacterial properties. It is given orally for mucosal and intestinal fungal infections in doses of 250 mg four times a day for 10 days. It is also of value in the prophylactic treatment of patients at risk, i.e.

transplant and cancer patients receiving immunosuppressive treatment.

In severe systemic fungal infections, miconazole may be given by intravenous infusion in doses of 600 mg 8-hourly, with frequent changes of the injection site to avoid phlebitis, as extended treatment may be necessary. Doses of 10–20 mg daily have been given by intrathecal injection. Miconazole is sometimes used for mycotic infections of the bladder, either by the direct installation of a dose of 100 mg, or by irrigation with 500 ml of saline containing 100 mg of miconazole.

Side-effects include nausea, fever, pruritus and rash. Combined use with astemizole or terfenadine should be avoided.

The use of miconazole for trichomonal infections is referred to on page 456.

Nystatin § (dose: 2 million units daily)

Brand name : Nystan §

Nystatin is an antifungal antibiotic that is not absorbed orally, and is too toxic for systemic therapy; it is used in the treatment of oral, intestinal and vaginal candidiasis. For oral candidiasis it may be given as pastilles containing 100 000 units, to be chewed four time a day, or in similar doses as a suspension to be used as a mouthwash. In intestinal candidiasis, doses of 500 000 units are given four times a day, a dose that can be doubled in severe infections. In the treatment of vaginal candidiasis, nystatin pessaries of 100 000 units, and vaginal cream are available (p. 457).

Side-effects are nausea and vomiting, with diarrhoea after high doses. Allergic contact dermatitis has been reported as occurring after the topical application of nystatin.

Terbinafine §▼ (dose: 250 mg daily)

Brand name: Lamisil §▼

Terbinafine is a new type of antifungal agent. Like the triazole derivatives, it acts by blocking the synthesis of ergosterol, but differs in action by inhibiting the fungal enzyme squalene epoxidase. In fungal infections of the skin it is given in doses of 250 mg daily for 2–6 weeks, but fungal infections of the nails may require treatment for up to 3 months. In athlete's foot terbinafine can be used as a 1% cream for application to the affected areas once or twice a day for 1–2 weeks. Side-effects of oral therapy are headache, myalgia, taste and gastrointestinal disturbances. Care is necessary in hepatic dysfunction, and when other therapy may affect liver enzyme activity.

Other antifungal agents used for candidiasis or dermatophyte infections are represented by **clotrimazole** § (Canestan §), **econazole** § (Ecostatin §, Pevaryl §), **isoconazole** § (Travogyn §) and **metronidazole** § (Flagyl §).

6

Cardiovascular drugs and blood-lipid lowering agents

The cardiovascular system is a closed circuit in which blood is circulated to maintain the micro-environment of the body cells, supplying oxygen and nutrients, and removing waste products. The driving force of the system is the heart, a remarkably efficient and reliable four-chambered pump with one-way valves. During a normal life-span it may beat about 2000 million times, and in health it has adequate reserves of power to cope with any physiological demands that may be made on it. It is a double-acting pump, part of which supplies the pulmonary circulation, and part the general circulation. Its efficiency depends on several factors, including the oxygen supply, the rate and strength of the cardiac muscle contractions, as well as the speed of conduction of the contractile impulses. In addition, cardiac efficiency is also linked with the pressure of the blood entering the heart (the pre-load) as well as that leaving it (the after-load).

Heart failure occurs when the cardiac output is no longer capable of coping with the physiological demands to maintain adequate supplies to the tissues, and frequent causes are hypertension, coronary artery disease and chronic obstructive airways disease. In the early stages of cardiac weakness, compensatory mechanisms come into play that increase the heart rate, and the decreasing efficiency of the heart may become manifest only after exercise and stress. Later, if the decline continues, blood begins to accumulate in the vessels, thus increasing the cardiac pre-load, fluid leaks from the vessels and begins to accumulate in the tissues as the renal efficiency wanes, and so leads to the oedema, cyanosis and congestion characteristic of heart failure. Treatment is aimed at breaking some link in the vicious circle of cardiac weakness–oedema–congestion–reduced renal efficiency–increasing cardiac weakness, by drugs that stimulate the heart to contract more powerfully, and by diuretics that promote the elimination of fluid, relieve the congestion, and so reduce the cardiac pre-load. Further support can be provided by some vasodilator drugs, which by lowering the general blood pressure reduce both the pre-load and after-load burden on the weakening heart (Fig. 6.1).

Poole-Wilson P A, Linday D 1992 Advances in the treatment of chronic heart failure. British Medical Journal 304: 1067–1070

CARDIAC THERAPEUTICS

In the treatment of congestive heart failure, digitalis has long held pride of place. Digitalis is the dried leaf of the foxglove, and was introduced into medicine by William Withering in 1785 for the treatment of dropsy (oedema) and is still used as digoxin, the active glycoside obtained from the Austrian foxglove. The mode of action of digoxin is complex but its cardiotonic action is the result of an increase in the intracellular concentration of calcium ions available to interact with the contractile myocardial fibres. In myocardial cells there is an ionic balance across the cell membrane, and for contraction to occur the membrane becomes transiently permeable to extracellular sodium and calcium ions, which enter by specific 'fast-sodium' and 'slow calcium' channels and trigger off the muscle contraction. The action of digoxin is linked with an increase in intracellular calcium, and also with the activity of adenosine triphosphatase (APTase), an enzyme concerned with the movement of potassium and sodium ions.

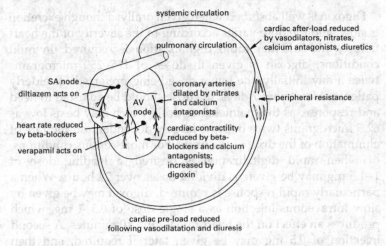

Figure 6.1   Sites of action of some drugs used in angina and heart failure.

Digoxin §

Digoxin is used in the treatment of congestive heart failure, especially in patients with atrial fibrillation and a high ventricular rate. Its mode of action is complex, as it reduces the ventricular rate, and so promotes improved ventricular filling and output. At the same time it has a positive inotropic action that improves cardiac efficiency and brings about a general improvement in the circulation. It also stimulates the vagus nerve, which depresses conduction through the atrio-ventricular node. With the circulatory improvement, blood flow through the kidneys is increased, and so digoxin has an indirect diuretic action that also helps to relieve oedema and congestion.

Points about digoxin

(a) Starting dose in mild heart failure 125–250 micrograms twice a day (loading dose not required).
(b) Maintenance dose often once a day.
(c) For rapid digitalization in severe heart failure 0.75–1 mg by intravenous infusion over 2 hours.
(d) Intramuscular injection is painful and not recommended.
(e) Nausea, vomiting and visual disturbances indicate reduction of dose.
(f) Specific antidote is Digibind.

Digoxin is well absorbed when given orally, although excretion is slow, and the dose varies according to the severity of the heart failure, and whether rapid digitalization is required. In mild conditions, digoxin is given in doses of 125–250 micrograms twice a day initially, the lower dose being preferred for elderly patients. After about 7 days, the dose should be adjusted to need and response, as the maintenance dose, which may be as low as 62.5 micrograms twice daily, is largely dependent on the rate of elimination of the drug in the urine. For more serious conditions, or when rapid digitalization is desired, a loading dose of 1–1.5 mg may be given as divided doses over 24 hours. When a particularly rapid response is required, digoxin may be given by slow intravenous injection as a single dose of 0.5–1 mg, which produces an effect on the heart rate within 10 minutes. A second injection of 0.5 mg may be given later if required, and then followed by standard oral maintenance doses.

Elderly patients require smaller doses of digoxin, partly because of the increased sensitivity of the myocardium to digoxin in such patients, and partly because of a decrease in the renal elimination of the drug. Children, on the other hand, tolerate relatively large doses of digoxin, and to permit easy adjustment of dose for these two groups of patients, tablets containing 62.5 micrograms of digoxin are available as **Lanoxin PG** (paediatric-geriatric). These tablets must be distinguished from the standard tablets which contain 250 micrograms of digoxin and are also available under the brand name **Lanoxin**.

Toxicity. The margin between the therapeutic and toxic doses of digoxin is small, and side-effects are relatively common; as a precaution, the heart rate should not be allowed to fall below 60 beats/minute. Nausea, vomiting and anorexia are early symptoms of digoxin overdose, as are abdominal pain and diarrhoea. Central toxic effects include headache, drowsiness, confusion, hallucinations and visual disturbances such as blurred and coloured vision.

More serious **side-effects** include disturbances of cardiac rhythm such as bradycardia, atrioventricular block and vent-ricular extrasystoles which are similar to the symptoms of the cardiac disease under treatment. It can be difficult at times to tell whether a patient is being overdosed or under-dosed with digoxin, so determinations of the plasma level of digoxin should be carried out if overdose is suspected. Toxicity is likely with plasma concentrations greater than 2 nanograms/ml, but marked individual variations may occur.

Hypokalaemia, which may follow the prolonged use of certain diuretics, is also associated with chronic digoxin toxicity, whereas hyperkalaemia occurs in acute overdose. Treatment is the immediate withdrawal of the drug, and correction of the potassium imbalance, but in very serious overdose, with life-threatening cardiac rhythm and conduction disturbances, the rapid reversal of the toxicity can be achieved by the use of a specific digoxin antidote (**Digibind**).

Digibind is a sheep-derived, digoxin-specific antibody preparation suitable for intravenous injection, and it acts by attracting digoxin away from its receptor sites in the myocardium, and binding it as an inert digoxin–antibody complex in the extracellular fluid. The complex is rapidly excreted in the urine, and the symptoms of digoxin toxicity begin to subside within an hour or even less. The dose of Digibind depends on the body load of digoxin, and it is considered that 40 mg of the antidote can detoxify about 600 micrograms of digoxin. Close cardiac control is essential during the use of Digibind, together with monitoring of the serum potassium levels, as symptoms of the original cardiac disease may return as the excess digoxin is mobilized and excreted.

Certain other digitalis glycosides, including **digitoxin**, are occasionally useful as alternatives to digoxin. Digitoxin is extensively bound to plasma proteins, and as enterohepatic reabsorption occurs, it has a long action. The maintenance dose varies from 50 to 200 micrograms daily.

Sympathomimetic drugs which have an inotropic action and increase the force of the heart beat are referred to on page 231. See also angiotensin-converting enzyme inhibitors (p. 197).

Enoximone § (dose: up to 24 mg/kg daily)

Brand name: Perfan §

Enoximone differs from the cardiac glycosides as it is a synthetic inhibitor of phosphodiesterase, an enzyme that plays an important part in the metabolism of the messenger substance, cyclic AMP. It has a selective action on the enzyme in the myocardium and vascular muscle which leads to a reduced breakdown of cyclic AMP and a rise in intracellular calcium.

Enoximone is used in the treatment of congestive heart failure not responding to other therapy, as it has an inotropic action on the heart, and its vasodilator action also reduces the cardiac workload. It is given by intravenous infusion in doses of 90 micrograms/kg/minute initially, with subsequent supportive doses of 5–20 micrograms/kg/minute up to a total dose if required of 24/mg/kg over 24 hours. It is also given by slow intravenous injection as an initial dose of 0.5–1 mg/kg, followed by 0.5 mg/kg every 30 minutes according to response, up to a maximum of 3 mg/kg.

Side-effects are hypotension, anginal pain, headache and occasional arrhythmias.

Milrinone § (dose: up to 1.13 mg/kg daily)

Brand name: Primacor §

Milrinone resembles enoximone in being a selective inhibitor of phosphodiesterase, and has similar actions, uses and side-effects. It is used for the short-term treatment of severe congestive heart failure that does not respond to conventional therapy. It is given initially by slow intravenous injection over 10 minutes in doses of 50 micrograms/kg, followed by doses of 375–750 nanograms/kg/minute by intravenous infusion, up to a maximum daily dose of 1.13 mg/kg. Treatment may be required for 48–72 hours. It should not be used immediately after myocardial infarction.

Xamoterol § (dose: 400 mg daily)

Brand name: Corwin §

Xamoterol is referred to here as it is used in the treatment of *mild* chronic heart failure in which breathlessness and fatigue are induced by exercise. It is a partial B$_1$ adrenoceptor agonist that improves myocardial contractility, and reduces the cardiac workload by lowering left ventricular pressure. Xamoterol is given in doses of 200 mg twice daily, and symptoms are said to improve steadily over some weeks. Half-doses should be given in renal impairment. Xamoterol should be withdrawn if the heart failure worsens.

Side-effects include gastrointestinal disturbances, dizziness and headache. It is contraindicated in severe heart failure, and caution is necessary in arrhythmias and obstructive airways disease.

DISTURBANCES OF CARDIAC RHYTHM

Disturbances of the normal rhythm of the heart not only lower cardiac efficiency, but in the more severe forms such as tachycardia they are among the principal causes of death in heart disease.

Cardiac arrhythmias are linked with abnormalities in the complex system that governs the contractile mechanism of the heart. The initiating contractile impulse arises in the sino–atrial (SA) node, or pacemaker, which is situated at the junction of the right atrium with the superior vena cava. The impulse excites the atrium to contract, then continues on to the atrioventricular (AV) node, and passes along the His–Pirkinje fibres to reach the ventricles, which are then stimulated to pump blood into the aorta and pulmonary artery. Relaxation then occurs, and the ventricles refill in readiness for the next contraction.

This complex system is controlled by the movement of sodium, potassium and calcium ions in and out of the cardiac cells. At rest, these cells are negatively charged, and the contractile impulse brings about a rapid depolarization (loss of charge) as positively charged sodium ions enter the cell (phase 0). A refractory period follows, during which calcium ions move into the cell, and at this stage the cell does not respond to further stimuli (phases 1–2).

A period of rapid initial repolarization sets in, during which potassium ions flow out of the cell (phase 3), which goes on to the final stage of repolarization, in which sodium ions pass out and potassium ions pass into the cell, which is then again able to respond to a contractile impulse. The cycle is referred to as the action potential.

Any disturbance of the action potential, either in the formation of the originating impulse or its subsequent conduction, or the repolarization of the cell, may give rise to arrhythmias. Thus disturbances at the AV node may prevent the impulse reaching the ventricles, and so cause AV block and bradycardia, while the ventricles, not receiving the full stimulus, beat at a lower and less efficient rate. The pacemaker may fail, and atrial fibrillation at a rate as high as 500 or more times a minute may occur, but ventricular fibrillation is a rapidly life-threatening condition.

In atrial fibrillation and flutter, digoxin is often used to control the heart rate, but in other disturbances of cardiac rhythm, a variety of drugs is used, some of which differ widely in their mode of action.

They have been classified as follows: Class I drugs which have a cell membrane stabilizing action that may be mediated by blocking the fast inward current of sodium ions and so reducing the rate of rapid depolarization (phase 0), or by reducing the conduction rate in cardiac cells. This group includes quinidine, procainamide, some local anaesthetics of the lignocaine type, disopyramide and phenytoin. Class II drugs are those that indirectly reduce the activity of the central nervous system on the myocardium by beta-receptor blockade, and are represented by the beta-adrenoceptor blocking agents of the propranolol type. Class III compounds act by extending the refractory period of phase 2 and extend the action potential, such as amiodarone. Class IV drugs are calcium antagonists, and have a selective action in blocking the movement of calcium ions in the SA and AV nodes. They may also have some membrane stabilizing activity, and are represented by verapamil.

Natel S 1991 Anti-arrhythmic drug classification: a critical appraisal. Drugs 41: 672–701

Points about some anti-arrhythmic drugs

(a) Type of arrhythmia determined by ECG before treatment.
(b) Adenosine in paroxysmal supraventricular tachycardia.
(c) Verapamil is used in supraventricular arrhythmias (not in patients recently treated with beta-blockers).
(d) Quinidine may be effective in both supraventricular and ventricular arrhythmias.
(e) Lignocaine and similar drugs in ventricular arrhythmias.
(f) Bretylium is used only in resuscitation.

Pritchett E L C 1992 Management of atrial fibrillation. New England Journal of Medicine 326: 1264–1271

Quinidine § (dose: 600 mg–1.6 g daily)

Quinidine is the old, original class I or membrane stabilising anti-arrhythmic agent. Although its use has declined as more potent drugs have been introduced, quinidine is still of value for the prevention of ventricular tachycardias not responding to other therapy. It is given in doses of 200–400 mg three or four times a day, after a test dose of 200 mg to detect any quinidine hypersensitivity. The dose should be adjusted to need, as some patients with recurrent arrhythmias may require very prolonged treatment. Quinidine may also be given in doses of 500 mg twice a day as a sustained release product (Kinidin).

Quinidine is well absorbed orally, and an effective plasma level may be reached within 3 hours which persists over 8 hours. A therapeutic response is linked with a plasma level of 2–5 microgram/ml.

Side-effects include nausea and a dose-limiting diarrhoea. Sensitivity reactions, sometimes referred to as cinchonism, are tinnitus, visual disturbances, fever, vertigo and confusion, and may occur in hypersensitive patients after even small doses.

Cumulative toxic effects of quinidine are ventricular tachycardia and fibrillation. It is contraindicated in heart block. Quinidine brings about a marked increase in the plasma concentration of digoxin if both drugs are given together, requiring a reduction of digoxin dosage to avoid toxicity. Care is also necessary if combined treatment with amiodarone is given.

Adenosine §▼ (dose: 3–12 mg by intravenous injection)

Brand name: Adenocor §▼

Adenosine is a natural nucleotide that takes part in many biological processes. It is used therapeutically for the control of paroxysmal supraventricular tachycardia, as it restores sinus rhythm by slowing down conduction through the atrioventricular node, but its use requires careful monitoring. Adenosine is given initially as a dose of 3 mg by rapid intravenous injection, followed if necessary after 1–2 minutes by a further dose of 6 mg. An additional dose of 12 mg may be required. Side-effects include bronchospasm, severe bradycardia and flushing, but they are usually transient, as adenosine has a very short plasma half-life. It is contraindicated in second–third degree heart block.

Garratt C J et al 1992 Adenosine and cardiac arrhythmias. British Medical Journal 305: 3

Amiodarone § (dose: 600 mg daily)

Brand name: Cordarone X §

Amiodarone is a class III anti-arrhythmic drug that acts mainly by extending the refractory period of the contractile fibres of both atria and ventricles. It is used only in arrhythmias that are resistant to other drugs. It is of particular value in the Wolff–Parkinson–White (WPW) syndrome, a resistant re-entry supraventricular tachycardia arising from a secondary AV pathway, as the extension of the refractory period may prevent the re-entry of such secondary impulses.

The oral dose of amiodarone is 200 mg three times a day for at least 1 week, as the initial response is slow, followed by maintenance doses of 200 mg daily or on alternate days. In severe conditions, amiodarone may be given by intravenous infusion over 30–120 minutes in doses of 5 mg/kg up to a maximum dose of 1.2 g in 24 hours under ECG control. It increases the response to digoxin and warfarin, and the doses of those drugs should be adjusted accordingly.

Side-effects are numerous and include photosensitivity with occasional skin discolouration, benign corneal microdeposits, and sometimes pulmonary alveolitis. Nausea, vomiting and vertigo occur less frequently. Amiodarone is an iodine-containing drug, and it is contraindicated in thyroid dysfunction and iodine sensitivity. Sinus bradycardia and AV block are other contraindications.

Disopyramide § (dose: 300–800 mg daily)

Brand names: Dirythmin §, Rythmodan §

Disopyramide has the membrane stabilizing action of quinidine (class I) but it also extends the refractory period (class III), and has some of the calcium-blocking activity of verapamil (class IV). It is used in ventricular arrhythmia and tachycardia, especially after myocardial infarction, and in the Wolff–Parkinson–White syndrome. It is also of value in paroxysmal atrial tachycardia, and in the maintenance of rhythm after electroconversion. A standard dose of disopyramide is 150–400 mg twice a day. When a rapid action is necessary, a dose of 2 mg/kg up to 150 mg may be given by *slow* intravenous injection under ECG control, followed by doses of 400 micrograms/kg hourly up to a maximum of 800 mg daily, before transfer to oral therapy in doses of 200 mg 8-hourly.

Side-effects of disopyramide include hypotension, AV block and myocardial depression. It has some anticholinergic properties, and may cause dryness of the mouth. Care is necessary in glaucoma and disturbances of the urinary tract.

It is contraindicated in complete heart block.

Flecainide § (dose: 200–400 mg daily)

Brand name: Tambocor §

Flecainide is a class I anti-arrhythmic agent of the lignocaine type, and is used mainly in the treatment of severe ventricular and supraventricular tachy-arrhythmias and related conditions.

Flecainide is given orally in doses of 100–200 mg twice a day, reduced later according to response, with initial doses of 100 mg twice daily for elderly patients. In acute conditions, flecainide is given by slow intravenous injection in doses of 2 mg/kg up to a maximum dose of 150 mg, followed by oral therapy as the condition improves. Reduced doses are necessary in cases of renal impairment.

Side-effects of flecainide include dizziness and blurring of vision, which are often transient, and nausea, although uncommon, may occasionally occur. Heart failure and AV block are contraindications.

Lignocaine §

Brand name: Xylocard §

Lignocaine has a membrane stabilizing action, and is a class I drug for the rapid control of ventricular tachycardia after an acute myocardial infarction. Treatment is commenced with a bolus dose of 50–100 mg by *slow* intravenous injection, repeated if necessary after 5 minutes, followed by decreasing doses of 4 mg–1 mg per minute as required. Response to lignocaine is linked with a drug plasma level of 1.5–5 micrograms/ml. Reduced doses should be given in hepatic disease and cardiac failure.

Adequate plasma levels cannot be obtained by oral therapy as there is a high loss by first-pass liver metabolism.

Side-effects include nausea, vomiting, confusion, and epileptiform convulsions. Lignocaine is contraindicated in AV block and severe myocardial depression.

Mexiletine § (dose: 600 mg–1 g daily orally; 100–250 mg initially by injection)

Brand name: Mexitil §

Mexiletine is a class I drug with the actions of lignocaine with the advantage of being active orally. It is used mainly to control ventricular arrhythmias following myocardial infarction, and is given by an initial dose of 400 mg, followed by doses of 200–250 mg, three to four times a day. In acute conditions, mexiletine is given as a bolus dose of 100–250 mg by intravenous injection over 10 minutes, followed by supportive doses of 500 micrograms/minute according to need. Effective plasma levels are in the range of 0.75–2 micrograms/ml.

Side-effects include hypotension, bradycardia, tremor, dizziness, diplopia, dysarthria and confusion, and may be severe enough to limit dosage. It is contraindicated in heart block.

Moracizine §▼

Brand name: Ethmozine §▼

Moracizine is a phenothiazine derivative with a class I-like type of membrane stabilizing antiarrhythmic activity. It is used in the control of ventricular fibrillation/tachycardia. It is given in doses of 200–300 mg 8 hourly, subsequently adjusted at intervals of 3 days with additional doses of 50 mg 8-hourly for maintenance. In severe conditions, an initial dose of 400–500 mg may be given. In common with related drugs, with moracizine there is a risk of a drug-induced worsening of the arrhythmia. Headache, dizziness, palpitations and dyspnoea are amongst the side-effects of moracizine.

Horowitz L N 1990 Role of moracizine in the management of ventricular arrhythmias. American Journal of Cardiology 65: 41D–46D

Phenytoin sodium §

Brand name: Epanutin §

Phenytoin is a class I drug, and has been used to control ventricular arrhythmias associated with digitalis toxicity. It is of little value in cardiac arrhythmias due to acute or chronic heart disease. Dose by *slow* intravenous injection is 3.5–5 mg/kg, repeated once if necessary after about 10 minutes.

Side-effects are bradycardia, hypotension and confusion.

Procainamide § (dose: 1–1.5 g orally; up to 1 g by intravenous injection)

Brand name: Pronestyl §

Procainamide has the membrane stabilizing (class I) action of quinidine, and also has some class III properties of extending the refractory period, with the advantage of being effective both orally and by injection in the control of ventricular arrhythmias. Procainamide is given orally in initial doses of 1 g, followed by doses of 250 mg 4–6-hourly for prophylaxis and maintenance, but for the control of acute arrhythmias it is given by slow intravenous injection under ECG monitoring in doses of 25–50 mg/minute up to a maximum of 1 g, although a dose of over 500 mg is seldom required. A therapeutic response is correlated with a plasma level of 4–8 micrograms/ml. A sustained release preparation containing 500 mg of procainamide is Procainamide Durules.

Procainamide may cause nausea, anorexia and diarrhoea, and other **side-effects** include fever, rash, pruritus and hypersensitivity reactions, as well as cardiac weakness. Prolonged treatment has led to the development of a syndrome resembling lupus erythematosus, requiring withdrawal of treatment.

Propafenone § (dose: 450–900 mg daily)

Brand name: Arythmol §

Propafenone is a class I anti-arrhythmic agent of the lignocaine type used in the prophylaxis and treatment of ventricular arrhythmias not responding to other drugs. It is extensively metabolized in the liver, response may be variable and treatment should be initiated in hospital under ECG control. Propafenone is given orally in doses of 150 mg three times a day, increased at intervals of 3 days as required, up to a maximum of 900 mg daily. The tablets should be taken after food, with a drink, and swallowed whole.

Side-effects include nausea, vomiting, dizziness, diarrhoea, blurred vision, bradycardia and other cardiac disturbances. Postural hypotension may occur in the elderly, who should be given lower doses. It is contraindicated in heart block and uncontrolled congestive heart failure and it should be avoided in patients with myasthenia gravis as it has anticholinergic poperties.

Tocainide § (dose: 600–2400 mg daily)

Brand name: Tonocard §

Tocainide is a class I drug chemically related to lignocaine, and with similar anti-arrhythmic properties.

It is used only in the treatment of severe or life-threatening ventricular arrhythmias, particularly those not responding to other therapy. In such acute conditions tocainide is given in doses of 400 mg three times a day or more up to a maximum of 2.4 g daily, for a plasma level of 6–12 micrograms/ml.

Side-effects of tocainide are numerous, and include gastrointestinal disturbances, tremor, dizziness, confusion and fibrosing alveolitis. Like procainamide, tocainamide may cause a lupus-like syndrome. Blood counts are essential during treatment, as serious side-effects are agranulocytosis and related blood disorders. Care is necessary in renal and hepatic impairment.

Verapamil § (dose: 120–360 mg daily)

Brand names : Cordilox §, Securon §, Univer §

Verapamil is a class IV drug, and influences the movement of calcium ions in myocardial cells, and depresses conduction in the atrio-ventricular node. It is well absorbed orally, but considerable first-pass liver metabolism occurs. Verapamil is used mainly in the treatment of supraventricular arrhythmias, and is given in doses of 40–120 mg, three times a day, but in paroxysmal tachy-cardias it may be given by slow intravenous injection in a dose of 5–10 mg, repeated if necessary after 5–10 minutes, and followed by oral therapy.

Side-effects are nausea, vomiting and constipation, but after intravenous injection myocardial depression, bradycardia, and heart block may occur. Verapamil *should not* be given intravenously (and preferably not orally) to a patient receiving or recently treated with a beta-adrenoceptor blocking agent, as hypotension and asystole may result. Verapamil is contraindicated in AV node disease, bradycardia and heart block. The use of verapamil as a calcium antagonist in angina is referred to on page 208.

Bretylium tosylate § (dose: 5 mg/kg, intramuscular)

Brand name: Bretylate §

Bretylium is a class II anti-arrhythmic drug (p. 178) that acts by displacing noradrenaline from storage sites. It is occasionally of value for resuscitation in resistant ventricular arrhythmias, and is given in doses of 5 mg/kg by intramuscular injection, repeated at intervals of 8 hours. Exceptionally bretylium may be given by *slow* intravenous injection in doses of 5–10 mg/kg, repeated at intervals of 1–2 hours up to a total dose of 30 mg/kg, followed by intramuscular therapy.

Side-effects include nausea, vomiting, and severe hypoten-sion, but noradrenaline and related pressor amines should not be used to restore the blood pressure.

DRUGS USED IN HYPERTENSION AND ANGINA

The blood pressure of the body is maintained and balanced by two forces, the pumping action of the heart and the resistance to blood flow by the peripheral vessels. This balance is mediated via the sympathetic nervous system, as when the blood pressure falls, the system is activated to release noradrenaline from the sympathetic nerve endings. Noradrenaline in turn stimulates the alpha receptors in the arterioles, leading to vasoconstriction and a rise in blood pressure. The beta-receptors in the heart are also activated and the cardiac output is increased by stimulating the heart rate and the contractile force of the myocardium. The initial fall in blood pressure is thus automatically compensated. Conversely, as the blood pressure rises, the activity of the sympathetic nervous system is reduced, less noradrenaline is released, and the elevated blood pressure falls.

In health, the cardiovascular system is so well adjusted that it responds immediately to any physiological demands made upon it, yet it is so well balanced that changes are merely transient, and the blood pressure returns to normal as soon as the impulse has passed.

In later life, the peripheral resistance tends to rise with changes that occur in the vascular connective tissues, the blood pressure also rises, and there is some loss in the ability of the cardiovascular system to respond to physiological stress.

When the blood pressure is permanently raised, the condition is referred to as 'hypertension'. Sustained hypertension, which may be asymptomatic, causes cardiovascular disease, renal damage, myocardial infarction and stroke, and because of the close control over blood volume by the kidneys, renal damage may increase the hypertension. An elevated blood pressure can be lowered by decreasing peripheral resistance or reducing the cardiac output, and a wide range of drugs is now used in the treatment of hypertension. The aim of treatment, which is indicated in patients with an average diastolic pressure over 100 mmHg, is to reduce the blood pressure to a level consistent with the age and general condition of the patient, although benefit in patients over 80 years of age is unlikely.

The ideal drug would lower the elevated blood pressure slowly and evenly, without any disturbance of the electrolyte balance. In addition it should not affect the controls that govern normal blood pressure changes, as too great or too sudden a reduction, especially in the elderly, could cause hypotension and an impairment of renal efficiency that might have serious consequences. Such an ideal drug still awaits discovery, and in practice reliance is placed on a range of drugs that act by different mechanisms. They include alpha- and beta-receptor blocking agents, sympathetic neurone blocking agents, centrally acting antihypertensive drugs, angiotensin-converting-enzyme inhibitors, calcium channel blocking agents and diuretics (Chapter 12). Ganglion blocking agents are obsolete, but one survives as trimetaphan (Arfonad) which is used to obtain hypotension during surgery.

Angina pectoris is the paroxysmal chest pain that occurs when the supply of oxygenated blood reaching the heart is insufficient to meet physiological requirements. The most common cause is atheromatous narrowing of the coronary arteries, although some forms of angina may be due to coronary spasm (Fig. 6.2). Angina is in effect a stress response to factors that increase cardiac output, such as exercise and emotion, and treatment is with drugs which reduce cardiac drive and oxygen demand. They have little or no effect on the coronary obstruction that is the basic cause of angina. Drugs in use include the nitrates, represented by glyceryl trinitrate, beta-blocking agents and calcium channel blocking agents.

BETA-ADRENOCEPTOR BLOCKING AGENTS

These drugs, often referred to simply as beta-blockers, prevent the access of catecholamines to the beta-adrenergic receptor sites in the heart, bronchi and other organs, and so indirectly inhibit the response to sympathetic stimulation. They protect the heart against excessive stimulation, whether induced by physical or emotional stress, and reduce the oxygen requirements of the myocardium. They are widely used in the treatment of hypertension, angina, and are also useful in cardiac arrhythmias, myocardial infarction and thyrotoxicosis. They are

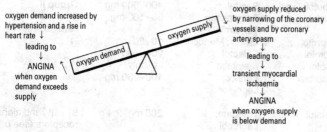

Figure 6.2 Diagram of oxygen balance in angina.

also used occasionally in migraine, to allay anxiety, and locally in glaucoma (p. 522).

As a group, the beta-blockers have the same basic action, but they can be divided into two main groups, those that have a general action on the β_1 and β_2 receptors, and those that have a more selective action on the β_2 receptors in the heart. Some also have a membrane stabilizing action (p. 178). Others such as acebutolol, carteolol, oxprenolol and pindolol, have a degree of 'intrinsic sympathomimetic activity' (ISA), which means that paradoxically they can to some extent stimulate as well as block some beta-receptors and so function as partial agonists. In practice, beta-blockers with some ISA activity tend to cause less bradycardia. Table 6.1 indicates the range of currently available beta-blockers, a few of which are referred to in some detail.

In hypertension, combined treatment with a beta-blocker and a thiazide diuretic may increase the response, and tend to reduce the hypokalaemia associated with such diuretics. Many

Table 6.1 Beta-adrenoceptor blocking agents, some of which are available in slow-release form

Approved name	Brand name	Daily dose range	Type
propranolol	Inderal; Apsolol; Berkolol	40–320 mg	**Group I** $\beta_1 + \beta_2$ or non-selective
betaxolol	Kerlone	20–40 mg	
nadolol	Corgard	40–240 mg	
oxprenolol	Trasicor; Apsolox; Betadren; Laracor	120–480 mg	
pindolol	Visken	7.5–45 mg	
sotalol	Beta-Cardone; Sotacor	160–480 mg	
timolol	Betim; Blocadren	15–60 mg	
acebutolol	Sectral	400–800 mg	**Group II** β_1 or cardioselective
atenolol	Antipressan; Tenormin	50–100 mg	
bisoprolol	Emcor; Monocor	10–20 mg	
celiprolol	Celectol	200–400 mg	
esmolol	Brevibloc	i.v. only	
metoprolol	Betaloc; Lopresor	100–200 mg	
labetalol	Trandate; Labrocol	200 mg–2.4 g	$\beta_1 + \beta_2$ and alpha receptors (see p. 231)

combined products are now available, designed mainly to simplify therapy and improve patient compliance. They are useful once control of the hypertension has been achieved, but are not intended for initial therapy.

Points about beta-blockers

(a) All have same basic action, but some (atenolol, nadolol and sotalol) are not lipid-soluble, and so less likely to cause sleep disturbances.
(b) All cause bradycardia and could precipitate incipient heart failure.
(c) May bring about histamine release and provoke asthma.
(d) Patients should be warned about postural hypotension, particularly after sleep.
(e) Coldness in the extremities may occur as the result of the reduced peripheral blood flow.
(f) Treatment should not be stopped abruptly — advise patients not to run out of supplies.
(g) No beta-blocker should be given to a patient recently treated with verapamil.

Some **side-effects**, such as bradycardia, sleep disturbances, bronchoconstriction and reduced peripheral blood flow are common to all beta-blockers in varying degrees. Sleep disturbances are less likely with atenolol, nadolol and solatol, as they are water-soluble, and so do not enter the brain as readily as the lipid-soluble blockers. Bronchoconstriction, which can be severe, is more likely to occur when Group I drugs are used and great care is necessary in initial treatment in patients with a history of asthma. Care is also necessary in patients with cardiac failure and heart block, and the reduced blood flow associated with beta blockade may also influence renal and hepatic efficiency. By the nature of their action, the beta-blockers interact with a wide range of other drugs, which may increase the bradycardia, myocardial depression and other side-effects.

It is of interest that some beta-blockers such as propranolol, sotalol, and timolol are used in the long-term secondary treatment of myocardial infarction, as early and prolonged treatment reduces the risk of re-infarction, and increases survival time.

The beta-blockers are also useful in preparing patients for thyroidectomy. If given for 4 days before operation, the clinical aspects of thyrotoxicosis can be temporarily reversed, and the gland becomes less vascular, thus facilitating surgery.

Propranolol § (dose: 40–320 mg daily)

Brand names: Inderal §, Apsolol §, Berkolol §

Propranolol was one of the first of the beta-adrenoceptor blocking agents. It inhibits the normal response to cardiac stimulation, and reduces the contractile force of the heart muscle. It is used in the control of angina, hypertension, thyrotoxicosis, cardiac arrhythmias of varied origin, and the prophylaxis of myocardial infarction and migraine.

Propranolol is given in angina in doses of 10–40 mg or more four times a day, increasing according to need. In hypertension, it is given in initial doses of 80 mg twice a day, increased at weekly intervals according to response, with maintenance doses varying from 160 to 320 mg daily, often in association with a thiazide diuretic.

For prophylaxis after acute myocardial infarction, treatment is commenced within 1–3 weeks with doses of 40 mg four times a day for a few days, after which the drug is given in doses of 80 mg twice a day.

In arrhythmic emergencies, propranolol may be given by slow intravenous injection, in doses of 1 mg per minute, up to a maximum of 10 mg, preceded by an injection of atropine 1–2 mg to reduce the bradycardial side-effects.

For migraine prophylaxis, propranolol may be given in doses of 40 mg or more three times a day, and in similar doses for the relief of tremor and palpitation associated with apprehension, stress and anxiety.

Although propranolol is generally well tolerated, **side-effects** include bronchospasm in susceptible patients, reduced peripheral blood flow, and gastrointestinal disturbances. In overdose, the bronchospasm may be severe, with bradycardia and hypotension. Propranolol is contraindicated in asthma, heart failure and heart block, and is not suitable for the treatment of hypertensive emergencies. It should not be given to patients receiving verapamil.

Acebutolol § (dose: 300–800 mg daily)

Brand name: Sectral §

Acebutolol has the actions and uses of propranolol, but is more cardioselective. It also has some intrinsic sympathomimetic activity, and so is less likely to cause bradycardia. In angina and hypertension, acebutolol is given in initial doses of 200 mg twice daily, gradually increased according to need, but doses of more than 1 g daily are seldom necessary. The response to treatment is usually prompt.

Acebutolol has the **side-effects** and contraindications of propranolol, and although it has less effect on the bronchial adrenoreceptors, it should be used with care in patients with obstructive airway disease. In common with related drugs, acebutolol should not be given to patients receiving intravenous verapamil, as asystole with hypotension may occur.

Atenolol § (dose: 50–100 mg daily)

Brand names: Antipressan §, Tenormin §

Atenolol is a cardioselective beta-adrenoceptor blocking agent with an extended action. It is given in hypertension in single doses of 50–100 mg daily, but the full response may not occur until after 1 or 2 weeks. It is often given with a thiazide diuretic to increase the effect. In angina, 100 mg daily as a single or divided dose is adequate, as larger doses are seldom more effective.

Atenolol is also of value in cardiac arrhythmias, and is then given in oral doses of 50–100 mg daily, but in acute conditions it is given by slow intravenous injection in doses of 2.5 mg, repeated at intervals of 5 minutes up to four doses. It may also be given by intravenous infusion in doses of 150 micrograms/kg. Marked bradycardia may follow intravenous use, which can be relieved by the injection of atropine (600 micrograms) as required. Atenolol is also used in the initial acute stage of myocardial infarction as a dose of 5 mg by intravenous infusion, followed by supportive oral doses of 50 mg twice daily.

Like acebutolol, it is less likely to provoke bronchospasm, but it should be used with care in asthma and related conditions. It is contraindicated in untreated heart failure and heart block.

Esmolol § (dose: 50–200 mg/kg intravenously)

Brand name: Brevibloc §

Esmolol differs from other beta-blockers in having a very brief action. It has cardio-selective properties, and is used in the short-term treatment of supraventricular arrhythmias and tachycardia, and in postoperative hypertension. It is given by intravenous infusion in doses of 50–200 micrograms/kg per minute, but the dosage must be carefully titrated according to individual need.

Labetalol § (dose: 200 mg–2.4 g daily)

Brand name: Trandate §

Labetalol differs from related drugs as it has the double action of blocking both alpha- and beta-adrenoceptors. Blockade of the alpha-adrenoceptors brings about a peripheral vasodilatation, with a fall in blood pressure and a reduction in peripheral resistance. The beta-blockers have little action on the peripheral circulation, as compensatory mechanisms come into play to offset any vasodilator response. With labetalol, the balance of alpha and beta blocking activity results in a smoother hypotensive response with fewer side-effects.

Labetalol is useful in hypertensive states generally in the hypertension of pregnancy after acute myocardial infarction and in hypertensive crisis. It is sometimes used for controlled hypotension in surgery. In labile hypertension it is given in initial doses of 100–200 mg twice daily with food, increased according to need. High doses are required only in severe conditions. It is not usually necessary to give combined treatment with diuretics. In acute conditions, labetalol can be given by slow intravenous injection in doses of 50 mg, repeated after 5 minutes up to a total dose of 200 mg, or by intravenous infusion in doses of 2 mg/minute up to a similar maximum. The bradycardia that may follow intravenous labetolol may be controlled by atropine in doses of 600 micrograms.

In the acute hypertension of pregnancy and after acute myocardial infarction, doses of 15–20 mg/hour by intravenous infusion may be given, increased according to need up to 150 mg/hour. In hypotensive surgery, doses of 10–20 mg are given by intravenous injection, with a second dose of 5–10 mg after 5 minutes if necessary.

Side-effects include dizziness and lethargy, and postural hypotension may occur after high initial doses. Care is necessary in heart block and asthmatic patients.

Oxprenolol § (dose: 40–480 mg daily)

Brand name: Trasicor §

Oxprenolol is a beta-adrenoceptor blocker of the propranolol type with similar actions and uses. It is given orally in doses of 40–160 mg or more three times a day, according to the condition, adjusted to individual needs and response. Oxprenolol may occasionally cause bronchospasm, and is contraindicated in heart block.

ALPHA-ADRENOCEPTOR BLOCKING AGENTS

Noradrenaline raises the blood pressure by acting on the alpha-adrenoceptors and a limited number of drugs function as post-synaptic alpha-adrenoceptor blocking agents. They bring about a reduction of peripheral vascular smooth muscle tone, and by that relaxant action they lower the peripheral resistance, but they have little effect on skeletal muscle, where the blood flow is controlled by the beta-receptors. They are of value in hypertensive crises, and are also used with beta-blockers and diuretics to obtain a smoother response in the control of hypertension. Prazosin was the first alpha-adrenoceptor blocking agent to be used therapeutically, but it has the disadvantage of causing marked first-dose hypotension.

Some newer drugs have a more selective $alpha_1$-adrenoceptor mediated action on prostatic and bladder smooth muscle, and are used for the symptomatic treatment of benign prostatic hyperplasia. (See prazosin p. 361, and alfuzosin p. 359.)

Points about alpha-adrenoceptor blocking agents

(a) Warn patients about hypotension, particularly first-dose hypotension.
(b) Subsequent postural hypotension may be increased by hot baths, long standing and large meals.
(c) Advise patients to rest at any feeling or onset of faintness.

Doxazosin § (dose: 1–16 mg daily)

Brand name: Cardura §

Doxazosin has a more selective and longer action than prazosin (p. 196), and in hypertension it is given in doses of 1 mg initially, slowly increased after 1–2 weeks to 2 mg daily, and subsequently further increased according to need up to a maximum of 16 mg daily. Combined treatment with a beta-blocker and a diuretic is common. Doxazosin may be given in standard doses to the elderly, and to patients with renal insufficiency.

Side-effects are headache, dizziness and postural hypotension.

Indoramin § (dose: 50–200 mg daily)

Brand name: Baratol §

Indoramin also has a more selective and extended action on the alpha$_1$-adrenoreceptors, and lowers the blood pressure by reducing peripheral resistance. In mild hypertension indoramin may be given alone in doses of 25 mg twice a day initially, slowly increased at intervals of 2 weeks up to a maximum of 200 mg daily, usually in association with a beta-blocker and/or a diuretic. Any incipient heart failure should be controlled by digoxin and diuretics before indoramin treatment is commenced. The use of indoramin in benign prostatic hypertrophy is referred to on page 360.

Side-effects include drowsiness, dizziness and dryness of the mouth. Care is necessary in epilepsy, parkinsonism, and hepatic and renal impairment.

Phenoxybenzamine § (dose: 10–20 mg or more daily)

Brand name: Dibenylene §

Phenoxybenzamine is an alpha-adrenoceptor blocking agent with an extended action that is used in the control of hypertensive episodes associated with phaeochromocytoma. It is given in doses of 10 mg initially, increased by 10 mg daily according to need, up to a total daily dose of 1–2 mg/kg (divided into two doses).

Side-effects include postural hypotension and dizziness. In some cases, the tumour may liberate both adrenaline and nor-adrenaline, and cause marked tachycardia and other arrhythmias, and combined treatment with a beta-adrenoceptor blocking agent such as propranolol may then be necessary to control such side-effects. There is some risk of contact sensitization with phenoxybenzamine, and care should be taken to avoid skin contact with the drug.

Metirosine § (dose: 1–4 g daily)

Brand name: Demser §

Metirosone is not an alpha-receptor blocking agent, but is referred to here as it has an action similar to that of phenoxybenzamine. It acts indirectly by blocking the formation of noradrenaline and other catecholamines from tyrosine by inhibiting the enzyme tyrosine hydroxylase.

It is used in the treatment of phaeochromocyoma, as well as in the pre-operative preparation of patients with that catecholamine-secreting tumour, but it is not suitable for the treatment of essential hypertension.

Metirosine is given in doses of 250 mg four times a day initially, increased if necessary up to 4 g daily according to laboratory reports of urinary catecholamine levels, which should fall by 50%. If required, combined treatment with phenoxybenzamine may be given.

Side-effects include sedation, diarrhoea and extrapyramidal symptoms. A fluid intake of at least 2 litres daily should be taken to avoid crystalluria.

Phentolamine § (dose: 5–10 mg by intravenous injection)

Brand name: Rogitine §

Phentolamine is a short-acting alpha-receptor blocking agent used in the diagnosis of phaeochromocytoma and in the control of the associated hypertensive crises. Such tumours release press or amines such as adrenaline into the circulation, and bring about a rise in blood pressure that can be distinguished from essential hypertension by the intravenous injection of phentolamine. Phentolamine temporarily neutralizes the vasoconstrictor action of adrenaline, with a consequent fall in blood pressure, which returns to the previous level within minutes. In essential hypertension, phentolamine causes no significant changes in the blood pressure. It has also been used in the hypertensive crisis that may follow the sudden withdrawal of clonidine.

Phentolamine is given in doses of 5–10 mg by intravenous injection, repeated as required, or by intravenous infusion of doses of 5–60 mg over 15–30 minutes according to need and response.

Side-effects include nausea, diarrhoea, tachycardia, hypotension and dizziness, but as phentolamine has some anti-arrhythmic properties, the tachycardia is unlikely to be severe. Combined treatment with a beta-blocking agent may be necessary during surgical removal of the tumour.

Prazosin § (dose: 500 micrograms–20 mg daily)

Brand name: Hypovase §

Prazosin lowers peripheral resistance by dilatation of the arterioles, brought about by a blockade of the postsynaptic alpha adrenoceptors. Unlike some other drugs, prazosin does not induce a reflex tachycardia, and is unlikely to cause or exacerbate bronchospasm. It is used in the treatment of all types of hypertension, and is given in doses of 500 micrograms two or three times a day initially, slowly increased according to need up to 20 mg daily. The initial dose of prazosin may cause hypotension with loss of consciousness, so the first dose should be taken in the evening, and in bed.

Prazosin is also used in congestive heart failure in maintenance doses of 4–20 mg daily, and in Raynaud's disease lower maintenance doses of 1–2 mg twice a day may be effective. In severe conditions, it may be given in association with a beta-blocker or a diuretic, but dosage requires careful adjustment, and that of prazosin should be reduced by half to avoid an excessive response. It may be used in patients with impaired renal function, as prazosin has little effect on renal blood flow or glomerular filtration rate, even during long-term administration. The use of prazosin in prostatic hypertrophy is referred to on page 361.

Side-effects are sedation, dizziness, hypotension and weakness. Nasal congestion, depression and palpitations have also been reported.

Terazocin § (dose: 1–10 mg)

Brand name: Hytrin §

Terazocin is an antihypertensive agent that produces peripheral vasodilatation by a selective blockade of post-synaptic alpha$_1$-adrenoceptors. It is used in mild to moderate hypertension, and is given initially as a 1 mg dose *at night*. That precaution is essential, as an acute hypotensive episode may follow the initial dose within 30–90 minutes, but recurrence is uncommon provided dose increases are kept low.

Subsequent doses may be slowly increased at weekly intervals up to 10 mg or more daily, but doses over 20 mg daily are unlikely to evoke an improved response. No adjustment in dose is necessary in the elderly, or in renal impairment. Lower doses of terazocin may be given with a thiazide diuretic.

Side-effects are dizziness, light-headedness, peripheral oedema and postural hypotension.

Thymoxamine § (dose: 160–320 mg daily)

Brand name: Opilon §

Thymoxamine is a selective alpha-adrenergic blocking agent with the actions and uses of that group of drugs. It is given in doses of 40 mg four times a day in the short-term management of primary Raynaud's disease. If there is no response after doses up to 320 mg daily, treatment should be discontinued.

Side-effects are nausea, diarrhoea and vertigo.

ANGIOTENSIN-COVERTING ENZYME INHIBITORS

The renin–angiotensin system is one of the most powerful systems of the body, as it is concerned with the maintenance of the arterial pressure and salt and water balance. Renin is the enzyme that controls the rate of formation of angiotensin I, which is inactive, but which is converted into the active angiotension II by the angiotensin-converting enzyme (ACE).

Angiotension II which is the most potent pressor substance known, has a direct vasoconstrictor action on the vascular smooth muscle of the arterioles and larger arteries, but it has less action on the venous system. It also stimulates the zona glomerulosa cells of the adrenal cortex to release aldosterone, and also has an indirect action of raising the blood pressure by reducing the excretion of salts and water.

ACE is present in many tissues apart from the blood vessels, and the conversion of angiotensin I to angiotensin II takes place largely in the lungs. As some forms of hypertension are associated with high plasma levels of renin, and in consequence of angiotensin II, a circle of activity is set up that brings about a rise in blood pressure and adds to the cardiac burden (Fig. 6.3). An interruption of that circle by inhibiting the formation of angiotensin II could lead to a reduction in blood pressure and a reduction of the cardiac load. One approach to the problem would be the discovery of a drug that could inhibit the activity of renin, and so break the circle at an early stage, and an orally active renin-inhibitor is under experimental investigation. At present, however, reliance is largely placed on drugs that act at a later stage by inhibiting the conversion of angiotensin I to angiotensin II, a group referred to as the ACE-inhibitors.

They bring about both arterial and venous vasodilatation, reduce arterial tone and venous return, and so increase cardiac efficiency and improve peripheral and renal circulation. The ACE-inhibitors are now in wide use, both in the early stages of heart failure as well as in the treatment of late and severe stages, particularly when beta-blockers or thiazide diuretics fail to control or relieve the heart failure. They are also of value in the treatment of hypertension. They differ to some extent in their duration of effect, and with some single daily doses are adequate.

The initial use of these drugs requires care, as with some patients there may be a very rapid and marked first-dose fall in blood pressure. The risk can be reduced to some extent by very low initial doses of the ACE-inhibitor, and the previous withdrawal of any diuretic therapy for a few days.

Patients should be kept supine for an hour or two after the first dose of an ACE-inhibitor, with frequent measurement of the

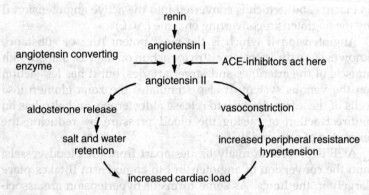

Figure 6.3   Point of action of ACE-inhibitors.

blood pressure. The duration of action of subsequent doses appears to be inversely related to the creatinine clearance, and as some ACE-inhibitors may cause renal impairment, adjustments of dose may be necessary. Renal efficiency should be checked before and during ACE-inhibitor therapy as ACE-inhibitor-induced renal impairment may become progressive.

The ACE-inhibitors have side-effects that are largely common in varying degree to all representatives of the group, and include headache, dizziness, oedema, fatigue, hypotension and occasional rash and pruritus. A delayed **side-effect**, often associated with extended treatment, is a persistent and non-productive cough, which may sometimes be severe enough to require withdrawal of the drug. The cause of the cough is unknown, but nurses should encourage patients to persist with treatment.

Berkin K E, Ball S G 1988 Cough and angiotensin converting enzyme inhibition. British Medical Journal 296: 1279–1280

> **Points about ACE-inhibitors**
>
> (a) First-dose hypotension may be marked.
> (b) Reduce risk by withdrawing diuretic therapy for a few days, and giving a low first-dose at night with the patient in bed.
> (c) Discontinue potassium-sparing diuretics or potassium supplements.

Captopril § (dose: 25–150 mg daily)

Brand names: Acepril §, Capoten §

Captopril is used in the treatment of severe hypertension resistant to other therapy, in mild to moderate hypertension, often in association with thiazide diuretics and beta-blockers, and in congestive heart failure. In severe hypertension, it is given in initial doses of 12.5 mg twice a day, 1 hour before food, together with a thiazide diuretic. Subsequent doses are slowly increased up to a maximum of 50 mg three times a day. In milder cases, a maintenance dose of 25 mg twice a day, supported by other therapy, is often sufficient. In severe heart failure, initial doses of 6.25–12.5 mg twice a day are given, increased if necessary up to

50 mg three times a day under close supervision. Lower doses are used in renal impairment, and for the elderly.

In all cases initial therapy requires care, as a marked hypotension may occur within an hour or two of the first dose, for which treatment should be immediately available. As a precaution, diuretic therapy should be withdrawn for a few days.

Side-effects include a pruritic rash which tends to disappear with continued treatment, loss of taste, cough and paraesthesia, but more serious side-effects are proteinuria, neutropenia and agranulocytosis, and urinary and blood tests are necessary during captopril treatment. Other reported side-effects include angio-oedema and urticaria.

As captopril decreases aldosterone release, a rise in serum potassium may occur, and care is necessary if potassium-sparing diuretics are used; these are best avoided (risk of hyperkalaemia), as is combined therapy with allopurinol and procainamide.

Cilazapril § (dose: 1–5 mg daily)

Brand name: Vascace §

Cilazapril is an ACE-inhibitor, and has the actions and general uses of that group of drugs in the treatment of hypertension. It differs by having a half-life that extends over 9 hours, so that single daily doses may be given. Diuretics should be withdrawn for 2–3 days before starting cilazapril. Initial doses of 0.5–1 mg daily are slowly increased to 2.5–5 mg daily according to response, and diuretic therapy can be reintroduced later if required. The **side-effects** are similar to those of other ACE-inhibitors, and care is necessary in congestive heart failure, ascites and aortic stenosis.

Enalapril § (dose: 5–40 mg daily)

Brand name: Innovace §

Enalapril is a pro-drug, and is slowly hydrolyzed following oral administration to enalaprilat, which is the active metabolite. It has the angiotensin-converting-enzyme inhibitory action of captopril, but the effect is more powerful and prolonged. Enalapril is used in all types of essential hypertension, including that not responding to other drugs, and in the supplementary treatment of congestive heart failure. It is also used in the treatment of hypertension due to renal artery stenosis.

Enalapril should be regarded as a second-line drug, mainly for use when other treatment is contraindicated or ineffective. Diuretics should be withdrawn before commencing enalapril therapy, as acute hypotension after the first dose has been reported, and initial treatment in hospital is advisable.

In hypertension, it is given in initial doses of 5 mg daily, increased up to a maximum of 40 mg daily. In the elderly, or when renal impairment is present, initial doses of 2.5 mg are used, and in such cases maintenance doses of 1–2 mg daily may be adequate. In congestive heart failure, initial doses of 2.5–5 mg are given in conjunction with digoxin and diuretics. Innozide § contains enalapril 20 mg with hydrochlorothiazide 12.5 mg.

Side-effects include hypotension, headache, dizziness, rash, nausea, diarrhoea and persistent cough. Renal function should be checked before and during treatment.

Fosinopril § (dose: 10–40 mg daily)

Brand name: Staril §

Fosinopril is an ACE-inhibitor with the general action, uses and side-effects of that group of drugs. It is used mainly in essential hypertension when other drugs are either ineffective or unsuitable. It is given in doses of 10 mg daily initially, rising to 20 mg daily or more to a maximum dose of 40 mg daily. Any diuretic treatment should be withdrawn some days before fosinopril is given and resumed only with care after 4 weeks if the blood pressure is not fully controlled.

Lisinopril § (dose: 2.5–40 mg daily)

Brand names: Carace §, Zestril §

Lisinopril is an analogue of enalapril, with similar actions, uses and side-effects. It has the advantage of a longer action that permits control of blood pressure by a single daily dose. Lisinopril is indicated in essential and renovascular hypertension of varying severity, and as adjunctive treatment in congestive heart failure. It is given in initial doses of 2.5 mg daily, increased according to need to 10–20 mg daily, up to a maximum of 40 mg daily if required. In diuretic-treated patients, such therapy should be withdrawn for 2–3 days before commencing lisinopril dosage. As with all ACE-inhibitors, care is necessary in renal insufficiency, and potassium-sparing diuretics should be avoided. Carace Plus § and Zestoretic § contain lisinopril 20 mg with hydrochlorothiazide 12.5 mg.

Perindopril § (dose: 2–8 mg daily)

Brand name: Coversyl §

Perindopril is a long-acting ACE-inhibitor that is effective in single daily doses. It is used for the control of essential and renovascular hypertension not responding to other drugs. Current treatment with diuretics should be withdrawn 3 days before commencing with perindopril in doses of 2 mg daily before food. Subsequent doses can be increased according to response up to a maximum of 8 mg daily. Renal function should be assessed before and during treatment, and if necessary the dose should be adjusted to the creatinine clearance.

   Side-effects include cough, headache and malaise.

Quinapril § (dose: 5–40 mg daily)

Brand name: Accupro §

Quinapril, like enalapril, is a pro-drug, and the active metabolite is quinaprilat. It has the actions of the ACE-inhibitors, and is useful in all grades of hypertension when other therapy is ineffective, or unsuitable because of side-effects. It is also used in congestive heart failure. In hypertension, quinapril is given as an initial dose of 5 mg, often given as a single daily dose. In congestive heart failure, an initial dose of 2.5 mg is given, with subsequent maintenance doses of 10–20 mg daily. In common with other ACE-inhibitors, patients receiving diuretics may experience a marked initial first-dose fall in blood pressure, which may be minimized by the previous temporary withdrawal of diuretic therapy. The serum levels of potassium should be monitored. Accuretic § is a mixed product containing quinapril 10 mg with hydrochlorothiazide 12.5 mg.

   Side-effects of quinapril are similar to those of the ACE-inhibitors generally.

Ramipril § (Tritace §) is an ACE-inhibitor with similar actions and uses, given in doses of 1.25–5 mg once daily.

Trandolapril §▼ (dose: 0.5–4 mg daily)

Brand names: Gopten §, Odrik §

Trandolapril is a pro-ACE-inhibitor, as it is hydrolyzed in the body to a long-acting metabolite. It is used like other ACE-inhibitors in the treatment of mild to moderate hypertension. In patients without congestive heart failure or renal or hepatic impairment, treatment is commenced with doses of 500 micrograms daily, doubled at intervals of 2–4 weeks according to response up to 2–4 mg as a single daily dose for maintenance. Any diuretic therapy should be withdrawn initially to reduce the incidence of hypotensive side-effects. Patients with reduced renal or hepatic efficiency should receive reduced doses. In congestive heart failure, trandolapril treatment requires hospital supervision. **Side-effects** include cough, headache, dizziness, hypotension and palpitations.

CALCIUM CHANNEL-BLOCKING AGENTS (CCBAs)

Muscle contraction is linked with an influx of calcium ions into the muscle cells via calcium channels in the cell membrane. The channels are normally occupied by calcium ions bound to high-affinity sites, and act as voltage-dependent ionic gates. When stimulated, calcium ions are released, the ionic gate opens, and calcium ions flow through the channels into the cell and stimulate muscle contraction.

Certain differences in these channels have been recognized, as some are designated receptor-operated channels (ROC) which are activated by acetylcholine and other agents, and voltage-operated channels (VOC), which are activated by depolarization of the cell membrane. The VOCs have been differentiated as long-lasting (L) channels and transient (T) channels, but the L channels appear to be the main sites of action of calcium channel-blocking agents, as the ROC and T channels are largely insensitive to such blockade.

When cardiac muscle is stimulated by the flow of calcium ions, the heart rate and myocardial oxygen demand increases, and when that response is excessive, cardiac irregularities, coronary artery spasm and angina may occur.

Drugs that could block the flow of calcium ions would clearly have wide applications in cardiovascular therapeutics, and research has resulted in the introduction of a group of drugs referred to as calcium channel-blocking agents (CCBAs). They all act by restricting the movement of calcium ions, and so reduce the sensitivity of cardiac muscle to contractile stimulations. They also reduce the blood pressure by a direct relaxant effect on vascular smooth muscle. By virtue of their action they are not indicated in heart failure, as they may further depress an already reduced cardiac efficiency.

The CCBAs in current use differ in their individual pattern of activity, as some are more effective in angina than in hypertension and some have no anti-arrhythmic activity. They have been divided into three groups: Class I represented by verapamil; Class II includes nifedipine and other dihydropyridine derivatives, and Class III, represented by diltiazem. It should be noted that some CCBA products have been specially formulated to provide a more sustained period of activity. These long-acting products must not be regarded as interchangeable, and a change from one type of product to another should not be made without good cause and careful assessment of the need for change.

Kenny J 1985 Calcium channel blocking agents and the heart. British Medical Journal 291: 1150–1152

Points about calcium channel blockers

(a) Some are used in angina; others in hypertension, as they differ in their pattern of activity.
(b) Not indicated in heart failure.
(c) Nimodipine is exceptional in its use in subarachnoid haemorrhage.
(d) Long-acting products should not be regarded as interchangeable.

Amlodipine § (dose: 5–10 mg daily)

Brand name: Istin §

Amlodipine has the general properties of the CCBAs, but it is eliminated more slowly and so has a longer action. It is used in the treatment of angina and hypertension in doses of 5 mg daily, increased if required to 10 mg daily. It can be used as the sole agent in the control of hypertension, or in combination with other antihypertensive agents such as diuretics and beta-blockers, usually without adjustment of dose.

Side-effects include flushing, headache, fatigue and dizziness. The hypotensive episodes and reflex tachycardia that sometimes occur with CCBAs are less likely with amlodipine by virtue of its slower action.

Diltiazem § (dose: 120–360 mg daily)

Brand names: Adizem §, Britiazem §, Dilzem §, Tildiem §

Diltiazem is a Class III calcium channel blocking agent, and differs from others by having little inotropic action on the heart, as it reduces conduction in the AV and SR nodes. It is used in the treatment of angina in doses of 60 mg three times a day, or twice a day for elderly patients, but the individual response may vary, and require doses up to 360 mg daily. Diltiazem may be effective in angina resistant to beta-blocker treatment. It is also used, mainly as a slow-release product, for the treatment of hypertension in doses of 90 mg or more twice a day. These slow release products are not necessarily bio-equivalent, and transfer from one product to another should not be made without good cause and re-assessment. Diltiazem should be used with care in patients with poor cardiac reserves, as its depressant action on cardiac conduction may precipitate heart failure. **Side-effects** are bradycardia, hypotension and ankle oedema, while headache and rash and less common. Adizem-SR, Adizem XL, Dilzem SR, Tildiem Retard and Tildiem LA are sustained action products.

Felodipine §▼ (dose: 5–20 mg daily)

Brand name: Plendil §▼

Felodipine is a more recently introduced CCBA, and has a pattern of activity similar to that of amlodipine. It is used in all degrees of hypertension, and is given in initial doses of 5 mg once daily, with subsequent adjustment according to response, up to a maximum of 20 mg daily. The **side-effects** of felodipine are similar to those of most other CCBAs, but rash and mild gingival hyperplasia may occur.

Isradipine § (dose: 5–20 mg daily)

Brand name: Prescal §

Isradipine is a calcium antagonist that has a higher affinity for calcium channels in arterial smooth muscle than for those in the myocardium and so is largely free from cardiodepressant side-effects. In hypertension isradipine is given in doses of 2.5 mg twice daily initially, increased after 3–4 weeks if the response is inadequate to 5 mg twice a day, or very occasionally up to 20 mg daily. Combined treatment with a beta-blocker/diuretic may permit the use of lower doses. Isradipine undergoes extensive first-pass liver metabolism, and reduced doses should be given to the elderly and in renal impairment.

Side-effects include dizziness, headache and tachycardia. Rash, weight gain and hypotension are less common.

Lacidipine §▼

Brand name: Motens §▼

Lacidipine is a recent addition to the range of Class II calcium channel-blocking agents. It is chemically related to nifedipine, and has similar properties, differing mainly in having a smoother and more prolonged action. In the treatment of hypertension it may be given alone, or together with other antihypertensive agents such as diuretics and beta-blockers. The standard dose is 4 mg, taken in the morning with food, but half-doses are indicated in the elderly. The development of full response is slow, and 3–4 weeks should elapse before an increase in dose to 6 mg daily is considered. Lacidipine is not excreted in the urine, so no modification of dose is required for patients with renal disease. The **side-effects** are those of calcium channel antagonists generally, but are usually transient, but chest pain may indicate myocardial ischaemia.

Heber M E 1990 Effectiveness of the once-daily calcium antagonist lacidipine, in controlling 24-hour ambulatory blood pressure. American Journal of Cardiology 66: 1228–1232

Nicardipine § (dose: 60–120 mg daily)

Brand name: Cardene §

Nicardipine has the general properties of the calcium channel-blocking agents, but differs from diltiazem and verapamil in not depressing myocardial contractility. It is used mainly for the prophylaxis and treatment of angina in patients with some cardiac dysfunction, and in hypertension to reduce the reflex tachycardia that may occur with beta-blocker therapy. It is also used alone in hypertension as it brings about a direct fall in blood pressure by lowering arteriolar resistance. Nicardipine is given in doses of 20 mg three times a day initially, increased at intervals of not less than 3 days up to a maximum of 120 mg daily.

Side-effects include dizziness, headache, flushing, palpitations, nausea and lower limb oedema, If any ischaemic pain occurs, or is worsened, within 30 minutes of the first dose, treatment should be discontinued.

Nifedipine § (dose: 30–60 mg daily)

Brand names: Adalat §, Calcilat §

Nifedipine is a typical member of the group of Class II calcium channel-blocking agents derived from dihydropyridine. These drugs have a mainly vasodilator action with little influence on cardiac conduction. Nifedipine is used both for the prophylaxis and treatment of angina, and in the treatment of hypertension, and is given in doses of 10 mg three times a day initially, slowly increased if required up to 60 mg daily. A liquid-filled capsule of 5 mg is available, and if a rapid effect is required, the patient should bite into the capsule, and retain the liquid in the mouth. Like other Class II CCBAs, nifedipine has little if any anti-arrhythmic activity or depressant action on the myocardium, and it may be given together with a beta-blocker. The antihypertensive effects may be additive, and care is necessary to control any marked hypotension that may follow combined therapy.

Adalat Retard and Nifensar XL are sustained action products.

Side-effects are basically similar to those of glyceryl trinitrate, and are usually transient, but lethargy and hyperplasia of the gums may sometimes occur. Nifedipine may cause or increase ischaemic pain in a few patients within minutes of initiating treatment, and in such cases the drug should be withdrawn.

Nimodipine § (dose: 360 mg daily)

Brand name: Nimotop §

Nimodipine is a calcium antagonist that crosses the blood–brain barrier and has a preferential action on the calcium channels in the cerebral vessels. It is used orally in subarachnoid haemorrhage following rupture of intracranial aneurysm to prevent the development of ischaemic neurological sequelae. Treatment should be commenced within 4 days of the onset of the haemorrhage with nimodipine in doses of 60 mg every 4 hours, and continued for 21 days. If cerebral oedema or ischaemia occurs, oral therapy should be replaced by the intravenous infusion of the drug in doses of 1 mg hourly initially, increased later to 2 mg hourly, and continued for 5 days. Care is necessary in cerebral oedema or increased intracranial pressure.

Side-effects are hypotension and gastrointestinal disorders.

Verapamil § (dose: 240–360 mg daily)

Brand names: Cordilox §, Securon §

Verapamil is the oldest of the calcium channel-blocking agents, and was used therapeutically before the nature of its function as a CCBA was understood. It is a Class I CCBA, and has a depressant effect on cardiac conduction mediated by the atrio-ventricular node, and so is of value in supraventricular arrhythmias and by injection in paroxysmal tachycardia (p. 185). It is also used in the control of angina and hypertension. In angina it is given in doses of 80–120 mg three times a day, and in hypertension up to 480 mg daily. Care is necessary in patients with poor cardiac reserves, as it may precipitate heart failure. For the same reason, combined treatment with a beta-blocker is contraindicated.

Securon SR and Univer are sustained action products.

Side-effects are nausea, headache and constipation. Verapamil is contraindicated in bradycardia, heart block and acute myocardial infarction.

ADRENERGIC NEURONE-BLOCKING AGENTS

These agents inhibit the release of noradrenaline and reduce stores of noradrenaline at nerve endings.

Drugs of this type, represented by guanethidine, bring about a reduction in peripheral resistance and heart rate, and lower an elevated blood pressure. Careful adjustment of dose or combined treatment with other drugs may be necessary to obtain a smooth and consistent response, as too rapid an action may cause postural hypotension. They are now used mainly in resistant hypertension not fully controlled by other drugs.

Guanethidine § (dose: 20–100 mg daily)

Brand name: Ismelin §

Guanethidine is used in the treatment of moderate to severe hypertension that has not responded to other treatment, usually in association with a beta-blocker and a thiazide diuretic. It is given initially in doses of 10 mg twice a day, increased at intervals of 3 days to maintenance doses of 25–50 mg daily.

Care is necessary in coronary or renal insufficiency, in peptic ulcer, and in recent cerebral or myocardial infarction, as the lowering of blood pressure may increase the risks of further clotting. Guanethidine is sometimes given in the control of hypertensive crisis, including toxaemia in pregnancy, in doses of 10–20 mg by intramuscular injection, repeated after 3 hours according to need.

Side-effects of guanethidine include diarrhoea, nasal congestion and postural hypotension, particularly in the elderly, and may require an adjustment of dose. The use of guanethidine in the treatment of glaucoma is referred to on page 523.

Bethanidine § (dose: 10–200 mg daily)

Brand name: Bendogen §

Bethanidine has a chemical relationship with guanethidine and has similar adrenergic neurone blocking properties, but of shorter duration. The initial dose in hypertension is 10 mg three times a day, increased by 5 mg every 2 days up to a maximum daily dose of 200 mg, often with a diuretic and a beta-blocker.

Side-effects such as diarrhoea are less common, and bethanidine is a useful alternative when guanethidine is not tolerated.

Debrisoquine § (dose: 20–120 mg daily)

Brand name: Declinax §

Debrisoquine resembles guanethidine in its type and pattern of activity, and is given in doses of 10 mg twice a day initially, increased at intervals of 3 days up to a maximum dose of 120 mg daily, in association with a beta-blocker and a thiazide diuretic.

Side-effects are similar to those of guanethidine, but diarrhoea is less common.

CENTRALLY-ACTING ANTIHYPERTENSIVE DRUGS

Some drugs used less frequently in the treatment of hypertension have both a central as well as a peripheral action. They reduce the central flow of impulses to the sympathetic nerves, as well as reducing the release of noradrenaline at adrenergic nerve endings, and so have an antihypertensive action mediated by more than one mechanism. Clonidine is an example of a drug with such a double action.

Points about centrally-acting antihypertensives

(a) Now used less frequently.
(b) Clonidine may cause hypertensive crisis if treatment is stopped suddenly.
(c) Methyldopa may be given during pregnancy, and in asthma and heart failure.

Clonidine § (dose: 150 micrograms–1.2 mg daily)

Brand name: Catapres §

Clonidine is occasionally useful in patients resistant to or unable to tolerate guanethidine or related drugs. It is given in initial doses of 50–100 micrograms three times a day, slowly increasing according to response, although doses of more than 1 mg daily are seldom necessary. Clonidine is also useful in the control of hypertensive crisis, and is given by slow intravenous injection in doses of 150–300 micrograms, repeated if required up to a maximum of 750 micrograms over 24 hours.

Clonidine reduces both the supine and standing blood pressure, and postural hypotension is not uncommon.

In all cases, treatment with clonidine should be withdrawn slowly, as sudden withdrawal may cause a rebound hypertension or precipitate a hypertensive crisis.

Side-effects are sedation, bradycardia, fluid retention and dry mouth. The use of clonidine in the prophylactic treatment of migraine is referred to on page 106.

Methyldopa § (dose: 0.7–3 g daily)

Brand names: Aldomet §, Dopamet §

Methyldopa has a complex action. It has some central effects, and also interferes with an enzyme system concerned with the production of noradrenaline. Instead of noradrenaline, the related methyl-noradrenaline is produced which acts as a 'false transmitter' of nerve impulses, so the result of treatment is an indirect reduction of peripheral resistance and a lowering of blood pressure.

Possibly as a result of this indirect action, postural hypotension or that induced by exercise, is less with methyldopa than with some more directly acting drugs. It also has the advantage of being less likely to cause bronchospasm, and is more suitable for asthmatic patients.

Methyldopa is given orally in all types of hypertension in doses of 250 mg three times a day, together with a thiazide diuretic, increased if necessary up to 3 g daily. In elderly patients, the maximum daily dose should not exceed 2 g. It is sometimes given intravenously in hypertensive crisis in doses of 250–500 mg repeated as required.

Side-effects include drowsiness, diarrhoea, fluid retention, a systemic lupus erythematosus-like syndrome and haemolytic anaemia. Blood and liver function tests are advisable during treatment. Methyldopa may interfere with certain laboratory urine tests, and give a false-positive diagnosis of phaeochromocytoma.

ANTIHYPERTENSIVE AGENTS WITH A MAINLY VASODILATORY ACTION

A few powerful drugs are available that reduce arteriolar resistance (as distinct from peripheral vasodilators (p. 217). They are used mainly in hypertensive crisis, but are sometimes of value in severe hypertension when given with a beta-blocker and a diuretic.

Diazoxide § (dose: 150 mg–1.2 g over 24 hours)

Brand name: Eudemine §

Diazoxide has a powerful antihypertensive action mediated by a selective vasodilator effect on the arterioles and a reduction in peripheral resistance. It is used mainly in hypertensive crisis, or when a very rapid control of severe hypertension is required.

It is given by rapid intravenous injection in doses of 1–3 mg/kg up to 150 mg. A maximum response occurs within about 5 minutes, and lasts about 4 hours. Further doses may be given as required up to a maximum of 1.2 g over 24 hours. The use of diazoxide requires care, as it may cause marked ECG changes, bradycardia and cerebral ischaemia. The solution is strongly alkaline, so injection requires care.

Diazoxide may cause a sudden hyperglycaemia, which can be controlled by insulin, or if less severe, by a sulphonylurea such as tolbutamide. Because of the powerful action and side-effects of diazoxide, close control is necessary throughout treatment.

The use of diazoxide in the treatment of hypoglycaemia is discussed on page 414.

Hydralazine § (dose: 50–100 mg daily)

Brand name: Apresoline §

Hydralazine has a direct relaxant action on the arterioles, and is used mainly in the supplementary treatment of the long-term control of moderate to severe hypertension. It is given in doses of 25 mg twice a day, increased according to need up to 100 mg daily, but care is necessary, as a too-rapid reduction in blood pressure may occur even with small doses. It is occasionally given by slow intravenous injection or infusion in doses of 5–10 mg in the control of hypertensive crisis.

Side-effects include nausea, tachycardia, fluid retention and postural hypotension. A syndrome similar to lupus erythematosus has occurred after high-dose therapy.

Minoxidil § (dose: 5–50 mg daily)

Brand name: Loniten §

Minoxidil is a powerful peripheral vasodilator for the treatment of severe hypertension resistant to other drugs. It is given in doses of 5 mg daily initially, slowly increased at intervals of 3 or more days up to a maximum of 50 mg daily. It must never be used alone, as it causes fluid retention and tachycardia, and combined administration with a diuretic of the frusemide type and a beta-blocker is essential.

Side-effects include nausea, weight gain and hirsutism. As with related drugs, it is contraindicated in phaeochromocytoma. (It is of interest that minoxidil is used locally for the treatment of alopecia areata, p. 541.)

Sodium nitroprusside § (dose: 0.3–1 micrograms/kg per minute by intravenous infusion)

Brand name: Nipride §

Sodium nitroprusside is a very powerful, short-acting antihypertensive agent, and produces a vasodilatation by a direct action on the arterioles and blood vessels. It is used in hypertensive crisis, to obtain controlled hypotension during surgery, and in heart failure.

Sodium nitroprusside is given in hypertensive crisis by intravenous infusion in initial doses of 0.3–1 micrograms/kg per minute, increasing up to a maximum of 8 micrograms/kg, with lower doses of 0.5–1.5 micrograms/kg for controlled hypotension in surgery. In heart failure doses of 10–15 micrograms/minute are given initially, increased every 5–10 minutes as required up to a maximum of 280 micrograms/minute. Constant monitoring of the blood pressure is essential, and sodium nitroprusside should be used only when such monitoring can be carried out.

As one of the products of its metabolism is cyanide, the plasma concentration of cyanide should be measured if treatment is prolonged.

Trimetaphan § (dose: 3–4 mg/minute by intravenous infusion)

Brand name: Arfonad §

Trimetaphan is a short-acting ganglion blocking agent, and is the surviving representative of a now obsolete group of antihypertensive drugs. It is used solely to obtain controlled hypotension during surgery, and is given by intravenous infusion in doses of 3–4 mg/minute initially, with subsequent doses according to need. Tachycardia and respiratory depression may occur, particularly when muscle relaxants are also used.

Trimetaphan brings about some histamine release, so care is necessary in asthmatics or allergic subjects. It is contraindicated in severe cardiac disease or atherosclerosis.

NITRATES USED AS VASODILATORS

The nitrates have a general vasodilator action, exerted mainly on the venous system, although in high doses they also dilate coronary and other arteries. Venodilatation leads to a pooling of blood in the peripheral veins, so the venous return to the heart is reduced, with a consequent reduction in the cardiac workload and oxygen demand. The nitrates also improve circulation in ischaemic areas, and are widely used in the prophylaxis and treatment of angina. Tolerance and a reduction of the therapeutic response may occur with the continued use of nitrates. The risk may be limited by dose adjustment, so that low blood nitrate levels occur for several hours each day, or by reducing the period for which skin patches are applied.

Glyceryl trinitrate § (dose: 300 micrograms–1 mg)

Glyceryl trinitrate (GTN) is a time-honoured drug for the treatment of angina pectoris, as it was introduced over 100 years ago. Its use is increasing, as newer methods of presentation are now available, such as a drug-impregnated skin patch which functions as a transdermal drug delivery system (p. 28).

GTN is used mainly in acute angina of effort, but as it is almost completely metabolized in the liver when given orally, it is usually taken as sublingual tablets containing 300 or 500 micrograms, which are best taken sitting down to offset any initial hypotension. The relief of angina is prompt, as the vasodilator action begins in about 2 minutes, and lasts up to 20–30 minutes. When GTN is used prophylactically it should be taken *before* any exertion that is likely to cause an anginal attack. Most patients need education on the sublingual use of GTN, either as tablets or spray, to get the optimal prophylactic action.

Headache is a common side-effect but tolerance may develop with continued use.

In refractory angina associated with severe ischaemia, glyceryl trinitrate is sometimes given by intravenous infusion in doses of 10 micrograms/minute, increased at intervals of 30 minutes up to a dose of 200 micrograms/minute. Nitrocine §, Nitronal § and Tridil § are brand products for such intravenous use after suitable dilution.

Glyceryl trinitrate tablets must be kept in airtight glass containers, and unused tablets should be discarded about 8 weeks after supply to the patient. Many cases of poor response to oral glyceryl trinitrate are due to the use of deteriorated tablets.

Sustac and **Nitrocontin Continus** are long-acting tablets for prophylactic use available in strengths of 2.6, 6.4 and 10 mg, and should be swallowed whole. Suscard is a buccal tablet presentation of GTN.

Coro-Nitro, Glytrin and **Nitrolingual** are rapidly acting oral spray products useful as alternatives to sublingual tablets. **Percutol** is an ointment containing glyceryl trinitrate. Deponit, Minitran, Nitro-Dur and Transiderm-Nitro are self-adhesive patches containing glyceryl trinitrate. They are intended for once-daily application to the skin and are designed to permit the slow release of the drug for the extended control of angina. They are also of value for patients who experience attacks at night. The patches should be changed every 24 hours, using a different skin area. These patches can also be used in association with venous cannulation for the short-term maintenance of venous patency.

Isosorbide dinitrate § (dose: 30–120 mg daily)

Brand names: Cedocard §, Isordil §, Sorbitrate §, Isoket §

Isosorbide dinitrate is a longer acting vasodilator used in the prophylaxis and treatment of angina pectoris. It is given sublingually in doses of 5–10 mg when a prompt action is required, and orally for prophylactic treatment in doses of 5–20 mg three or four times a day. Alternatively, it may be given for the prevention and treatment of acute angina as a sublingual spray (Imtack) in doses of 1.25–3.75 mg.

Some sustained-release oral products are available when an extended action is required. Isosorbide dinitrate is also used in the treatment of left ventricular heart failure, and is then given in larger doses up to a maximum of 240 mg daily. In severe conditions, it may be given by intravenous infusion in doses of 2–10 mg hourly.

Side-effects including tolerance are similar to those of glyceryl trinitrate.

Isosorbide mononitrate § (dose: 40–120 mg daily)

Brand names: Elantan §, Ismo §, Monit §, Mono-Cedocard §

Isosorbide mononitrate is used for the prophylaxis and treatment of angina, and is also useful in congestive heart failure. It is given in doses of 10–20 mg three times a day, slowly increased according to individual need up to a maximum of 120 mg daily.

The mononitrate is the metabolic derivative of the dinitrate, to which the action of the dinitrate is mainly due. It is well absorbed orally, and largely escapes first-pass metabolism in the liver.

Side-effects include headache, dizziness, flushing and palpitations, which are usually transient, but may be relieved by a temporary reduction of dose. **Pentaerythritol tetranitrate** § (Mycardol §) is also used in the prophylaxis of angina.

Points about nitrate vasodilators

(a) Glyceryl trinitrate given sublingually; tablets must be kept in glass airtight containers and rejected if more than 2 months old.
(b) Patches to be applied to a hairless skin area where little movement occurs, and replaced daily at a slightly different site.
(c) Isorbide mono/dinitrate more stable, and can be used for prophylaxis.
(d) Tolerance may occur; risk may be reduced by giving low doses, or by the temporary removal of a skin patch.

PERIPHERAL VASODILATORS

Although peripheral vasodilators are relatively ineffective in the treatment of hypertension, they are considered here as they have some applications in the treatment of peripheral vascular disorders associated with vascular spasm or occlusion, particularly Raynaud's disease. Their value is limited as the vasodilator effect may be more marked in the healthy peripheral vessels, and the blood flow through damaged vessels may be improved to a lesser extent.

Cinnarizine (dose: 225 mg daily)

Brand name: Stugeron Forte

Cinnarizine is an antihistamine with some peripheral vasodilatory activity, and is given in doses of 75 mg two or three times a day in the treatment of peripheral vascular disorders and Raynaud's disease.

It has the **side-effects** of the antihistamines, and care is necessary if hypotension is present. The use of cinnarizine as an antiemetic is referred to on page 333.

Nicofuranose (dose: 1.5–3 g daily)

Brand name: Bradilan

Nicotinic acid, part of the vitamin B complex (p. 483) has some transient vasodilatory side-effects such as flushing and hypotension. Nicofuranose is a derivative of nicotinic acid with a less intense and more prolonged vasodilator action, and it is given in the treatment of peripheral vascular disorders in doses of 750 mg three times a day, although doses up to 1 g three times a day have been used. As the action is slow, the risk of hypotension as a side-effect is correspondingly reduced.

Nicotinyl tartrate (dose: 100–200 mg daily)

Brand name: Ronicol

Nicotinyl tartrate is partly metabolized to nicotinic acid, and has a similar vasodilator action. It is used in peripheral vascular disorders, and given in doses of 25–50 mg four times a day. It may cause some flushing and dizziness, but symptoms of hypotension are usually mild.

Inositol nicotinate (dose: 3–4 g daily)

Brand name: Hexopal

Inositol nicotinate has vasodilator properties as it is partly metabolized to nicotinic acid. It is sometimes used in cerebral vascular disease as well as disorders of the peripheral circulation in doses of 0.5–1 g three or four times a day.

Oxpentifylline § (dose: 800 mg–1.2 g daily)

Brand name: Trental §

Oxpentifylline is chemically related to theophylline, but it is used only as a vasodilator in peripheral vascular diseases. It is given in doses of 400 mg two or three times a day, and following response, doses of 200 mg three times a day may be given for maintenance.

Side-effects include nausea, dizziness and flushing, and care is necessary in hypotensive patients. Oxpentifylline may potentiate the action of some antihypertensive agents, and an adjustment of dose of such drugs may be required.

Co-dergocrine § (Hydergine §) is a cerebral vasodilator used only for senile dementia in doses of 4.5 mg daily.

BLOOD-LIPID LOWERING AGENTS

Hyperlipidaemia is a broad term referring to a general rise in the level of blood lipids which is also a broad term that includes cholesterol, triglycerides and phospholipids. Cholesterol, derived from dietary fats, is the substance from which steroids are formed by biosynthesis; triglycerides are present in many animal and vegetable fats and are derivatives of glycerin and fatty acids that function as an energy source; phospholipids are components of cells of the nervous system. Blood lipids are present in the plasma as protein complex particles (lipoproteins) and have a core of cholesterol and triglycerides, and an outer shell of phospholipids and protein. They differ according to the varying amounts of their constituents, and are classified as chylomicrons, very-low-density lipoproteins (VLDL), low-density lipoproteins (LDL) and high-density lipoproteins (HDL).

The HDL contain a high proportion of protein with small amounts of triglycerides; the LDL contain more cholesterol; the VDL contain more triglyceride than cholesterol, whereas the chylomicrons consist almost entirely of triglycerides. The chylomicrons transport dietary fat to the liver where the VLDL are formed, and when these VLDL enter the circulation much of their triglyceride content is removed by the action of the enzyme lipoprotein lipase, and they become low density lipoproteins. These LDL are involved in the transport of cholesterol to the peripheral tissues. The HDL are formed in the liver and small intestines, and function as cholesterol scavengers, as they pick up any free cholesterol in the circulation and return it to the liver for excretion or conversion to bile acids. Attempts have been made to classify the hyperlipidaemias according to variations in the levels of the different lipoprotein levels, and the Fredrickson/WHO classification is outlined in Table 6.2.

The most common form of hyperlipidaemia is a rise in the blood level of cholesterol (hypercholesterolaemia) and although diet and smoking play an important role in its development, genetic factors may also have an influence. It leads to the formation of lipid deposits (atheromas) in the arterial linings, particularly the coronary arteries, resulting in atherosclerosis and ischaemic heart disease. As the blood supply to the heart is

Table 6.2 Fredrickson/WHO classification of hyperlipidaemias

Type	Frequency	Notes
I	Rare	High triglyceride levels; symptoms may occur in childhood with symptoms of acute pancreatitis
IIa	Common	High cholesterol levels, high risk of CHD
IIb	Common	High cholesterol and triglyceride levels, high risk of CHD
III	Uncommon	High cholesterol and triglyceride levels, with risk of diabetes, high risk of CHD and peripheral vascular disease
IV	Common	High risk of peripheral vascular disease
V	Uncommon	High triglyceride and chylomicron levels with risk of diabetes

restricted, and becomes insufficient to meet the oxygen demands of the body, the ischaemia may be manifested by angina and myocardial infarction. Ischaemic heart disease is the main cause of death in industrial countries. A lowering of the cholesterol levels in hypercholesterolaemia, particularly when the level rises above 6.5 mmol/l, reduces the risks of ischaemia heart disease, and may also reduce the rate of the progressive atherosclerosis. A rise in the HDL may also have a protective effect by reducing tissue stores of cholesterol.

The main treatment of hyperlipidaemia is a strict low-fat diet, weight reduction and cessation of smoking. Drug treatment should be regarded as adjunctive, and is mainly indicated for patients unable to tolerate, or who do not respond to such dietary restrictions. The range of drugs used includes ion-exchange resins, lipase-stimulating drugs derived from fibrinic acid, enzyme inhibitors and nicotinic acid derivatives.

Points about blood-lipid lowering agents

(a) Exchange resins bind intestinal bile acids and so act indirectly on lipid formation.
(b) The fibrate group of drugs reduce blood levels of lipids partly by enzyme activity.
(c) The statins inhibit the synthesis of cholesterol in the liver.
(d) They can all cause a myositis-like syndrome.
(e) The nicotinic acid derivatives are also peripherol vasodilators and may cause undesirable flushing.

 O'Connor P et al 1990 Lipid lowering drugs. British Medical Journal 300: 667–672

BILE ACID BINDING AGENTS

Cholestyramine § (dose: 12–24 g daily)

Brand name: Questran §

Bile acid binding agents are anion exchange resins. They act by binding to and preventing the re-absorption of bile acids, and so

Table 6.3 Table of blood-lipid lowering agents

Type of drug	Approved name	Brand name	Daily dose	Main lowering effect on
Bile acid binding resins	cholestyramine colestipol	Questran Colestid	12–24 g 10–30 g	Cholesterol
Fibric acid derivatives	bezafibrate ciprofibrate clofibrate fenofibrate gemfibrozil	Bezalip Modalim Atromid-S Lipantil Lopid	400–600 mg 100–200 mg 2 g 300–400 mg 1–5 g	Cholesterol and triglycerides
HMG CoA reductase inhibitors	fluvastatin lovastatin pravastatin simvastatin	Lescol Lipostat Zocor	20–40 mg 10–40 mg 10–40 mg	Cholesterol
Nicotinic acid derivatives	acipimox nicofuranose	Olbetam Bradilan	500–1200 mg 1.5–3 g	Cholesterol and triglycerides
Unclassified	omega-triglycerides probucol	Maxepa Lurselle	10 g 1 g	Triglycerides

interrupt the normal enterohepatic recirculation of those acids. The insoluble bile acid–resin complex is excreted in the faeces. The bile acids that the body requires are then derived from stores of cholesterol in the liver, and those stores are replaced in turn from cholesterol-containing low-density lipoproteins (LDL). With the extended use of anion exchange resins, the plasma levels of cholesterol and LDL are slowly reduced. They are used mainly in the treatment of the more common hyperlipidaemias (IIA and IIb), particularly in patients who have not responded to other therapy, but prolonged treatment is necessary.

Cholestyramine is given orally as a powder, often sprinkled on food, in doses of 8 g initially, slowly increased to over 3–4 weeks up to 24 g or more, in single or divided doses. Some patients may find treatment more acceptable if the drug is taken as a drink with fruit juice or soup. Nausea, flatulence and abdominal disturbances are the main side-effects. It is of no value in biliary obstruction, as in that state no bile acids reach the intestinal tract.

Cholestyramine may reduce the absorption of certain other drugs such as digoxin and warfarin and thiazide diuretics, and any combined therapy should be given at least 1 hour before cholestyramine, or 4 hours afterward to prevent any interference with absorption. With prolonged treatment, the absorption of fat-soluble vitamins may be reduced, and supplementary treatment may be required.

Cholestyramine is also used in doses of 4–8 g daily in the treatment of pruritus associated with partial biliary obstruction, and in standard doses in the treatment of diarrhoea caused by Crohn's disease, ileac resection and radiotherapy.

Colestipol (Colestid) is another anion exchange resin used in hyperlipidaemia, and is given in doses of 10 g initially, slowly increased up to 30 g daily.

THE FIBRATE GROUP OF LIPID-LOWERING AGENTS

The fibrates, of which clofibrate was the first to be introduced, reduce the plasma levels of both cholesterol and triglycerides. The mode of action is not yet clear, but they appear to increase the activity of lipoprotein lipase, augment the removal of triglycerides from chylomicrons, and promote the uptake of cholesterol by high density lipoproteins. They are used in the treatment of most forms of hyperlipidaemia in patients who have not responded to other therapy, but reduced doses should be given in renal insufficiency, and they are contraindicated in severe renal and hepatic impairment and gall bladder disease, and in pregnancy.

Gemfibrozil differs chemically from other fibrates, and is used mainly when response to other drugs is inadequate. The side-effects of the fibrates include abdominal discomfort, flatulence and nausea. An uncommon reaction that may occur with any member of the group is a myositis-like syndrome.

Bezafibrate § (dose: 600 mg daily)

Brand names: Bezalip §; Bezalip-Mono §

Bezafibrate is a typical member of the fibrate group, and is used in the treatment of most types of hyperlipidaemia with the exception of Type I. It is given in doses of 200 mg three times a day, preferably after food, although doses of 200 mg twice daily may be adequate in hypertriglyceridaemia. Bezalip-Mono is a delayed release product containing 400 mg of bezafibrate, for administration at night. The **side-effects** are those of the fibrates generally. Bezafibrate is contraindicated in severe renal and hepatic disease, biliary cirrhosis and gall bladder dysfunction.

Clofibrate § (dose: 1–1.5 g daily)

Brand name: Atromid-S §

Clofibrate is used in the treatment of most types of hyperlipidaemia with the exception of Type I. It is given in doses of 500 mg three times a day after food. It has the disadvantage of increasing the biliary excretion of cholesterol, and may promote gall stone formation, and is now used mainly in patients who have undergone cholecystectomy. **Side-effects** are abdominal discomfort, nausea and flatulence.

Gemfibrozil § (dose: 0.9–1.5 g daily)

Brand name: Lopid §

Gemfibrozil is usually given in doses of 600 mg twice a day and is effective in most types of hyperlipidaemia (except Type I) that have not responded to other treatment. It is also used for the prevention of coronary heart disease in men in the 40–55 year age group with hyperlipidaemia unresponsive to diet or drug therapy. It differs structurally from other fibrates, and blood counts and liver function tests are necessary before long-term treatment with gemfibrozil is considered. Annual eye examinations are also recommended. The **side-effects** are those of the fibrates, including dizziness, blurred vision and painful extremities. Other fibrates are listed in Table 6.3.

THE STATINS (ENZYME INHIBITORS)

This group of drugs offers a different approach to the treatment of hyperlipidaemia, as they have a direct action on the biosynthesis of cholesterol in the liver. The rate-limiting enzyme in the cascade of reactions involved in cholesterol synthesis is hydroxymethylglutaryl co-enzyme, a reductase (HMG-CoA-reductase). An inhibitor of that enzyme would interrupt the hepatic synthesis of cholesterol at an early stage. Such an interruption w+ould in turn lead to a compensatory increase in the number of active LDL receptors in the liver, and so further increase the take-up and removal of cholesterol from the circulation. Currently available inhibitors of HMG-CoA-reductase are fluvastatin (Lescol), pravastatin (Lipostat) and simvastatin (Zocor). See Table 6.3. They are given in doses of 10–40 mg daily in the treatment of primary hypercholesterolaemia (Type IIa). They tend to have more effect than the exchange resins in lowering LDL levels, but are less active than the fibrates in lowering triglyceride levels. **Side-effects** include gastrointestinal disturbances, headache and rash. Myositis is an uncommon side-effect, but it and other reactions may occur more frequently during combined therapy with fibrates and nicotinic acid, and liver function tests should be performed before such combined therapy is considered. Multiple treatment with an exchange resin, on the other hand, may have an additive effect, but when so given the resin should be given some hours before the statin to avoid loss of the drug by resin-binding.

NICOTINIC ACID AND DERIVATIVES

Nicotinic acid and related compounds reduce the plasma concentrations of cholesterol and triglycerides. They act by reducing the release into the circulation of some non-esterified fatty acids present in adipose tissue, thus reducing the amount of such acids available for take-up in the liver for cholesterol synthesis and LDL formation.

Nicotinic acid (dose: 3–6 g daily)

Nicotinic acid is given in large doses of 1–2 g three times a day. Such doses may cause intense flushing, and treatment is best commenced with small initial doses of 100–200 mg three times a day for 2–4 weeks before increasing the dose slowly to a therapeutic level. The flushing, which appears to be mediated by prostaglandins, may also be relieved in some cases by the administration of aspirin in doses of 300 mg about half an hour before the dose of nicotinic acid.

Other **side-effects** include dizziness, nausea, abdominal discomfort, pruritus and urticaria. **Nicofuranose** (Bradilan, dose 0.5–1 g three times a day) is a related compound that is converted to nicotinic acid in the body, and has a similar action in hyperlipidaemia. It may be better tolerated than nicotinic acid.

Acipimox § (dose: 500–1200 mg daily)

Brand name: Olbetam §

Acipimox is chemically related to nicotinic acid and has a similar but longer hypolipidaemic action. It is used mainly in lipid disorders associated with raised triglyceride levels and is given in doses of 250 mg two or three times a day with food. Doses should be reduced in renal impairment.

Side-effects include flushing, which tends to disappear as treatment is continued, rash and gastrointestinal disturbances.

Probucol § (dose: 1 g daily)

Brand name: Lurselle §

Probucol is an unrelated drug that is thought to act by increasing the clearance of LDL from the circulation, probably by promoting the incorporation of LDL into lipoproteins. It also has some antioxidant properties, and may retard the appearance of fatty streaks in the arterial walls that are associated with the development of atherosclerosis. It is used mainly to supplement dietary measures in the common hyperlipidaemias. It is given in doses of 500 mg twice daily with food, as food appears to increase the absorption of the drug, but extended therapy is necessary to obtain the maximum response. Care is necessary in ventricular arrhythmias, or following recent myocardial damage, and in such cases an ECG should be carried out before probucol is given.

Fish oil concentrate

Brand name: Maxepa

The low incidence of coronary heart disease in Greenland Eskimos has been linked with their dietary intake of polyunsaturated fish oils. These oils contain eicosapentaenoic acid (EPA) and decosahexonoic acid (DHA), sometimes referred to as the omega-3-fatty acids, and differ from the 6-fatty acids in Western diets.

A fish oil concentrate containing EPA 18% and DHA 10% (and merely negligible amounts of vitamins A and D) is used in some hyperlipidaemias as it brings about a sustained fall in plasma triglyceride levels. It is given in doses of 5 ml twice daily with food in severe triglyceridaemia, and in patients at risk of ischaemic heart disease. It also inhibits platelet aggregation, and care is necessary in patients already receiving anticoagulants.

7

Drugs acting on the autonomic nervous system

The autonomic or involuntary nervous system controls the internal functions of the body, and is concerned with the activities of the gastrointestinal tract, the heart and vascular system, the eyes, the suprarenal and other secretory glands. It maintains the physiological equilibrium of the body, yet at the same time it is not completely independent of the central nervous system, as factors which affect the higher centres may also influence some physiological functions of the body. The effect of fear and anger on the pulse-rate is an example of this interdependence.

PARASYMPATHETIC AND SYMPATHETIC SYSTEMS

Anatomically, the autonomic nervous system consists of two parts, the sympathetic and parasympathetic nervous systems. Each organ controlled by the autonomic nervous system can be stimulated or inhibited according to physiological needs. The functions of the sympathetic and parasympathetic nervous systems can be regarded as having basically opposite effects, and this difference is reflected in the anatomical details of their structure.

The sympathetic part consists of a series of short nerve fibres, running out from the thoracic and lumbar parts of the spinal cord, and a chain of attached nerve ganglia. From these ganglia other and longer nerve fibres (the post-ganglionic fibres) pass out to the smooth muscle of the visceral organs.

The parasympathetic nervous fibres originate in the midbrain, medulla and sacral portions of the spinal cord, and these preganglionic fibres also pass out to ganglia, from which post-ganglionic fibres link with the organs concerned. In general, the parasympathetic ganglia are near to the organs supplied, so the post-ganglionic fibres are short; whereas the sympathetic fibres are correspondingly long.

Transmitters and receptors

The study of the mechanism by which the nerves of this autonomic nervous system finally affect the organs of the body with which they are connected has led to considerable advances in therapeutics.

Briefly, when an impulse passes out from the spinal cord and reaches a ganglion, a messenger substance, acetylcholine, is liberated, which carries the impulse across to the post-ganglionic nerve. As soon as the impulse has passed, the released acetylcholine is immediately broken down by an enzyme, cholinesterase, and is inactivated.

The impulse continues along the post-ganglionic fibres, and in the case of parasympathetic nerves, acetylcholine is released again when the impulse reaches the point where the nerve joins the organ concerned, i.e., the myoneural junction.

The acetylcholine acts on a receptor of the organ to produce the necessary response. This response is limited in duration and intensity by the rapid destruction of the acetylcholine by the tissue enzymes, as it is when released in the ganglia.

Noradrenaline

A similar process takes place in the sympathetic nervous system up to the junction of nerve and tissue. At this point, instead of acetylcholine, another neurotransmitter substance, noradrena-

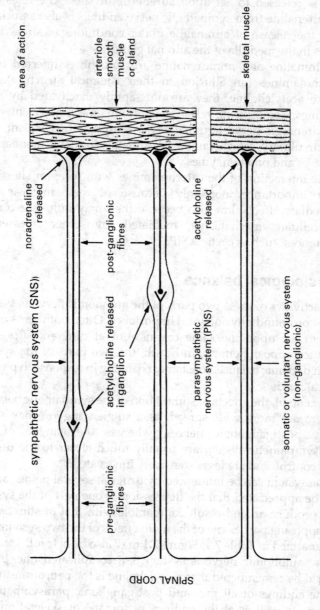

Figure 7.1 Neurotransmitter systems.

line, is released to act upon adrenoceptor sites. The release of noradrenaline from sympathetic nerve endings is also associated with the release of adrenaline under conditions of stress from stores in the medulla of the adrenal gland.

Adrenaline and noradrenaline are sometimes referred to as catecholamines (an allusion to their chemical structure), but unlike acetylcholine, they are not rapidly inactivated by local enzymes. Some of the released noradrenaline may re-enter the noradrenergic nerve terminals by a re-uptake mechanism, and the circulatory catecholamines are metabolized by monoamine oxidases and other enzymes.

The interaction of the catecholamines with receptor sites is of great importance, not only because of their intrinsic and immediate effects, but also because they may influence certain intracellular mechanisms mediated by other messenger substances, such as cyclic AMP.

Physiological balance

The activities of these two parts of the autonomic nervous system are of profound physiological importance. Often both parts of the system act upon the same organs, but at different sites, and produce opposite effects. In health, the two parts of the system are in dynamic balance, constantly changing in response to physiological needs.

In general, the effects of stimulation of the sympathetic nervous system are more wide-spread, as a single ganglion may serve many post-ganglionic nerves, whereas the ganglia of the parasympathetic system are usually much closer to the organs they control, and are less extensively innervated.

The system can be influenced by drugs at several points, and it will be appreciated that the depression of one part of the system will produce an end-result comparable with that of stimulating the opposing part. Some of the main effects of the two systems are summarized in Table 7.1. Figure 7.1 may also be helpful.

The autonomic nervous system is a complicated one, but it should be remembered that acetylcholine is the neurotransmitter at the endings of all pre- and post-ganglionic parasympathetic nerves, as well as at the endings of somatic or skeletal muscle nerves, *and* at the endings of those post-ganglionic sympathetic nerves serving sweat glands and the blood vessels of

Table 7.1 Main effects

Organ	Sympathetic stimulation	Parasympathetic stimulation
Heart	Rate increased	Rate slowed
Blood vessels	Constricted	Dilated
Lungs (bronchial muscles)	Relaxed	Contracted
Gastrointestinal tract	Activity decreased	Increased
Urinary system:		
Bladder	Relaxed	Contracted
Sphincter	Contracted	Relaxed
Eye	Pupil dilated	Constricted

skeletal muscles. Noradrenaline is the neurotransmitter at the endings of all post-ganglionic sympathetic nerves *except* those serving sweat glands and skeletal muscle blood vessels.

Because parasympathetic nerves liberate acetylcholine at nerve endings, they are sometimes referred to as cholinergic nerves. As the sympathetic nerves liberate noradrenaline, they have been termed adrenergic nerves.

SYMPATHOMIMETIC DRUGS (Fig. 7.2)

Sympathomimetic drugs are those that act on the adrenoceptors, and elicit a response similar in some respects to those produced by the natural messenger substance noradrenaline. They may act directly on the adrenoceptors, or indirectly by releasing stored noradrenaline from nerve endings. Dopamine, a precursor of noradrenaline is primarily a neurotransmitter in the central nervous system (p. 254). The adrenoceptors are of two main types, the alpha-adrenoceptors and the beta-adrenoceptors, and an organ may possess both types of receptor. Some sympathomimetic agents may therefore have more than one type of action.

The alpha-receptors are concerned mainly with peripheral and visceral vessels, and stimulation leads to vasoconstriction of the skin and viscera, thus increasing the amount of blood available to other organs.

The beta-receptors have been divided into two groups: the β_1 and β_2 receptors. The β_1-receptors occur mainly in heart muscle, and when stimulated bring about an increase in cardiac force and rate. The β_2-receptors have a wider distribution, as they are found in vascular, bronchial and uterine smooth muscle. Stimulation of

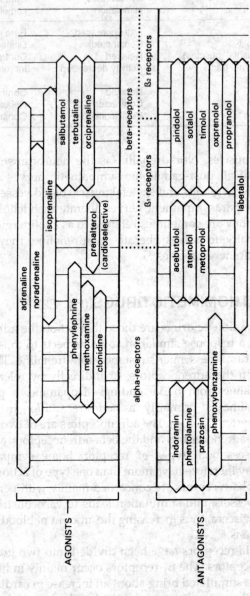

Figure 7.2 Some sympathomimetic agonists and antagonists, and an indication of their range of andrenoceptor affinity.
Note: Agonists imitate the natural responses to nerve stimulation; antagonists block such responses.

those receptors results in relaxation, with vasodilatation and bronchodilatation.

Sympathomimetic drugs that have an affinity for and act upon adrenoceptors are referred to as agonists, but drugs that have an affinity for but no action upon receptor sites are known as antagonists, or adrenoceptor blocking agents. Beta-adrenoceptor blocking agents play an important part in the control of hypertension and angina, and are discussed in Chapter 6.

Points about sympathomimetics

(a) Different agents may act more or less selectively on different receptors.
(b) Type of response varies accordingly.
(c) Injection of inotropic sympathomimetics (dobutamine, dopamine, dopexamine) requires care, as the response may vary markedly with an increase in dose.
(d) Vasoconstrictor sympathomimetics now used less frequently in shock.

SYMPATHOMIMETIC DRUGS WITH A MAINLY PRESSOR ACTION

Adrenaline § (dose: 200–500 micrograms by subcutaneous or intramuscular injection).

Adrenaline (epinephrine) is the natural hormone, formerly obtained from the suprarenal gland, but now made synthetically. It acts on both adrenoceptors, but is now used less frequently as more selective drugs are available. It has a powerful bronchodilator action, but in severe status asthmaticus, salbutamol is now preferred as it has fewer cardiac side-effects. In anaphylactic shock, which is characterized by cardiovascular collapse, and a sudden fall in blood pressure, with bronchospasm and pulmonary oedema, adrenaline remains the keystone of treatment.

Anaphylactic shock, although uncommon, may occur in a patient who has become sensitized in some way, possibly to a drug, a food or an insect sting or even to an allergen desensitizing injection. It is an emergency requiring prompt treatment to restore the blood pressure, and adrenaline should be given by intramuscular or subcutaneous injection as soon as possible as a 0.5 ml dose of adrenaline solution (1–1000), repeated every 10 minutes as required. (The value of subcutaneous injections have been questioned, but in the early stages of anaphylaxis vasodilation is marked, and subcutaneous absorption of adrenaline may be rapid, as shown by the response to self-treatment in emergency by pre-filled automatic injection devices. If treatment is delayed and shock occurs, the intravenous injection of adrenaline may be required.)

An antihistamine such as chlorpheniramine should also be given by slow intravenous injection to maintain the response, and continued for 24 hours or more to prevent a relapse. Hydrocortisone may also be given intravenously in a dose of 100 mg, as further supportive therapy, although the action is slow, and may not be apparent for some hours.

For individuals known to be at risk from insect stings, syringes pre-filled with adrenaline solution for injection, and an adrenaline aerosol inhalation product (Medihaler-epi) are now available for emergency use. Adrenaline is occasionally used in the treatment of cardiac arrest by the direct intracardiac injection of 10 ml of a 1–10 000 solution.

Adrenaline is also used for its vasoconstrictor action by its inclusion as an additive to some local anaesthetic solutions to delay absorption and prolong the action, but care is necessary that such adrenaline-containing solutions are not injected into tissues where they could cause ischaemic necrosis.

For the use of adrenaline in the treatment of glaucoma see page 522.

Noradrenaline § (dose: 8–12 micrograms per minute by intravenous infusion)

Brand name: Levophed §

Noradrenaline differs from adrenaline chiefly by exerting its action mainly on the alpha-receptors. It raises the blood pressure by a more general vasoconstriction, although it also has some minor cardiac stimulant action. It has been used in the treatment of shock in doses of 8 micrograms or more per minute by slow intravenous infusion of a well-diluted solution, but the dose and rate of administration require considerable care, as the response may fluctuate. Great care must be taken to avoid extravasation, as the intense local vasoconstriction so caused may result in necrosis and gangrene.

Noradrenaline is also used occasionally as a special solution of 200 micrograms for intracardiac injection in cases of cardiac arrest. Like adrenaline, noradrenaline is also added to some local anaesthetic solutions (1 in 80 000 or less) to prolong the anaesthetic action.

The use of noradrenaline and other vasoconstrictor drugs in the treatment of shock is declining, as it is now considered that the general vasoconstriction and rise in blood pressure that it causes may reduce the blood supply to essential organs such as the kidney to a dangerous extent. In any case, vasoconstrictors in shock are of little value if much blood loss has occurred, and reliance is now placed on the restoration of blood volume by expanders, and the use of more selectively acting cardiac drugs such as **dopamine** and **dobutamine**, often in association with high doses of **hydrocortisone** or other corticosteroid.

Dobutamine § (dose: 2.5–10 micrograms/kg per minute by intravenous infusion)

Brand name: Dobutrex §

Dobutamine is a sympathomimetic agent that acts mainly on the β_1-receptors, and has a more selective cardiac action than some related drugs.

It is used in the treatment of cardiogenic shock associated with myocardial infarction and cardiac surgery, and in heart failure due to organic heart disease.

Dobutamine is given by the slow intravenous drip infusion of a dilute solution in doses of 2.5–10 micrograms/kg per minute according to need and response, followed by slow withdrawal after the condition has been controlled. Its administration requires constant supervision as higher doses may exacerbate heart failure.

Side-effects include nausea and headache, but the onset of tachycardia is indicative of overdose.

Dopamine § (dose: 2–5 micrograms/kg per minute by intravenous infusion)

Brand name: Intropin §

Dopamine is a natural substance from which noradrenaline is formed, and both compounds have some properties in common.

Like dobutamine, dopamine acts on the β_1-receptors, but it has a more potent inotropic action, i.e. it increases the force more than the rate of the heart beat. It increases the cardiac output and tends to correct any haemodynamic imbalance without causing excessive tachycardia. It also appears to act on some 'dopaminergic receptors' in the kidney, so that with small doses renal vasodilatation occurs, renal blood flow increases, and renal efficiency is maintained.

Dopamine is used in the treatment of cardiogenic shock, and of shock unresponsive to the replacement of fluid loss, but its use requires considerable care. It is given in initial doses of 2–5 micrograms/kg per minute by intravenous infusion in 5% glucose injection, preferably into a large vein to avoid tissue necrosis, but the action of the drug is very brief, and continuous control of administration is essential. The dose may be increased according to response, and in exceptional cases a dose as high as 50 micrograms/kg per minute has been given, although large doses may cause vasoconstriction and tend to exacerbate heart failure. A reduction in urine flow is an indication that the dose of dopamine should be reduced. Once the condition is under control, the drug should be slowly withdrawn over some hours as hypotension and anuria may follow sudden withdrawal. As with related drugs, preliminary restoration of a depleted blood volume is necessary.

Dopexamine §

Brand name: Dopacard §

Dopexamine is a synthetic catecholamine, related to dopamine, but with a much more powerful action on the β_2-adrenoceptors. It is indicated in the short-term treatment of acute exacerbations of heart failure, and for support after cardiac surgery. The mode of action is basically that of producing systemic and pulmonary vasodilatation, which results in a reduction in the ventricular afterload, but at the same time it has some inotropic activity that maintains the blood pressure. It also brings about an increase in the renal blood flow. Dopexamine is given by intravenous infusion under careful control in doses of 500 nanograms/kg/minute initially, increased at intervals of 10–15 minutes by increments of 1 microgram/kg/minute up to a maximum of 6 micrograms/kg/minute, adjusted to need and response, including measurement of cardiac output. The half-life of dopexamine is 6–7 minutes, so any excessive response is likely to be short-lived if treatment is withdrawn.

Side-effects include tachycardia, nausea and anginal pain.

Isoprenaline § (dose: 180–840 mg daily)

Brand name: Saventrine §

Isoprenaline is closely related chemically to adrenaline and noradrenaline, but differs in acting almost exclusively on the beta-adrenoceptors, and in being active orally. It is used in the treatment of bradycardia, heart block, and to control attacks of Stokes–Adams syndrome mainly as short-term treatment in emergencies.

Isoprenaline is given orally in doses of 10–30 mg or more three times a day, but in the emergency treatment of heart block and cardiogenic shock it is given by slow intravenous injection in doses of 5–10 micrograms/min under ECG control.

Side-effects include palpitation, nausea, tremor and tachycardia, and the drug is now less widely used. Its bronchodilator properties are referred to on page 243.

Metaraminol § (dose: 2–10 mg by subcutaneous or intramuscular injection; 15–100 mg by intravenous infusion)

Brand name: Aramine §

Metaraminol has the general vasoconstrictor properties of noradrenaline and is used in the severe hypotension of shock, including myocardial infarction, haemorrhage, trauma and surgery. It is given in doses of 15–100 mg by intravenous infusion, after dilution with 500 ml of normal saline or 5% glucose solution.

Side-effects include cardiac irregularities.

Methoxamine § (dose: 5–20 mg by injection)

Brand name: Vasoxine §

Methoxamine is a sympathomimetic agent that has a selective

action on the alpha-adrenoceptors. It brings about a prolonged constriction of the peripheral blood vessels with a consequent rise in the arterial pressure, but it may also markedly reduce renal blood flow. It has little direct action on the heart, although a reflex bradycardia may occur.

Methoxamine is used for its pressor action to maintain blood pressure during spinal anaesthesia, and during and after anaesthesia with halothane or cyclopropane. It is given by intramuscular injection in doses of 10–15 mg or more, repeated if necessary after about 15 minutes. In emergencies, methoxamine may be given by slow intravenous injection in doses of 3–5 mg; intravenous doses up to 10 mg are given to control paroxysmal tachycardia.

Side-effects include nausea, vomiting, headache and bradycardia. Care is necessary in cardiovascular disease.

Ephedrine (p. 243) is also given by intramuscular injection to prevent hypotension in spinal anaesthesia in doses of 15–30 mg; to reverse such hypotension it is given by slow intravenous injection in doses of 3–6 mg.

Phenylephrine (dose: 2–5 mg by injection)

Phenylephrine is chemically related to adrenaline, but it has a more specific action on the alpha-adrenoceptors, and has a pressor action similar to that of methoxamine. It is used in acute hypotensive states such as circulatory failure, spinal anaesthesia and drug-induced hypotension, and is given in doses of 2–5 mg by subcutaneous or intramuscular injection, or in doses of 100–500 micrograms by slow intravenous injection. Alternatively, phenylephrine may be given in doses of 5–20 mg by intravenous infusion at a rate not greater than 180 micrograms/minute. Phenylephrine has also been used to control paroxysmal supraventricular tachycardia in doses up to 500 micrograms by slow intravenous injection.

Side-effects of phenylephrine include nausea, vomiting, headache; care is necessary in cardiovascular disease, and in patients receiving guanethidine or a related antihypertensive drug.

Phenylephrine is also used in ophthalmology as a mydriatic, and to lower intra-ocular pressure in open angle glaucoma (Ch. 23).

Xamoterol § (dose: 400 mg daily)

Brand name: Corwin §

Xamoterol is a sympathomimetic agent that acts on the $beta_1$-receptors. It is used in the treatment of *mild* chronic heart failure, when breathlessness and fatigue are increased by exercise. It inhibits noradrenaline-induced activity, and so reduces the myocardial stimulation that might otherwise exacerbate the cardiac weakness. Xamoterol is given initially in doses of 200 mg daily, increased after a week to 200 mg twice a day. It is contraindicated in severe heart failure, and in patients receiving ACE therapy, or frusemide in doses above 40 g daily.

Side-effects are headache, dizziness, hypotension, bronchospasm and gastrointestinal disturbance.

SYMPATHOMIMETICS USED AS BRONCHODILATORS

Certain sympathomimetic agents (β_2 agonists) are widely used in the treatment of bronchial asthma and obstructive airway disease generally. In such conditions, the airways are both hypersensitive and inflamed and the bronchoconstriction may be due to a variety of trigger factors including allergens, dust and upper respiratory tract infections as well as drugs such as aspirin and some beta-blocking agents. Plugging of the airways with mucus and oedema of the bronchial mucosa may add to the obstruction.

In the treatment of reversible airway disease and related conditions, reliance is largely placed on synthetic sympathomimetic drugs with a selective stimulant action on the β_2-receptors, represented by salbutamol. Although cardiac stimulation is less likely to occur with these more selectively acting drugs, they usually possess some residual β_1-adrenoceptor activity, and may cause cardiac disturbances such as tachycardia in sensitive patients. Such disturbances are less likely to occur when the drug is given by oral inhalation from a metered-dose, pressurized aerosol, and such inhalation is the preferred method of administration, as the drug is delivered directly to the bronchi, and is effective more rapidly, and with fewer side-effects, *provided* the aerosol is operated correctly.

Patients often require repeated instruction in the use of

metered-dose aerosols, and nurses can play an important part in such inhalation therapy by emphasizing the importance of synchronising breathing with inhalation, as well as warning against excessive use (see Fig. 1.4 p. 24). Failure to respond initially to inhalation therapy is more likely to be due to faulty technique rather than drug failure, whereas a failure to respond after previous control has been achieved should be investigated, as it may indicate that a deterioration of the airway disease has occurred that requires alternative therapy.

The use of corticosteroids in obstructive airway disease is referred to on page 374.

Points about bronchodilators

(a) Two main types — β_2-adrenoceptor stimulants and antimuscarinics (anticholinergics).
(b) Some are given by inhalation, and patients should be given detailed instructions on the use of inhaler devices.
(c) Antimuscarinics have a slow action useful in chronic conditions.
(d) Hypokalaemia is a potential risk with β_2-adrenoceptor stimulants, and may be increased by combined therapy. Plasma potassium levels should be monitored in severe asthma.

Salbutamol § (dose: 6–32 mg daily orally; 100–200 micrograms by oral inhalation as required; 500 micrograms by intramuscular injection)

Brand names: Salbulin §, Ventodisks §, Ventolin §, Volmax §

Salbutamol is a sympathomimetic agent with a selective stimulant action on the β_2-adrenoceptors and it is one of the most widely used drugs for the treatment of reversible airways disease generally. It is also effective in preventing exercise-induced bronchospasm.

Salbutamol may be given orally in doses of 4 mg three or four times a day, reduced to 2 mg for elderly patients, but for the rapid relief of acute bronchospasm it is given by oral inhalation from a pressurized aerosol in doses of 100–200 micrograms (1–2 puffs) as required. Such inhalation doses may also be given for the prophylaxis of exercise-induced bronchospasm or for maintenance therapy in acute conditions. The drug may also be administered by the inhalation of a powder from inhalation capsules, and some sustained-release oral products are available that are useful in the treatment of nocturnal asthma. Another development is the breath-actuated Aerolin Autohaler, which is claimed to respond to an inspiratory flow rate as low as 30 L/minute and provide 100 micrograms of salbutamol per inhalation.

In severe acute bronchospasm, salbutamol may be given by subcutaneous or intramuscular injection in doses of 500 micrograms, repeated 4-hourly as required; by slow intravenous injection in doses of 250 micrograms; or by intravenous infusion in doses of 5–20 micrograms/minute according to need, together with corticosteroid therapy.

In status asthmaticus and severe conditions salbutamol is sometimes given by the inhalation of a nebulized solution, delivered as a mist in oxygen-enriched air (to prevent hypoxaemia) from an intermittent, positive pressure ventilator. Such ventilator treatment requires strict control, as the dose varies from 2.5 to 5 mg or more 4-hourly, or 1–2 mg hourly, doses much larger than those given by aerosol inhalation.

Salbutamol is usually well tolerated, but fine tremor, tension, headache and tachycardia may occur, although the latter is less common with aerosol inhalation. Caution is necessary in hypertension, ischaemic heart disease and hyperthyroidism. Hypokalaemia is a potential risk with salbutamol, as with other β_2-adrenoceptors, especially in severe asthma, and may be increased by theophylline, diuretics and corticosteroids. It is now recommended that plasma potassium levels should be monitored in severe asthma. A recently introduced derivative is **salmeterol** § (Serevent §), which has a longer action, and in doses of 50 micrograms by inhalation, is suitable for twice daily maintenance treatment.

The use of salbutamol to prevent premature labour is referred to on page 453.

Terbutaline § (dose: 7.5–15 mg daily orally; 250–500 micrograms by oral inhalation as required; 250–500 micrograms by injection)

Brand names: Bricanyl §, Monovent §

Terbutaline is a sympathomimetic agent with the actions, uses and side-effects of salbutamol. In reversible airways disease it is given in doses of 5 mg two or three times a day; for the control of intermittent bronchospasm and for the prophylaxis of exercise-induced conditions, terbutaline may be given by aerosol in doses of 250–500 micrograms (1–2 puffs) 4-hourly as needed. In the maintenance treatment of chronic obstructive airways conditions, the total daily inhalation dose should not exceed 2 mg (8 puffs).

In acute and severe obstructive states, terbutaline is given by subcutaneous, intramuscular or slow intravenous injection in doses of 250–500 micrograms up to four times a day. Alternatively, it may be given by continuous intravenous infusion in doses of 1.5–5 micrograms/minute according to need and response, together with supportive oxygen therapy to avoid hypoxia. As with salbutamol, in severe and acute conditions terbutaline may also be given by the inhalation of a nebulized solution. Bambuterol §▼ (Bambec §▼) is a terbutaline pro-drug. It has similar actions and uses, but a more prolonged effect. It is given as a single dose of 10–20 mg at night.

Terbutaline is sometimes used as a myometrial relaxant in the control of premature labour (p. 453).

Orciprenaline § (dose: 40–80 mg daily orally; 750–1500 micrograms by oral inhalation)

Brand name: Alupent §

Orciprenaline is a sympathomimetic agent with the broncho-dilator properties of salbutamol, but it has a less selective action on the β_2-adrenoceptors, and is more likely to cause tachycardia. In reversible obstructive airways disease it is given orally in doses of 20 mg four times a day or by aerosol inhalation in doses of 750–1500 micrograms (1–2 puffs), up to a maximum of 12 puffs a day.

Side-effects of orciprenaline are similar to those of related drugs, but tremor, palpitations and cardiac irregularities are more common.

Fenoterol § (Berotec), **pirbuterol** § (Exirel), **reproterol** § (Bronchodil), **tuobuterol** § (Respacal) and **rimiterol** § (Pulmadil) represent other selective β_2-adrenoceptor stimulants with the actions, uses and side-effects of salbutamol.

Isoprenaline § (dose: 10–60 mg daily orally; 240 micrograms–1.9 mg daily by oral inhalation)

Brand names: Medihaler-iso §, Medihaler-iso Forte §

Isoprenaline is a sympathomimetic agent that acts on both β_1- and β_2-adrenoceptors and so has cardiac side-effects that are undesirable in the treatment of bronchospasm. Its use has declined since the introduction of the more selectively-acting bronchodilators of the salbutamol type.

Isoprenaline is given by aerosol inhalation in doses of 80–240 micrograms (1–3 puffs) up to eight times in 24 hours.

Side-effects include nervousness, weakness, palpitations, tremor, tachycardia and other cardiac irregularities.

The use of isoprenaline in bradycardia and heart block is referred to on page 237.

Ephedrine § (dose: 45–160 mg daily)

Ephedrine is a plant alkaloid introduced as an orally active drug with some of the bronchodilator properties of adrenaline, but it has now been largely replaced by salbutamol and related drugs.

Ephedrine is used to some extent in the prophylaxis of bronchospasm in doses of 15–60 mg three times a day. It has central stimulant properties, and **side-effects** include restlessness, insomnia and tachycardia. It relaxes the detrusor muscle of the bladder, and may cause acute retention of urine in cases of prostatic hypertrophy.

A single dose of 60 mg at night has been used in the treatment of enuresis (p. 358).

Ipratropium § (dose: 216–576 micrograms daily by aerosol inhalation)

Brand name: Atrovent §

Although ipratropium is referred to here, it is not a sympathomimetic agent but an anticholinergic (antimuscarinic) drug with a slower but more prolonged bronchodilator and antispasmodic action than those of the salbutamol group. Such agents reduce bronchospasm by blocking those muscarinic receptors in the lungs that normally control bronchomuscular tone.

Ipratropium is used mainly in the treatment of chronic bronchitis and related conditions of airways obstruction in patients no longer responding to bronchodilators of the salbutamol type. It is given by aerosol inhalation as a single dose of 40–80 micrograms (2–4 puffs) initially, followed by doses of 20–40 micrograms three or four times a day. Combivent is an aerosol product providing doses of ipratropium 20 micrograms and salbutamol 100 micrograms.

Dry mouth is an occasional **side-effect** and care is necessary in prostatic hypertrophy. Ipratropium is sometimes given by inhalation of a nebulized solution, but it has occasionally caused a paradoxical broncho-constriction, and such treatment requires close hospital supervision. Oxitropium (Oxivent) is an anticholinergic agent with similar properties used as a metered dose inhaler in doses of 200 micrograms (two puffs) two or three times a day.

Aminophylline (dose: 300–1200 mg daily)

Aminophylline and the closely related theophylline are included here as they have a relaxant effect on smooth muscle and are used in the relief of bronchospasm and to stimulate respiration. In the treatment of reversible airways disease, aminophylline is given orally in doses of 100–300 mg up to four times a day after food, but in practice the gastric irritant effects often prevent the administration of adequate doses.

In severe conditions such as acute bronchial asthma and status asthmaticus, aminophylline may be given by *slow* intravenous injection in doses of 250–500 mg over 20 minutes, followed if necessary by doses of 500 micrograms/kg/hour. Intramuscular injections are painful and are not recommended. The plasma concentrations of theophylline/aminophylline should be monitored, as the therapeutic window (p. 15) is narrow. Optimum level is 10–20 mg/litre.

Side-effects include gastrointestinal irritation with nausea and vomiting, headache, insomnia and confusion.

In general, the oral dosage of aminophylline and theophylline is complicated by individual variations in absorption and metabolism of the drug, with variations in response. These difficulties can be reduced to some extent by the use of long-acting oral preparations such as Phyllocontin Continus, Lasma, Neulin SA, Pro-Vent, Slo-phyllin, Theo-Dur and Uniphyllin Continus. These preparations of theophylline may provide an effective plasma level over 12 hours. **Choline theophyllinate** (Choledyl), dose 100–400 mg up to four times a day after food, is a derivative said to be better tolerated than the parent drug.

Caution. The long-acting products should not be regarded as interchangeable, and a patient stabilized on one preparation should not be transferred to another without good cause, as variations in the plasma level of theophylline may occur.

DRUGS USED IN THE RESPIRATORY DISTRESS SYNDROME

Premature infants often have respiratory difficulties, as they are deficient in the endogenous lung surfactants that promote normal lung expansion on inspiration. In such deficiency, increased respiratory effort is required to expand the alveoli and promote gas exchange and oxygenation. The condition is referred to as the respiratory distress syndrome (RDS) and if the respiratory effort weakens with continued distress, pulmonary failure may develop. RDS can now be relieved by the use of pulmonary surfactant products obtained from animal lung and containing phospholipids. They are given by endotracheal tube in the newborn, preferably within 8 hours of birth, who are receiving mechanical ventilation. Continuous monitoring of the arterial oxygenation and heart rate are necessary, as rapid changes may occur. Care must be taken to avoid blocking of the endotracheal tube by mucous. Dosage and details of administration vary with the product used, and the manufacturer's data sheet should be studied. The following products are available:

Beractant §▼; Survanta §▼; Colfosceril §▼; Exosurf §▼; Curosurf §▼; Alec §▼.

 Morley C J et al 1987 Ten-centre trial of artificial surfactant in very premature babies. British Medical Journal 294: 991–996

PARASYMPATHOMIMETIC OR CHOLINERGIC DRUGS

The cholinergic drugs are those that produce effects on various body organs similar to those that follow normal stimulation of the parasympathetic nervous system and can be divided into two groups:

1. those that have a direct action similar to that of acetylcholine on the parasympathetic receptors, and so are also referred to as parasympathomimetic drugs;

2. those drugs, known as anticholinesterases, that act by inhibiting the destruction of normally released acetylcholine by the enzyme cholinesterase, and so indirectly have a similar action to group 1 drugs; their action is usually more intense and prolonged than those in group 1.

GROUP 1

Although acetylcholine is the natural transmitter substance in cholinergic nerves, the wide variety of responses that it evokes, as well as its transient action because of its rapid enzymatic destruction, make it of little value therapeutically. In practice, reliance is largely placed on group 2 drugs, but a few choline derivatives and certain plant alkaloids with selective group 1 activity remain in limited use.

Carbachol (dose: 6 mg daily; 250 micrograms by subcutaneous injection)

Carbachol, or carbamylcholine, has some of the properties of acetylcholine, but it is more resistant to enzymatic breakdown, and so has a more prolonged action. It is used mainly in the treatment of acute and chronic retention of urine, as it increases bladder tone by stimulating detrusor muscle contraction.

Carbachol is given orally in doses of 2 mg three times a day before food in chronic retention, but in acute conditions it is given by subcutaneous injection in doses of 250 micrograms, repeated after 30 minutes, and again after a similar interval if required.

Side-effects of carbachol are those of general parasympathetic stimulation, and include nausea, vomiting, blurred vision, sweating and involuntary defaecation. Bradycardia and peripheral vasodilatation leading to hypotension may also occur and for that reason carbachol should not be given by intramuscular or intravenous injection. Carbachol has also been used as a miotic in the treatment of glaucoma as 3% eye-drops (p. 522).

Bethanechol (dose: 30–120 mg daily; 5 mg by subcutaneous injection)

Brand name: Myotonine

Bethanechol has the actions, uses and side-effects of carbachol, but cardiovascular disturbances are less likely to occur. It is given in doses of 10–30 mg three or four times a day before food in urinary retention, or in a dose of 5 mg by subcutaneous injection, repeated after 30 minutes, in acute conditions. It is sometimes given by injection in the treatment of postoperative paralytic ileus. Like carbachol, it should not be given by intramuscular or intravenous injection.

GROUP 2

The anticholinesterases permit the accumulation of acetylcholine at nerve endings and have a wide range of activity as well as side-effects. They may, however, increase some actions of acetylcholine more than others, so some are of value in urinary disorders, and others are used in myasthenia gravis. It should be noted that atropine, a potent anticholinergic drug, can oppose some but not all of the actions of anticholinesterases.

Neostigmine § (dose: 75–300 mg daily; 1–2.5 mg by injection)

Brand name: Prostigmin §

Neostigmine is a synthetic anticholinesterase that mainly increases the action of released acetylcholine on skeletal muscle, with less action on smooth muscle. It is used mainly in the treatment of myasthenia gravis, a condition characterized by a variably progressive muscular weakness. It may be due to an immunologically-induced receptor site abnormality that interferes with normal acetylcholine-mediated muscle contraction, or to a reduction in the number of active receptors. The condition may be alleviated by neostigmine in doses of 75–300 mg daily, given as divided doses modified according to individual need and response, and given at 4-hourly intervals. In more severe conditions, neostigmine may be given by subcutaneous or intramuscular injection in doses of 1–2.5 mg at intervals according to need, up to 2-hourly and a maximum of 20 mg daily.

Neostigmine is also given by injection in doses of 0.5–1 mg in the treatment of paralytic ileus and postoperative urinary retention. It also reverses the action of non-depolarizing muscle relaxants, and is used in anaesthesia to cut short the action of the tubocurarine-like muscle relaxants (p. 265).

Side-effects of neostigmine are linked with its cholinergic activity, and include nausea, vomiting, salivation, colic and diarrhoea, and may be severe enough to require control by atropine in doses of 500 micrograms three times a day. Bradycardia and hypotension may be indicative of excessive dosage, and it should be noted that overdose of neostigmine may have the reverse effects of reducing neurotransmission and increasing the muscle weakness, an effect that must be distinguished from a deterioration of the myasthenic condition. Neostigmine is contraindicated in the mechanical obstruction of the intestinal or urinary tract.

Distigmine § (dose: 5–20 mg daily; 500 micrograms by intramuscular injection)

Brand name: Ubretid §

Distigmine has the actions and uses of neostigmine, with the advantage of a longer duration of action that may extend over 24 hours. In myasthenia gravis it is given in an oral dose of 5 mg initially on an empty stomach (to promote absorption) half an hour before breakfast, and increased at intervals of 3 days or so according to response up to a maximum of 20 mg daily.

Distigmine is also useful in the treatment of urinary retention in patients with neurogenic bladder associated with upper motor neurone lesions, and is given in doses of 5 mg daily or on alternate days, preferably half an hour before breakfast. It is sometimes given by injection in doses of 500 micrograms for the prevention and treatment of postoperative urinary retention and intestinal atony.

Side-effects of distigmine are similar to those of prostigmine, but although usually milder, may be more prolonged. If side-effects are severe, treatment with 500 micrograms or more of atropine by injection may be required.

Pyridostigmine § (dose: 300–720 mg daily)

Brand name: Mestinon §

Pyridostigmine has the uses and side-effects of prostigmine, and although less potent, it has a slow and prolonged action. It is useful in those myasthenic states where a less intense action is required, and for night-time use when early morning muscle weakness is a problem. It is given orally in doses of 30–120 mg, taken at intervals during the day linked with need and response, up to a total of 300–720 mg or occasionally more daily.

It does not relieve the symptoms of myasthenia gravis so completely as neostigmine, but its reduced gastrointestinal side-effects may be an advantage. Like related drugs, pyridostigmine is sometimes used in postoperative paralytic ileus and urinary retention in doses of 60–240 mg as required.

Edrophonium § (dose: 10 mg by intravenous injection)

Brand name: Camsilon §

Edrophonium has the basic properties of neostigmine, but differs markedly in having a very brief action. It is correspondingly valuable in the diagnosis of myasthenia gravis as, in patients with that disease, a dose of 2 mg intravenously followed, if there is no adverse reaction after 30 seconds, by a further dose of 8 mg, brings about an immediate, definite but transient increase in muscle power. The effect lasts for about 5 minutes, after which the muscle weakness returns.

Edrophonium is also of value in distinguishing between overdose and underdose of an anticholinesterase or cholinergic drug such as neostigmine. If dosage is inadequate, an intravenous injection of the test dose of 10 mg intravenously will result in an immediate but temporary improvement of the myasthenia, whereas in cases of excessive therapy, the symptoms will be equally rapid but briefly intensified.

Edrophonium has few **side-effects**, but it has occasionally caused respiratory muscle weakness and great care is required in asthmatic patients.

Side-effects of cholinergic drugs

The side-effects of cholinergic drugs and anticholinesterases are associated with their general effects of augmenting the action of released acetylcholine or preventing its enzymatic breakdown. The actions of acetylcholine on autonomic ganglia and on the neuro-muscular junction are sometimes termed nicotinic, as they resemble the actions of nicotine on those sites. The actions of acetyl-choline on parasympathetic nerve endings, and on the sympathetic nerve endings serving the sweat and endocrine glands and the blood vessels of the skeletal muscles are termed muscarinic, as they mimic the effects of the fungal alkaloid muscarine.

The distinction is useful, as the main side-effects of the anticholinesterases are generally due to their muscarinic proper-ties, and include increased salivary and bronchial secretions, increased gastrointestinal activity with nausea, vomiting, colic and diarrhoea, and bradycardia. Atropine antagonises these muscarinic side-effects; in other words, atropine antagonises all the effects of cholinergic drugs with the exception of the effects on autonomic ganglia and neuromuscular junctions.

In cases of overdose with cholinergic drugs, atropine is given in doses of up to 1–2 mg by intravenous injection, repeated according to need. It should be noted that certain organophosphorus insecti-cides are extremely powerful anticholinesterases with a long action, and can cause severe poisoning and death from respiratory failure. Prompt treatment with atropine is essential, and very large doses of up to 50 mg over 24 hours may be required (p. 581).

ANTICHOLINERGIC OR PARASYMPATHOLYTIC AGENTS

Drugs that inhibit the action of acetylcholine by occupying

receptor sites at various points of the parasympathetic nervous system, as well as those of certain sites in the sympathetic system (p. 246) are referred to as anticholinergic drugs.

The oldest is the alkaloid atropine, but many synthetic anticholinergic drugs with some of the properties of atropine are in use.

Attempts have been made to classify the anticholinergic drugs into three groups, (1) those used mainly for their smooth muscle relaxant and antispasmodic and antisecretory properties, (2) those used for their effects on the central nervous system in the treatment of parkinsonism, and (3) those used in ophthalmology. In this chapter they will be divided into natural drugs, synthetic drugs, and those used almost exclusively in the treatment of Parkinson's disease. Those used in ophthalmology are discussed in Chapter 23.

Atropine § (dose: 250 micrograms–2 mg daily orally; 500 micrograms–1 mg intravenously)

Atropine is the alkaloid originally obtained from belladonna, although it is also prepared synthetically. It brings about a reduction in smooth muscle tone and gastrointestinal activity, and is given orally in doses of 500 micrograms three times a day, increased if required up to 2 mg daily, for the relief of gastrointestinal spasm, and in biliary and renal colic.

Atropine is used pre-operatively by injection in doses of 300–600 micrograms to decrease bronchial and salivary secretions. It increases the heart rate by its action on the vagus, and so prevents the bradycardia induced by some inhalation anaesthetics. It is also used in the treatment of bradycardia in myocardial infarction by intravenous doses of 300 micrograms–1 mg, up to a maximum of 3 mg over 24 hours. Atropine is also administered by intravenous injection in doses of 600 micrograms–1.2 mg in association with neostigmine to reverse the action of muscle relaxants of the tubocurarine type. Its use in ophthalmology is referred to in Chapter 23.

Side-effects of atropine include dryness of the mouth, dilatation of the pupils, dry skin and bradycardia. It is contraindicated in prostatic hypertrophy and glaucoma, and should be used with care in the elderly and in cardiac insufficiency. (Note: Belladonna extract, a survivor of older therapy, is still used in some mixed products for the treatment of gastrointestinal disorders associated with smooth muscle spasm).

Glycopyrronium §

Brand name: Robinul §

Glycopyrronium is a synthetic antimuscarinic agent used like atropine in premedication to reduce salivary secretions. It is given by intramuscular or intravenous injection in doses of 200–400 micrograms. It is also used together with neostigmine as Robinul–Neostigmine to reverse the effects of the non-depolarising muscle relaxants such as tubocurarine (p. 265).

Hyoscine (dose: 200–600 micrograms orally or by subcutaneous injection)

Hyoscine, also known as scopolamine, is an alkaloid closely related to atropine, and has some similar properties. It differs in having a depressant effect on the cerebral cortex, and so it has some hypnotic properties, although sometimes the hyoscine-induced drowsiness may be preceded by a brief period of excitement. Hyoscine is mainly used for premedication in doses of 200–600 micrograms by subcutaneous injection, together with 20 mg of papaveretum or 10 mg of morphine to reduce secretions and facilitate induction. Such combined treatment has also been used in obstetrics to produce analgesia and amnesia.

Hyoscine has a depressant action on the vomiting centre, and it is widely used in the treatment of travel sickness and vertigo. It is given in oral doses of 600 micrograms (150–300 micrograms for children of 6–12 years) about 20 minutes before starting a journey, with subsequent doses three or four times a day as required. **Scopoderm** TTS § is a patch dressing containing 500 micrograms of hyoscine, for the prevention of travel sickness. It should be applied to a hairless area of the skin about 5 hours before the start of the journey. The slow absorption of the drug from the patch is said to provide an action extending over 72 hours, with the advantage of reduced side-effects. Only one patch should be used at a time, and care should be taken to wash the hands after the application and removal of the patch. The use of hyoscine in ophthalmology is referred to in Chapter 23.

Side-effects of hyoscine are anticholinergic, and include dryness of the mouth, blurred vision and urinary difficulties. It should be used with caution in the elderly, and is contraindicated in glaucoma. **Hyoscine butylbromide** (Buscopan) is a derivative of hyoscine used in the treatment of acute gastrointestinal spasm. It should be given by intramuscular or intravenous injection in doses of 20 mg, repeated as required. Tablets of 20 mg are available, but the response is unreliable as absorption is poor.

Homatropine

A derivative of atropine used mainly in ophthalmology as a rapidly acting mydriatic (Chapter 23).

SYNTHETIC ANTICHOLINERGIC AGENTS

With the synthetic anticholinergic or antimuscarinic drugs many of the side-effects of atropine have been reduced. They do not pass the blood–brain barrier easily, and so are less likely to have central effects such as confusion or visual disturbances. On the other hand, they are less lipid-soluble, absorption after oral administration may be poor, and marked differences may exist between oral doses and those given by injection.

These anticholinergic agents are used mainly in the treatment of gastrointestinal disorders associated with smooth muscle spasm, and by delaying gastric movement they help to prolong the action of antacids. They are also used in urinary frequency and enuresis, as they increase bladder capacity by a stabilizing action on the detrusor muscle. Anticholinergic drugs may cause confusion in the elderly as well as urinary hesitancy, and care is necessary in glaucoma.

Propantheline is a representative of this group of drugs. Those anticholinergic agents used mainly in the treatment of Parkinson's disease are referred to on page 256.

Propantheline § (dose: 45–90 mg daily)

Brand name: Pro-Banthine §

Propantheline has the peripheral action of atropine on the

response to released acetycholine, and it is used in the treatment of gastrointestinal disturbances associated with smooth muscle spasm, and in biliary and urinary tract spasm. It is also used in urinary frequency and enuresis, as it reduces the contractions of an unstable detrusor muscle.

Propantheline is given in doses of 15 mg three time a day before meals, with a 30 mg dose at night, subsequently adjusted as required with a maximum dose of 120 mg daily. In the treatment of enuresis, a bed-time dose of 15–45 mg has been used.

Side-effects of propantheline are similar to those of atropine, but in general are less severe.

Other antispasmodics used mainly in gastrointestinal disturbances are referred to in Chapter 11.

PARKINSON'S DISEASE

As anticholinergic drugs have been used for many years in the treatment of parkinsonism, it is convenient to review current therapy here, although some newer drugs act by a different mechanism. Originally described in 1817 as the 'shaking palsy', Parkinson's disease or parkinsonism is due to a progressive degeneration of a regulatory system in the substantia nigra-corpus striatum and associated areas of the midbrain.

Both dopamine and acetylcholine are concerned in this regulatory system, and the degeneration of the pigment-containing cells and dopaminergic neurones in the nigra-striatal system leads to an over-activity of the cholinergic neurones. The normal balance between the two neurotransmitter substances is disturbed and the loss of dopamine results in the tremor of the hands, weakness and rigidity of muscles, excessive salivation and the depression so characteristic of parkinsonism, which is basically a dopamine-deficiency disease. It should also be noted that some psychotropic drugs have as a side-effect an adverse effect on the cerebral dopamine-acetylcholine balance either by blocking dopamine receptors or reducing dopaminic stores, and so cause a drug-induced parkinsonism.

The treatment of parkinsonism is aimed at restoring the disturbed balance between dopaminergic and cholinergic activity, but at present drug treatment is palliative, not curative, and does not prevent the slow degenerative nature of the disease, and patients should be warned accordingly. At the same time, many of the symptoms of parkinsonism can be brought under some control by suitable therapy, but treatment must be adjusted for the individual patients, as the response is often variable, and some patients may tolerate one drug better than another. Regrettably, more than 10% of patients fail to respond to any treatment.

Patients should be advised to maintain muscle function and reduce stiffness by gentle exercise, and to minimise any dose-limiting side-effects by taking all drugs after food. They should also be warned about the abrupt changes in response that can occur, the so-called 'on–off' effects, which can be particularly demoralizing to a patient who has not been warned about such fluctuations.

The drugs used to control the symptoms of parkinsonism fall into two main groups, the anticholinergic drugs, and those that act by increasing the level of dopamine in the cerebral tissues. As a rule, the anticholinergic drugs are the first choice for mild parkinsonism, and they are also preferred for drug-induced and post-encephalitic parkinsonism. For more severe conditions a dopaminergic drug such as levodopa is more effective but sometimes combined therapy will evoke the best response. Bromocriptine and amantadine are unrelated drugs that are sometimes useful as alternative or supplementary therapy.

In general, the anticholinergic agents relieve tremor and salivation, whereas dopaminergic drugs are often more effective in controlling rigidity and akinesia. As a rule, treatment with the former should be commenced with and increased by small doses, as they may cause confusion, particularly in elderly patients and may precipitate glaucoma and urinary retention.

Points about drugs used in parkinsonism

(a) Two main types — antimuscarinics/anticholinergics and dopaminergics.
(b) Antimuscarinics are useful initially in patients with mild symptoms; they relieve tremor more than rigidity.
(c) Dopaminergics are basically replacement therapy: value in later stages limited by fluctuations in response — the 'on–off' effect.
(d) Some other drugs act by stimulating surviving dopamine receptors.

ANTICHOLINERGIC DRUGS

Benzhexol § (dose: 2–15 mg daily)

Brand names: Artane §, Broflex §

Benzhexol relieves the muscular rigidity more than the tremor of parkinsonism, but it has little influence on dyskinesia. It is given in doses of 1–2 mg daily initially, slowly increased by incremental doses of 2 mg until 6–15 mg are given daily in divided doses. Patients with post-encephalitic parkinsonism tend to require and tolerate larger doses, whereas reduced doses should be given to elderly patients. Combined therapy with levodopa may evoke a better response, and in some cases permit a reduction in the dose of benzhexol, but any change of dose should be carried out slowly. Benzhexol is also used in the treatment of drug-induced parkinsonism, but it should not be used for the tardive dyskinesia associated with long-term antipsychotic therapy, as it may exacerbate the symptoms.

Side-effects of benzhexol are those common to the anticholinergic drugs, and include dryness of the mouth, visual disturbances, occasional tachycardia and confusion. Benzhexol may sometimes cause severe mental disturbances, requiring withdrawal of the drug if adjustment of dose is ineffective.

Benztropine § (dose: 500 micrograms–6 mg daily)

Brand name: Cogentin §

Benztropine is mainly effective in controlling the tremor and rigidity of parkinsonism, and the muscle relaxation obtained reduces the discomfort and restlessness at night. It differs from benzhexol in having a sedative action in normal doses, and may be more suitable for elderly patients. Benztropine is also useful in controlling the symptoms of drug-induced parkinsonism. The initial dose is 500 micrograms–1 mg daily, increased very slowly to a maximum of 6 mg daily according to response. In conditions where a prompt action is required, benztropine may be given by intramuscular or intravenous injection in doses of 1–2 mg, repeated according to need.

Side-effects of benztropine are similar to those of benzhexol.

Related anticholinergic drugs

Many anticholinergic drugs have been used in the control of parkinsonism, but as response may be variable, treatment is largely on an individual basis. Table 7.2 lists some available drugs, some of which have some antihistaminic as well as anticholinergic properties.

Table 7.2 Anticholinergic drugs for parkinsonism

Approved name	Brand name	Daily dose range
benzhexol	Artane, Broflex	2–15 mg
benztropine	Cogentin	0.5–6 mg
biperiden	Akineton	2–6 mg
orphenadrine	Biorphen, Disipal	150–400 mg
procyclidine	Arpicolin, Kemadrin	7.5–30 mg

DOPAMINERGIC DRUGS

Levodopa § (dose: 250 mg–8 g daily)

Brand names: Brocadopa §, Larodopa §

Although parkinsonism is due to a deficiency of dopamine, which is a key neurotransmitter in the central nervous system, dopamine cannot be used therapeutically as it is poorly absorbed when given orally, and does not pass the blood–brain barrier. Levodopa, the natural precursor of dopamine, differs in being well absorbed, but much of a dose is converted in the liver to dopamine by the enzyme dopa-decarboxylase, so that very little unchanged levodopa reaches the central nervous system for conversion into centrally acting dopamine.

The dopamine that consequently appears in the peripheral tissues is responsible for many of the side-effects of levodopa therapy, and in practice levodopa is often given with a dopa-carboxylase inhibitor such as benserazide or carbidopa (p. 258). Such combined use largely prevents the hepatic conversion of levodopa to dopamine, and permits a greater proportion of an orally administered dose of levodopa to reach the brain for localized conversion to the active drug. It also permits a reduction in the dose of levodopa, a smoother control of symptoms and fewer side-effects.

In the treatment of idiopathic parkinsonism, levodopa is given in initial doses of 125–250 mg daily in divided doses, after food,

followed by small increases in dose at intervals of 2–4 days up to
a total daily dose of 2.5–8 g. For combined therapy, 10–25 mg of
benserazide or carbidopa[1] may be given and with such combined
therapy, a daily dose of 1 g of levodopa may be adequate. In all
cases, long-term treatment extending over some years is necessary, with doses adjusted to the individual patient at a level that
provides optimum relief with acceptable side-effects.

The 'on-off' response

Some patients do not respond to levodopa therapy, and with
those that respond there may be sudden variations in response as
treatment is continued, the so-called 'on-off' response, with a
reduction in mobility which may last from 2–4 hours. The mechanism of these variations is not clear, and although it may be
related to blood levels of levodopa, adjustment of dose frequency
has little effect. With extended treatment over some years, the
response to levodopa may become less satisfactory, and may be
linked with an altered receptor sensitivity as well as with the
progressive nature of the disease. It has been suggested that
ferrous sulphate should not be given with levodopa, as the two
compounds may react to form a poorly absorbed complex.

Side-effects of levodopa are numerous. Nausea and
anorexia are common, and cardiovascular responses such as
postural hypotension, faintness and dizziness may occur, as may
flushing, palpitations and sweating. With longer treatment,
agitation, aggression, hallucinations and other psychiatric
disturbances may occur. Involuntary movements are common at
the optimum dose levels. The urine and other body fluids may be
discoloured during levodopa therapy but such changes are of no
significance.

Some side-effects have been attributed to the unmasking of
underlying conditions as the disease is brought under control.
Levodopa is contraindicated in severe psychiatric disturbances,
and in closed-angle glaucoma.

---

[1]*Note.* Combined products are **Sinemet** and **Sinemet Plus**, containing levodopa
100 mg with carbidopa 10 and 25 mg, respectively (co-careldopa). **Madopar 62.5**
contains levodopa 50 mg with benserazide 12.5 mg; **Madopar 125** and **Madopar
250** contain 100 and 200 mg of levodopa with benserazide 25 mg and 50 mg,
respectively (co-beneldopa).

Amantadine § (dose: 100–200 mg daily)

Brand name: Symmetrel §, Mantadine §

Amantadine is a synthetic compound, and was originally used as an antiviral agent in the prophylaxis of influenza. By chance it was given to a patient with Parkinson's disease who commented on the subsequent relief of rigidity and tremor.

The drug has since proved useful in the treatment of the less severe forms of parkinsonism, and although the mode of action is not clear, amantadine may increase the release of dopamine from still functioning dopaminergic neurones in the nigrostriatum. It improves the hypokinesia and rigidity of parkinsonism, and also the tremor to some extent, but tolerance may occur, and not all patients respond well to amantadine. It is given in doses of 100 mg daily, later increased to 100 mg twice a day, (the second dose not later than 4 p.m.), often in association with anticholinergic therapy. Larger doses may cause confusion. Amantadine is not suitable for the treatment of drug-induced parkinsonism.

Side-effects include insomnia, nausea, skin discolouration and occasional oedema. Treatment should not be stopped abruptly.

Bromocriptine (dose: 10–80 mg daily)

Brand name: Parlodel §

Bromocriptine differs from other drugs used in the treatment of parkinsonism. It evokes a response similar to that to levodopa, but by a different mechanism as it is a dopamine receptor agonist. Its action is therefore independent of any surviving dopaminergic neurones. It is mainly used for patients who cannot tolerate adequate doses of levodopa, and is given in initial doses of 1–1.25 mg with food at night for 3–7 days, slowly increased at weekly intervals up to 40–100 mg or more daily, as three divided doses, with food. Combined therapy with levodopa is sometimes used, but careful balancing of the doses of bromocriptine and levodopa is required, as confusion and abnormal movements may occur with such combined treatment.

Side-effects of bromocriptine are numerous, and include nausea, headache, postural hypotension, drowsiness and confusion. Tolerance may be reduced by alcohol. With higher doses, hallucinations and other psychiatric disturbances may occur, and pleural effusions have been reported.

It should be noted that the doses of bromocriptine used for the treatment of parkinsonism are very much higher than those used for the suppression of lactation (p. 380).

Lysuride § (dose: 200 micrograms–5 mg daily)

Brand name: Revanil §

Lysuride, like bromocriptine, is a dopamine agonist, and its stimulating effect on dopamine receptors is independent of dopamine stores or surviving dopaminergic neurones. It is given initially in doses of 200 micrograms, with food, at night, followed by weekly increments of 200 micrograms according to response up to a maximum dose of 5 mg. Lysuride may also be given in association with levodopa.

Side-effects include hypotension, about which warning should be given, dizziness, drowsiness, nausea, malaise and psychotic disturbances.

Pergolide § (dose: 50 micrograms–3 g daily)

Brand name: Celance §

Pergolide resembles both bromocriptine and lysuride in being a dopamine agonist, and acts by stimulating dopamine receptors but differs in having a longer action. It is used mainly as a supplement to levodopa therapy and is given in doses of 50 micrograms daily initially, increased at intervals of 3 days by increments of 250 micrograms up to a maintenance divided dose of 3 g daily. The side-effects are similar to those of bromocriptine, and patients should be warned that hypotensive side-effects may be disturbing during the initial days of treatment. Abrupt withdrawal may precipitate hallucinations.

Selegiline § (dose: 5–10 mg daily)

Brand name: Eldepryl §

Selegiline is an inhibitor of monoamine oxidase-B, and has a selective action in preventing the enzymatic breakdown of levodopa. It is used mainly in association with levodopa in the more severe forms of parkinsonism, as combined therapy may permit a reduction of dose, and a smoother response. Such treatment may possibly retard further dysfunction of the dopaminergic-striatal neurones, and the antidepressant action of selegiline may play a part in the symptomatic improvement.

Selegiline is given in morning doses of 5 mg, increased if necessary to 10 mg, but a reduction in the associated dose of levodopa by up to 50% may be necessary to prevent an increase in levodopa-linked side-effects. It should be noted that unlike conventional monoamine oxidases used in the treatment of depression, selegiline does not cause the so-called 'cheese reaction' or episodes of hypertension.

Side-effects include nausea, hypotension, confusion and agitation.

Apomorphine §▼ (dose: 3–30 mg daily by injection)

Brand name: Britaject §▼

Apomorphine is a powerful dopamine receptor agonist, but its emetic properties have hitherto prevented its use in parkinsonism. Some of the difficulties have been overcome to some extent by pre-medication of the patient with domperidone, and the administration of apomorphine by subcutaneous injection or continuous subcutaneous infusion in doses of 3–30 mg daily. It is mainly used in the treatment of refractory on–off periods not responding to other treatment, and under close hospital control. Success requires well-motivated patients who are able to co-operate with the method of administration.

DRUG-INDUCED PARKINSONISM

It should be noted that some powerful neuroleptics such as chlorpromazine and related drugs, that function as dopamine-antagonists, may cause extra-pyramidal side-effects resembling the symptoms of parkinsonism. Such symptoms may also occur with metoclopramide, particularly in children and young adults. Such side-effects can be reduced by the use of one of the antimuscarinic agents used in the treatment of parkinsonism, such as procyclidine, but they should not be used prophylactically as they may cause tardive dyskinesia.

8

Neuromuscular blocking agents and other muscle relaxants

Skeletal or striped muscle differs from smooth muscle both anatomically and physiologically. Although acetylcholine is liberated at the nerve-endings of both types of muscle, it is only in smooth muscle that atropine functions as an acetylcholine antagonist, and has a relaxant effect, and a different type of drug is required to produce relaxation of skeletal muscle.

Such drugs fall into two groups, those that act at the spinal level, and those that act on the neuromuscular junction. The latter, known as neuromuscular or myoneural blocking agents, are widely used to produce muscle relaxation during surgical anaesthesia, as otherwise large doses of anaesthetic with associated side-effects would be required to produce a comparable degree of relaxation. As such drugs also relax the respiratory muscles, controlled respiration is essential during the period that the relaxant is acting.

These neuromuscular blocking agents can be further divided into two groups, the non-depolarizing drugs represented by tubocurarine, and the depolarizing agent suxamethonium. Both types produce relaxation, but by different mechanisms.

When a nerve impulse reaches a voluntary muscle, acetylcholine is released to act at the receptor site on the membrane of the muscle end-plate (p. 228). The outside of this motor end-plate is positively charged, the inside has a negative charge, and the plate is referred to as being polarized. Acetylcholine released at the end-plate alters the charge, depolarization occurs, and the muscle relaxation is initiated. The action is brief, as the acetylcholine is rapidly destroyed by cholinesterases.

Non-depolarizing relaxants act by competing with acetylcholine for membrane receptor sites, and so produce relaxation by inhibiting normal muscle contraction. Depolarizing muscle relaxants, such as suxamethonium, appear to have an initial action similar to acetycholine but differ from the non-depolarizing relaxants in having a much shorter action. The action of depolarizing muscle relaxants cannot be reversed by other drugs, and except for short procedures, the longer-acting non-depolarizing muscle relaxants are usually preferred.

Points about muscle relaxants used in anaesthesia

(a) Two types, depolarizing and non-depolarizing. Suxamethonium is the only example of the latter, and has a brief action.
(b) Depolarizing muscle relaxants have a longer action; some have side-effects associated with histamine release.
(c) The action of depolarizing agents can be reversed by neostigmine, which must be preceded by atropine.
(d) Patients given a muscle relaxant must have assisted or controlled respiration until the relaxant has been metabolized or antagonized.

NON-DEPOLARIZING OR COMPETITIVE MUSCLE RELAXANTS

Tubocurarine §

Brand names: Tubarine §, Jexin §

Curare, an extract from a South American plant, was once used as an arrow poison, and produced its lethal effects by paralysing the respiratory and other muscles. Tubocararine, the principal alkaloid of curare, is now used as a long-acting non-depolarizing muscle relaxant in surgical anaesthesia. It is given by intravenous injection in doses of 15–25 mg; the action commences rapidly, reaches a maximum in 3–5 minutes, and declines after about 20 minutes. Relaxation can be maintained if required by supplementary doses of 5 mg up to a total intravenous dose of 45 mg.

The relaxant action of tubocurarine is potentiated by some inhalation anaesthetics, as well as by gentamicin and related aminoglycoside antibiotics. The hypotension caused by halothane may also be increased. It is now used less frequently.

Side-effects of tubocurarine include a transient fall in blood pressure and an erythematous rash of the neck and chest. Although the rash appears to be linked with histamine release, histamine-associated bronchospasm is very uncommon; nevertheless, the drug should be avoided in allergic patients.

The action of tubocurarine can be reversed if required to shorten the recovery period or offset the respiratory depression by the intravenous injection of **neostigmine** in doses of 1–3 mg, followed if necessary by a second dose after 20–30 minutes. Such doses may cause side-effects such as bradycardia and excessive salivation, so neostigmine must be given *after* atropine in a dose of 600 micrograms–1.2 mg by intravenous injection.

Tubocurarine has also been given in doses of 75–150 micrograms/kg intravenously, repeated as required, to control the spasms of tetanus.

Atracurium §

Brand name: Tracrium §

Atracurium is a widely used non-depolarizing muscle relaxant with a duration of action over 15 to 35 minutes. Unlike related drugs, the duration of activity is independent of urinary excretion or enzymatic metabolism, as the drug decomposes spontaneously at body temperature with the formation of inert break-down products. Atracurium is therefore of value when renal or hepatic impairment is present, and repeated doses do not have a cumulative effect. The initial intravenous dose is 300–600 micrograms/kg body-weight; supplementary doses are 100–200 micrograms/kg as required.

The drug is also given by continuous intravenous infusion in doses of 5–10 micrograms/kg/minute for long operative procedures. The relaxant action is increased by halothane and aminoglycoside antibiotics.

Flushing is a **side-effect** and although it is associated with histamine release, bronchospasm is uncommon. Atracurium should not be mixed in the same syringe as thiopentone, as rapid inactivation will result. As with tubocurarine, the action of atracurium can be reversed by neostigmine.

Gallamine triethiodide §

Brand name: Flaxedil §

Gallamine is a synthetic relaxant that resembles tubocurarine in its general properties, but it has a less prolonged action, and larger doses are necessary to produce comparable effects. It is now used less frequently. The average adult dose of gallamine is 80–120 mg intravenously; relaxation occurs within 2 minutes, continues for about 20 minutes, and can be maintained by a second dose of 40–60 mg. As with tubocurarine, the action is increased by some anaesthetics and aminoglycoside antibiotics.

Gallamine should be used with care in hypertension and cardiac conditions where its tachycardial **side-effects** are undesirable, and as it is largely excreted in the urine, it should not be used in severe renal insufficiency. The action of gallamine can be reversed by neostigmine, preceded by an injection of atropine to reduce bradycardia and excessive salivation.

Mivacurium §

Brand name: Mivacron §

Mivacurium is a non-depolarizing short-acting muscle relaxant with the action and uses of atracurium. It is given intravenously in doses of 70–150 micrograms/kg over 5–15 seconds to facilitate intubation, followed by maintenance doses of 8–10 micrograms/kg/minute by intravenous infusion. A reduction in the infusion dose rate may be necessary when mivacurium is given with some inhalation anaesthetics such as enflurane. A slow initial injection rate up to 60 seconds is advisable in asthmatic patients and those with heart disease, as histamine release may follow the rapid injection of mivacurium.

Pancuronium bromide §

Brand name: Pavulon §

Pancuronium is chemically related to the steroids, but has a muscle relaxant action similar to tubocurarine. The onset of action is more rapid, but the duration rather less, and with few side-effects. There is little risk of histamine release or blood pressure changes with pancuronium, and it is often considered the first choice relaxant in poor risk patients, although it should be used with care in severe renal disease. It has also been used in intractable status asthmaticus and tetanus. The initial dose is 50–100 micrograms/kg intravenously, followed by later doses of

10–20 micrograms/kg as required. The relaxant effect can be reversed by neostigmine, together with atropine.

Vecuronium §

Brand name: Norcuron §

Vecuronium is a muscle relaxant with a short to medium duration of action. It is given in initial intravenous doses of 80–100 micrograms/kg, with supplementary doses of 30–50 micrograms/kg. Much of the drug is eliminated in the bile. As with related compounds, the action of vecuronium is increased by a wide range of other drugs including inhalation and intravenous anaesthetics, aminoglycoside antibiotics and beta-adrenergic blocking agents. Cardiovascular side-effects are uncommon, and there is little risk of histamine release. As with tubocurarine, the action can be reversed by neostigmine, although spontaneous recovery from vecuronium is rapid. Rocuronium § (Esmeron §) is a new muscle relaxant with similar actions and uses.

DEPOLARIZING MUSCLE RELAXANTS

The depolarizing muscle relaxants are characterized by their brief action, although an extended effect can be obtained by repeated doses. Unlike the non-depolarizing relaxants, the action cannot be reversed by neostigmine, and recovery is spontaneous.

Suxamethonium §

Brand names: Anectine §, Scoline §

Suxamethonium, also known as succinylcholine, is a depolarizing muscle relaxant that acts by simulating the action of acetylcholine on the motor end plate that initiates muscle relaxation, but it evokes a longer response as it escapes the extremely rapid enzymatic breakdown of acetylcholine that normally occurs. When given by intravenous injection in doses of 20–100 mg, it induces a rapid relaxation of muscle, from which spontaneous recovery takes place after 5 minutes.

Suxamethonium is of value in procedures in which merely a brief relaxation is required, such as the passing of an endotracheal tube, but an extended action can be obtained by giving further doses of 2–5 mg/minute by intravenous infusion.

Suxamethonium causes an initial painful muscle fibrillation (with muscle pain after recovery), and it should be given after anaesthesia has been induced by an intravenous anaesthetic such as thiopentone.

The action of suxamethonium may be intensified by other drugs such as aminoglycoside antibiotics, narcotic analgesics, and the bradycardia induced by the drug may be increased by halothane and cyclopropane (but not by thiopentone), and premedication with atropine may be indicated. In a few exceptional patients, suxamethonium sometimes has a paradoxically long action, with marked apnoea, requiring extended assisted respiration.

It is contraindicated in severely injured patients, in severe eye injuries, in burned patients, and in severe hepatic disease.

The mode of action differs from that of non-depolarizing agents such as tubocurarine; in consequence, neostigmine does not antagonize the action of suxamethonium, and if given, may increase the relaxant action.

SKELETAL MUSCLE RELAXANTS

It is convenient to consider here some muscle relaxants that are used in spastic conditions and the relief of muscle spasm. Unlike the relaxants used in surgery, most drugs in the group act on the central nervous system, and not by neuromuscular blockade.

Points about skeletal muscle relaxants

(a) Most act via the central nervous system.
(b) Dantrolene differs in acting directly on skeletal muscle.
(c) Botulinum toxin is used to control blepharospasm by localized muscle paralysis

---

Baclofen § (dose: 15–100 mg daily)

Brand name: Lioresal §

Baclofen is an antispastic agent that acts at the spinal level, and affords relief in muscle spasticity associated with multiple sclerosis, tumours of the cord and similar conditions. It has little effect on muscle power, so that relief of spasticity is not accompanied by a corresponding increase in muscular function.

Baclofen is given initially in doses of 5 mg three times a day, after food, with subsequent doses slowly increased according to response up to a maximum of 100 mg daily. Careful adjustments of dose is essential, especially in the elderly, to minimize muscle weakness in any unaffected limbs.

Side-effects include nausea, drowsiness, fatigue and confusion. Care is necessary in psychiatric illness, epilepsy and cardiovascular disease. Abrupt withdrawal of baclofen should be avoided, as visual hallucinations and convulsions may be precipitated.

Dantrolene § (dose: 50–400 mg daily)

Brand name: Dantrium §

Dantrolene is a skeletal muscle relaxant that acts by blocking the muscle contraction response at a site beyond the myoneural junction, probably by interfering with the release of calcium ions from the sarcoplasmic reticulum, and so is largely free from side-effects on the central nervous system. It is used mainly in severe spastic conditions associated with stroke, spinal cord injury, cerebral palsy and multiple sclerosis, and is given in initial doses of 25 mg daily, slowly increased to a maximum of 100 mg four times a day. Careful adjustment of dose to response is necessary, and although for many patients a dose of 75 mg three times a day is the optimum, response to treatment may be slow, and if the drug is ineffective after 6 weeks, it should be withdrawn. Nausea and fatigue are usually transient side-effects.

Dantrolene is potentially hepatotoxic, and liver function tests are necessary before and during treatment. Care is necessary in obstructive pulmonary disease and myocardial impairment, and it is contraindicated in hepatic disease. As dantrolene has some central activity, patients should be warned not to drive until dose and response have been stabilized. The use of dantrolene in the treatment of malignant hyperthermia is referred to on page 39.

Diazepam § (dose: 2–15 mg daily)

Brand names: Atensine §, Valium §

Diazepam, widely used in psychiatry (p. 60) also has a muscle relaxant action that appears to be mediated by depressing excessive motor activity at a spinal or possibly a supra-spinal level. It is used in a variety of conditions associated with muscle spasm, in cerebral spasticity, and to control the spasms of tetanus and relieve status asthmaticus.

Diazepam is given orally in muscle spasm in doses of 2–5 mg three times a day, but in cerebral spastic conditions up to 60 mg daily in divided doses may be necessary. In acute conditions, diazepam may be given by deep intramuscular injection (from which absorption may be erratic) or by slow intravenous injection in doses of 10 mg, repeated after 4 hours. In the treatment of tetanus, a dose of 100–300 micrograms/kg is given by slow intravenous injection at intervals of 1–4 hours as required, or by continuous intravenous infusion in doses of 3–10 mg/kg over 24 hours. In status epilepticus, diazepam is given by slow intravenous injection in doses of 10–20 mg, repeated according to need, or by intravenous infusion up to a maximum of 3 mg/kg over 24 hours. It is also given rectally as a solution in doses of 10 mg, repeated if necessary.

Side-effects of diazepam include drowsiness, dizziness, and occasional confusion, but intravenous injections may not only cause hypotension, but also severe respiratory depression requiring the support of mechanical ventilation. Intravenous injections may also cause a local thrombophlebitis.

Related benzodiazepines, represented by **chlorodiazepoxide, ketazolam** and **medazepam** also have muscle relaxant properties that are useful in muscular–skeletal disorders, especially when an emotional component is present.

Other relaxants

Mild muscle relaxants used in muscle spasm include **carisoprodol** (Carisoma) dose 1.5 g daily; **chlormezanone** (Trancopal) dose 600 mg daily; **methocarbamol** (Robaxin) dose 6 g daily; **meprobamate** (Equanil; Tenavoid), dose 1.2 g daily; and **orphenadrine** (Norflex) dose 300 mg daily. Some of these mild relaxants are included in various mixed preparations with a mild analgesic such as paracetamol.

Drugs used in the relief of tremor, chorea, tics and other muscle movements include propranolol (p. 190), primidone (p. 81) and benzhexol (p. 256). Tetrabenazine § (Nitoman §) is used mainly in Huntington's chorea in doses of 12.5 mg twice daily, increased to 25 mg three times a day if required. Piractam § (Nootropil ▼) is a new drug used in the adjunctive treatment of cortical myoclonus. It is given in initial doses of 2.4 g three times a day, increased as required at intervals of 3–4 days up to a maximum of 20 g daily.

Dysport §

Dysport is a muscle relaxant of a very unusual type and limited use as it is a preparation of *Clostridium botulinum* Type A toxin. Such toxins, which are the cause of botulism, prevent the release of acetylcholine at parasympathetic nerve endings, and cause death by respiratory muscle paralysis. Yet very small doses can produce a localized muscle paralysis, and Dysport is used in the treatment of blepharospasm. The condition is characterized by repeated blinking with local irritation and photophobia, leading to uncontrollable closure of the eyelid. Dysport, injected in doses of 120 units into the appropriate muscles of the eye, produces a localized muscle weakness and relief of spasm. The onset of action is slow, and is not fully developed for 1–2 weeks, but relief is sustained for 2–3 months. Further injections are required at 8-week intervals, as muscle function returns as new neuromuscular junctions are slowly formed. **Side-effects** are linked mainly with the spread of action to facial muscles. Severe dysphagia has followed the use of Dysport in torticollis. Botex is a similar product, given in doses of 1.25–2.5 units.

The chemotherapy of malignant disease

The normal system of cell division (mitosis), which is greatest during sleep, is to some extent under hormone control, as adrenaline, which is liberated during the daytime as a result of exercise, has a general inhibitory effect on mitosis. Other substances, thought to be glycoproteins, and termed chalones, are present in cells, and may also act as inhibitors of mitosis.

Chalones appear to be lost when cells are damaged by injury, or as a result of normal body wear and tear, as in that of the skin and intestinal mucosa, and during the initial stages of healing mitosis proceeds unchecked, until with the development of new tissue the lost chalones are replaced, and mitosis gradually ceases as the healing process is completed.

It is possible that chalones or their absence may play a part in the development of cancer, as an extended disturbance of the chalone-replacing process could lead to uncontrolled cell replication, a concept supported by the finding that some animal tumours appear to be associated with a deficiency of chalones. Other factors such as cyclic AMP also play a part, but much remains to be known about the control mechanism of cell division, and the causes of its breakdown.

When cells escape from the normal rigid control of growth their subsequent rate of growth and type of development may change profoundly. The integration with other cells is lost, and specific differences of structure and function become blurred as undifferentiated growth proceeds with varying rapidity. These growths, referred to generically as tumours, neoplasms or cancers, are of two main types, the benign and the malignant.

Benign tumours consist chiefly of differentiated cells that resemble to some extent those of the cells of the originating tissues, and are characterized by a slow rate of growth, and by the presence of a surrounding capsule. They may cause pain by obstruction or by pressure on a nerve, and can often be dealt with surgically.

Malignant tumours or cancers are poorly differentiated, are not encapsulated, and develop rapidly. As a result of that rapid growth, penetration of the cancerous cells into adjacent tissues soon occurs, and if these renegade cells reach the blood or lymphatic system, they can travel to other parts of the body and set up new centres of abnormal growth, referred to as metastases.

Once such metastatic development has taken place, it is usually too late for surgical removal of the primary tumour to be effective, and much reliance is placed on chemotherapy to treat malignant tumours.

CHEMOTHERAPY

With the advances in phamacology, hopes have long been held that a new drug would be found with a selective action on all abnormal, rapidly dividing cells found in cancerous conditions. Such an ideal drug is unknown and may long remain a pharmacologist's dream, yet the possibility of killing infective bacteria in the body was once thought equally remote.

The aim of treatment with chemotherapeutic agents is to destroy malignant cells with as little effect as possible on normal cells, but few cytotoxic drugs have such a selective action, and many of the side-effects of cytotoxic drugs are linked with the nature of their action as they have adverse effects on all rapidly dividing cells. The response to cytotoxic therapy basically depends on an increased sensitivity or slower recovery of malignant cells as compared with normal cells. However, cytotoxic drugs are usually most active against rapidly dividing cells, so any resting cells at the time of treatment may escape destruction and develop later, and drugs that have a wide range of activity against malignant cells at all stages of development are still required. Developments in cytotoxic therapy may eventually involve the use of monoclonal antibodies and response modifiers such as interleukin.

The drugs in current use in the treatment of malignant disease differ both in their nature and in their action, as some interrupt the cell cycle at several points, and others may have a more selective action, but they all act at some active phase of the cell cycle (Fig. 9.1). They can be divided into five main groups: the alkylating agents, the antimetabolites, the cytotoxic antibiotics, the vinca alkaloids, and an ill-defined group of unrelated substances that have a cytotoxic action.

The alkylating agents are a varied group of chemical substances that cause the DNA strands to break, or cross-link abnormally, so that normal replication of DNA and cell growth is prevented.

The antimetabolites act by a different mechanism, as they inhibit malignant cell growth by combining with enzymes concerned with nucleic acid synthesis and cell development. Their action is less specific, as those enzymes are also concerned with normal cell growth.

The cytotoxic antibiotics act in ways similar to the alkylating agents, as they break down the system of DNA/RNA replication, and interfere with protein synthesis. The vinca alkaloids have an inhibitory effect on the metaphase stage of cell division. Some of these activities may overlap and combined therapy may sometimes have an additive effect, and increase the destruction of malignant cells without necessarily adding to the overall toxic effect. Several multiple dosage schemes are now in use, often referred to by the initial letters of the drugs concerned, as in the MVPP, MOPP and ABVD regimens.

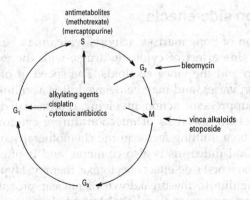

Figure 9.1 Cell cycle and points of cytotoxic drug attack. G_0 = resting stage; S = DNA synthesis; M = mitosis.

In general, cytotoxic drugs are most effective in leukaemias, in Hodgkin's disease and malignant lymphomas, and are useful in the control of myelomatosis, and mammary and ovarian carcinoma. The hormone treatment of mammary and prostatic carcinoma is referred to on pages 382 and 384.

As many cytotoxic drugs have short half-lives, attempts have been made in some cases to improve administration and extend the period of action by the use of a continuous low-dose infusion system. It is considered that by such intravenous infusion, more tumour cells would be exposed to the action of a cytotoxic drug during the more sensitive phases of the cell growth cycle. In addition, such extended low-dose therapy might reduce the nausea and vomiting associated with high peak cytotoxic drug concentrations. The introduction of portable infusion and bolus pumps has extended cytotoxic treatment to ambulant and home-based patients, and devices such as Parker Micropump can be programmed to control the rate of intravenous infusion or allow the patient to self-inject bolus doses at pre-determined periods. These systems may be developed to synchronize chemotherapy with circadian rhythms of the body, as well as increasing pain control by timed injections of potent analgesics. To obtain the maximum response close cooperation between all those involved in cytotoxic therapy is required, and nurses in particular may have to play an increasingly important part securing the patient's cooperation and understanding to achieve the maximum benefit from this interesting development in drug administration.

Common side-effects

Depression of bone marrow activity, which may be severe, is a common **side-effect** of cytotoxic drugs, with the exceptions of bleomycin and the vinca alkaloids. The speed of onset of such depression varies, and may be delayed. It is also linked with an immunosuppressant action involving cell-mediated immunity, thus increasing the risks of infection during cytotoxic therapy, and may be a limiting factor in the chemotherapy of malignant disease. Oral mucositis is also common, and is often for many patients the worst side-effect of cytotoxic therapy. Hyperuricaemia may occur due to the breakdown of nuclear proteins, and the calcium balance may also be disturbed, leading to hypercalcaemia. Alopecia is another common side-effect, although it is often reversible when therapy is withdrawn. Nausea and vomiting may be severe with some cytotoxic drugs, and intense nausea without vomiting may also occur; these side-effects may cause some patients to refuse further therapy. Domperidone, nabilone, metoclopramide, ondansetron and tropisetron are of great value as anti-emetics during cytotoxic therapy (pp. 333 and 336). Cytotoxic drugs are, by their nature, extremely toxic to embryonic tissues, and should not be used during pregnancy.

Handling cytotoxic drugs

Some cytotoxic drugs, especially the alkylating agents and certain antibiotics, are known to cause contact dermatitis and irritation of the skin and mucous membranes. That should be taken as a general warning, as it is *not repeated* when referring to individual drugs. Commonsense precautions should always be taken during the preparation and administration of cytotoxic drugs, using protective clothing. Contact or spillage should be dealt with by immediate washing and dilution with water if it occurs. For detailed guidance, the Report on Guidelines for the handling of cytotoxic drugs should be consulted: *Pharmaceutical Journal*, 1983, 233: 230.

Great care must also be taken to avoid extravasation or leakage during intravenous injection, as severe local damage may occur. Extravasation can largely be avoided by a good injection technique, and careful choice of injection site with an adequate venous blood flow. A further injection of 10 ml or so of saline should be made after the drug has been injected. During an intravenous injection, the patient should be asked repeatedly about any discomfort or pain at the injection site.

If extravasation occurs or is suspected, the injection should be stopped immediately, but the needle or cannula should not be withdrawn, but used to remove as much of the injection fluid as possible. It may be advisable to inject some normal saline to reduce the concentration of the drug in the perivenous tissues.

Folinic acid may be injected in cases of methotrexate extravasation, sodium bicarbonate injection 8.4% may be of value in extravasation caused by doxorubicin, epirubicin and mustine, and the use of hyaluronidase has been suggested following the extravasation of the vinca alkaloids.

Points about cytotoxic drugs

(a) Four main types: alkylating agents, antimetabolites, cytoxic antibiotics and vinca alkaloids.
(b) All (except bleomycin and vincristine) depress bone marrow activity, and regular blood counts are necessary.
(c) Severe nausea and vomiting are common side-effects.
(d) Patients should be warned about temporary hair loss.
(e) Many are skin irritants; care must be taken to avoid contact with cytotoxic drugs or solutions.

ALKYLATING AGENTS

Mustine hydrochloride §

Mustine, also known as nitrogen mustard, was one of the first alkylating agents, but it is now used less frequently as better tolerated compounds have become available. It is used mainly in association with a vinca alkaloid in the treatment of Hodgkin's disease, especially when the condition has become resistant to irradiation therapy. Mustine has also been used in lymphosarcoma and related conditions, and in mycosis fungoides.

Mustine is very irritant, and is given by fast intravenous infusion as a dilute solution in normal saline as a single dose of 400 micrograms/kg, or as four daily doses of 100 micrograms/kg. Great care must be taken not to allow any of the solution to escape into the perivenous tissues or on to the skin. Mustine causes severe nausea and vomiting, and marked bone marrow depression.

Busulphan §

Brand name: Myleran §

Busulphan is orally active, and although chemically unrelated to the nitrogen mustards, has a similar but more selective depression of the bone marrow. It is used mainly in the treatment of chronic myeloid leukaemia, particularly in those patients who have become resistant to other forms of treatment.

Busulphan brings about a marked reduction in the excessive number of immature white cells, an increase in the haemoglobin level, and a considerable subjective improvement. It is given orally in doses of 2–4 mg daily initially, or on a basis of doses of 0.5–2 mg daily. Close haematological control is essential at all times, as marked myelosuppression may occur, with loss of bone marrow function. Hyperpigmentation may occur in some patients.

Carmustine §

Brand name: BiCNU §

Carmustine is an alkylating agent related to mustine, and is used as secondary therapy in Hodgkin's disease in combination with other drugs. It is also of value in multiple myeloma and some brain tumours. The dose is based on skin area, and an initial dose is 200 mg per square metre by slow intravenous injection every 6 weeks. Rapid infusion may cause an intensive but transient flushing of the skin and conjunctiva. Subsequent doses depend on the haematological response.

Side-effects include nausea and vomiting, often dose-related, but the most severe side-effect is delayed myelosuppression, and the effects on the bone marrow may be cumulative.

Chlorambucil §

Brand name: Leukeran §

Chlorambucil is an orally active alkylating agent. It is used in chronic lymphocytic leukaemia, in the long-term treatment of Hodgkin's disease and various malignant lymphomas, as well as in combined therapy. The average dose is 100–200 micrograms/kg daily for 6 weeks unless remission occurs earlier. Further suppressive treatment with lower doses of 100 micrograms/kg may be given daily, but a rest period is usually necessary between courses.

Nausea, gastrointestinal disturbances and rash may occur, but the depression of the bone marrow is less severe than that of related drugs. It is frequently reversible if the drug is withdrawn.

Cyclophosphamide §

Brand name: Endoxana §

Cyclophosphamide can be regarded as a pro-drug derivative of mustine, as toxicity and irritancy have been reduced by combination with an organic phosphorus derivative. Following administration, the combination is broken down by microsomal enzymes to release the active drug. Cyclophosphamide is used in the treatment of Hodgkin's disease, lymphosarcoma, carcinoma of the breast, lung and ovary, and in the control of various leukaemias. It also has marked immunosuppressant properties.

Cyclophosphamide may be given orally, by slow intravenous injection or fast-running intravenous infusion, or injected directly into body cavities when used for the treatment of malignant pleural or ascitic effusions.

Treatment may be commenced with a daily intravenous or oral dose of 100–300 mg daily, and up to a total dose of 6–8 g has been given, depending on the response or in doses of 2–6 mg/kg daily. Maintenance oral doses range from 100 to 300 mg daily. For the treatment of effusions, a single dose of 600 mg may be injected, but such localized injections may have little advantage over the standard intravenous therapy.

Side-effects of cyclophosphamide include nausea, haemorrhagic cystitis, bone marrow depression and loss of hair, although re-growth of hair usually occurs later. The haemorrhagic cystitis, which may be severe, is due to a locally toxic metabolite (acrolein), and can be reduced to some extent by a high fluid intake. It can be further controlled by the intravenous use of **mesna** (Uromitexan), given at the same time as cyclophosphamide, as it reacts with the acrolein and reduces its urothelial toxicity. Further treatment may be given orally. The dose of mesna is based on the dose of the cytotoxic agent.

Estramustine §

Brand name: Estracyt §

Estramustine represents a combination of mustine with oestradiol. Following oral administration, it is concentrated in prostatic tissues, and is used in the treatment of prostatic carcinoma, especially in conditions not responding to other therapy.

The initial dose is 560 mg daily with meals, followed by maintenance doses of 140 mg once or twice a day. It should not be taken with milk products.

Side-effects include nausea, angina and occasional gynaecomastia. Peptic ulcer, severe liver and cardiac disease are contraindications.

Ifosfamide §

Brand name: Mitoxana §

Ifosfamide is a derivative of cyclophosphamide, with similar actions, uses and side-effects. It is often used in combination with other drugs in multiple therapy. It is given by intravenous infusion in total doses of 8–10 per square metre, given in divided doses over 5 days.

Ifosfamide may cause haemorrhagic cystitis, and a high urinary output together with mesna administration (see cyclophosphamide) intravenously are essential.

Side-effects nausea, renal damage and alopecia. Central nervous system toxicity may result in confusion and require therapy.

Lomustine §

Brand name: CCNU §

Lomustine is an alkylating agent, but it may also have an inhibitory action on some essential enzymatic process. It is used in the treatment of brain and lung tumours, Hodgkin's disease and malignant melanoma, but usually as part of a multiple therapy scheme, or to supplement radiotherapy. When given as the sole therapy, the standard dose based on skin area is 120–130 mg per square metre as a single oral dose every 6–8 weeks, but smaller doses are used in combined therapy.

Side-effects include nausea and vomiting, followed by anorexia, which can be reduced by giving the drug in smaller doses at 2-week intervals.

The onset of bone marrow depression may be slow and its duration prolonged, and it may become irreversible after extended treatment.

Melphalan §

Brand name: Alkeran §

Melphalan represents a combination of mustine with an amino acid and the compound has the general cytotoxic properties of the nitrogen mustard group.

The drug is effective orally, and is used mainly in the treatment of myelomatosis and advanced breast cancer.

Myelomatosis is characterized by an excessive formation of plasma cells by the bone marrow, and this excess is not only damaging in itself, but may erode bone, and bring about skeletal changes. Melphalan can suppress this proliferation of cells by a general depression of bone marrow activity, and repeated courses of treatment may be necessary to obtain the maximum response. A rest period between each course is necessary to allow the blood count to recover.

In myelomatosis it is given orally in doses of 150 micrograms/kg or more daily for 4–6 days, together with prednisone 40 mg daily, repeated at intervals of 6 weeks. Larger doses are given in advanced breast cancer.

Melphalan is also used by the regional perfusion technique in the treatment of malignant melanoma. By this method a large dose of the drug, from 70–100 mg, may be circulated through the tumour.

Thiotepa §

Thiotepa is pharmacologically related to other alkylating agents, and has been used in the treatment of mammary and ovarian cancer, for superficial cancers of the bladder and to control pleural effusions. It has also been used by intrathecal injection in the control of malignant meningeal disease.

Thiotepa is less irritant than mustine, and may be given by intramuscular injection in divided doses of 15–30 mg three times a week for 2 weeks. A rest period of 6–8 weeks should elapse before a second course is given to allow the bone marrow activity to recover. For bladder instillation, a dose of 60 mg dissolved in 60 ml of water is used, and the solution should be retained for 2 hours.

For malignant pleural effusions, thiotepa has been given in doses of 10–30 mg by instillation at weekly intervals.

Side-effects are those common to most alkylating agents.

Treosulfan §

Treosulfan is an alkylating agent used in the treatment of ovarian carcinoma, often to supplement surgery. It is given in oral doses of 250 mg four times a day for 1 month, followed by a similar rest period before therapy is resumed. After the first course of treatment, the dose should be adjusted in accordance with the effects on bone marrow activity.

Side-effects include nausea and vomiting, and alopecia may occur. The drug is supplied in capsules, which should be swallowed whole, as if chewed, stomatitis may occur. Excessive doses may cause irreversible bone marrow depression.

ANTIMETABOLITES

Cytarabine §

Brand names: Cytosar §, Alexan §

Cytarabine, also known as cytosine arabinoside, functions as an antimetabolite by interference with the synthesis of deoxyribonucleic acid. It acts at the S-phase of the cell cycle. It is used in acute myeloblastic leukaemia and other leukaemias in children and adults. By the nature of its action, it is a powerful depressant of bone marrow function and haematological control during treatment is essential.

Cytarabine is used in initial doses of 2 mg/kg daily for 7–10 days, given by intravenous injection and subsequent doses are adjusted according to response. Intermittent therapy has also been used. Children tend to tolerate higher doses. Remission, once achieved, can be maintained by doses of 1 mg/kg given once or twice weekly by subcutaneous injection. As with many other cytotoxic drugs, cytarabine may induce severe hyperuricaemia following the destruction of the nuclei of the neoplastic cells.

Fluorouracil §

Fluorouracil acts by blocking the enzyme synthesis of DNA and RNA and so inhibits cell division.

It is used mainly in the palliative treatment of breast and gastrointestinal carcinoma, often in association with other drugs. It may be given orally in maintenance doses of 15 mg/kg weekly, or by intravenous injection and infusion. The dose is highly individual, but the total daily dose should not exceed 1 g. Folinic acid may enhance the cytoxic activity of fluoruracil, and it is given by slow intravenous injection in doses of 200 mg/m^2 immediately before the intravenous injection of the drug.

Side-effects include nausea, gastrointestinal disturbance, leucopenia and alopecia.

Mercaptopurine §

Brand name: Puri-Nethol §

Mercaptopurine is related to adenine, a constituent of nucleic acid, and acts by interfering with the synthesis of nucleic acid, and with the development and proliferation of the cancer cells. It has a valuable suppressive action in acute leukaemia and some cases of chronic myeloid leukaemia, particularly in children, but it is of no value in other malignant conditions.

Mercaptopurine is given orally in doses of 2.5 mg/kg daily, and there may be a time-lag of 3 weeks before any effect can be detected. It produces a remission of the disease of varying duration, but the response to a second course of treatment may be less dramatic.

Side-effects include liver damage and hyperuricaemia, and the dose should be reduced in patients receiving allopurinol as otherwise interference with the metabolism of mercaptopurine may occur.

Methotrexate §

Brand name: Matrex §

Methotrexate acts at the S-phase of the cell cycle, and inhibits the enzymatic synthesis of folic acid, purines and pyrimidine, and by blocking those metabolic processes it inhibits further cell development. Methotrexate is used in the treatment of a variety of neoplastic conditions, both alone, and as part of a multiple therapy scheme. Dosage varies accordingly.

It has been given alone for maintenance therapy in acute lymphoblastic leukaemia in doses of 15–30 mg/m^2 once or twice weekly, orally or by intramuscular injection. More intensive treatment with higher doses has been used in the treatment of various lymphomas, but in association with folinic acid, a scheme referred to as Folinic Acid Rescue. Folinic acid (Leucovorin; Refolinon) suppresses some of the side-effects of methotrexate, particularly myeolosuppression and mucositis, and treatment should be started 8–24 hours after beginning methotrexate therapy. It is given in divided doses up to a total of 120 mg over 24 hours by intramuscular or intravenous injection, followed by doses of 15 mg orally or by intramuscular injection 6-hourly for 48–72 hours.

Blood counts, renal and liver function tests are essential during methotrexate therapy. Pulmonary toxicity may also occur, and the development of cough or dyspnoea should be reported immediately. Treatment with NSAIDs should be avoided, as such agents decrease the excretion of methotrexate and so increase its toxic effects. The use of methotrexate in rheumatoid arthritis is referred to on page 427, and in psoriasis on page 539.

Jolivet J et al 1983 The pharmacology and clinical uses of methotrexate. New England Journal of Medicine 309: 1094–1104

Thioguanine §

Brand name: Lanvis §

Thioguanine has an action similar to that of mercaptopurine although its main use is in the treatment of acute myeloid leukaemia and chronic granulocytic leukaemia. It is active orally, and is given in doses of 2–2.5 mg/kg daily for 5–20 days, followed by maintenance doses of 2 mg/kg daily according to response. Thioguanine is a powerful myelosuppressive drug, and close haemotological control during therapy is essential.

CYTOTOXIC ANTIBIOTICS

Some cytotoxic antibiotics are available, which act mainly by preventing normal DNA and RNA replication and protein synthesis. They also have a radiomimetic action and combined radiotherapy should be avoided to reduce excessive toxicity. The side-effects of these drugs are similar to those of other cytotoxic agents.

Aclarubicin §

Brand name: Aclacin §

Aclarubicin is an anthracycline antibiotic with cytotoxic properties. It binds to DNA, and may prevent replication, and differs from doxorubicin in being less cardiotoxic, possibly because it is eliminated more rapidly. It is also less likely to cause alopecia. Aclarubicin is used mainly in relapsed acute non-lymphatic leukaemia and in patients resistant to other therapy, and is given in doses of 175–300 mg/m² by intravenous infusion over a period of 3–7 days. Maintenance doses of 25–100 mg/m² are given at intervals of 3–4 weeks according to the haematological response.

The cardiac efficiency should be monitored by ECG during treatment. Care is necessary in its use, as it is a tissue irritant.

Side-effects of nausea and vomiting appear to be dose-dependent, but leucopenia and thrombocytopenia may limit aclarubicin therapy.

Idarubicin § (Zavedos §) is a related drug with similar properties and uses, but used mainly to induce remission in acute non-lymphoblastic leukaemia.

Actinomycin D §

Brand name: Cosmegen §

Actinomycin D, also known as dactinomycin, inhibits cell growth by forming a stable complex with DNA. It is used mainly in the treatment of Wilm's tumour, rhabdomyosarcoma, and carcinoma of the uterus and testes. In Wilm's tumour, combined treatment with radiotherapy often evokes the best response. The standard adult dose is 500 micrograms by intravenous injection daily for 5 days. A second course may be given after an interval of 4 weeks. For children, doses of 15 micrograms/kg daily for 5 days have been given; alternatively a dose of 400–600 micrograms/m² body surface area may be injected daily for up to 5 days.

Actinomycin D is very irritant to the soft tissues and great care must be taken to avoid extravasation. **Toxic effects**, which may not be noted until a few days after a course of injections has stopped, include gastrointestinal disturbances, general malaise, severe bone marrow depression, skin eruptions and stomatitis.

Bleomycin §

Bleomycin acts by binding to and causing the breakdown of DNA strands. It differs from other antibiotics as it is taken up selectively by certain tissues, particularly the skin, and is mainly used in the treatment of squamous cell skin cancers. It is also useful in Hodgkin's disease and other lymphomas, in choriocarcinomas, mycosis fungoides and malignant effusions. It has the great advantage of not causing any significant depression of bone marrow activity, so the blood picture is not disturbed.

Bleomycin may be given by intramuscular or intravenous injection, and doses of 15–30 mg twice weekly have been used. Remissions in Hodgkin's disease have been maintained with weekly doses of 5 mg. In malignant effusions, a solution of 60 mg in 100 ml of saline is instilled after drainage.

The most serious **side-effect** is an occasional delayed progressive pulmonary fibrosis often associated with a total dose greater than 300 mg. There is also a risk with such patients of respiratory failure under general anaesthesia. Other side-effects include increased pigmentation of the skin as well as mucositis. Chill and fever and other hypersensitivity reactions may occur within a few hours, and as a precaution the simultaneous injection of hydrocortisone has been recommended.

Doxorubicin §

Doxorubicin appears to interfere with the synthesis of nucleic acids by forming a stable complex with DNA. It is most active at the S-phase. It has wide applications in the treatment of neoplastic conditions, and it has been used with success in acute leukaemia, lymphomas, soft tissue and osteogenic neoplasams, and in breast and lung carcinomas. It may be used alone, or as part of a multiple drug regimen.

A standard adult dose of doxorubicin, given by a free-running intravenous infusion is 60–75 mg/m^2 of body surface area, repeated at intervals of 3 weeks up to a total dose of not more than 500 mg/m^2. It has also been used for the treatment of papillary tumours of the bladder by the instillation of 100 ml of a solution containing 50 mg doxorubicin.

Side-effects of the drug are vomiting, buccal ulceration, myelodepression, tachycardia and alopecia, but the most serious side-effect, especially with higher doses, is cardiac myopathy that can lead to irreversible heart failure. Treatment should be carried out under ECG monitoring. Doxorubicin is largely excreted in the bile, and a raised bilirubin level indicates that dosage should be reduced. **Epirubicin** (Pharmorubicin) is an analogue said to be less cardiotoxic.

Mitomycin §

Mitomycin is a cytotoxic antibiotic that suppresses the synthesis of nucleic acids, and is most active at the late G and early S phases of the cell cycle. It has a wide range of activity, but is used mainly in breast and upper gastrointestinal cancer. It is given in doses of 10–20 mg/m^2 as a single dose by a fast-running intravenous infusion, repeated after 6–8 weeks. It has also been given in divided doses of 2 mg/m^2 daily for 5 days, repeated after a 2-day interval. Later doses are given when the leucocyte and platelet counts have returned to an acceptable level, as prolonged use may cause irreversible bone marrow damage. Mitomycin has also been used in bladder cancer by the instillation of a solution containing 10–40 mg of the drug. The **side-effects**, apart from myelosuppression, include lung fibrosis and renal damage.

Plicamycin §

Brand name: Mithracin §

Plicamycin, formerly known as mithramycin, and once used as a cytotoxic agent, retains a limited place in the treatment of hypercalcaemia of malignancy. The development of hypercalcaemia in such cases is due to the formation and release by the tumour of a peptide with properties similar to those of the parathyroid hormone, which both mobilizes bone calcium and reduces its renal excretion. The muscle weakness, nausea and vomiting of such hypercalcaemia can be relieved temporarily by plicamycin in doses of 25 micrograms/kg by intravenous infusion in 5% glucose solution, given daily for 3–4 days. The duration of response is variable, but bone marrow depression limits the course of treatment, and sodium etidronate (p. 398) is usually preferred.

Other **side-effects** of plicamycin are gastrointestinal disturbances and epistaxis.

VINCA ALKALOIDS AND OTHER PLANT PRODUCTS

The vinca alkaloids, obtained from a particular periwinkle inhibit cell division at the metaphase or M stage of chromosome separation, and so inhibit further cell development. They are irritant substances, and should be handled with great care. They should never be given by intrathecal injection, as such use has resulted in fatal neurological damage.

Vincristine §

Brand name: Oncovin §

Vincristine is of importance in the management of acute leukaemias, malignant lymphomas, Wilm's tumour and rhabdomycosarcoma. It is given by intravenous injection at weekly intervals in doses of 50–150 micrograms/kg in children, but in adults a weekly dose of 25–75 micrograms/kg has been given. Doses must be adjusted to individual need and toxic dose levels is narrow.

Vincristine is exceptional in causing very little myelodepression, but neuromuscular damage may occur, with peripheral paraesthesia, which may be dose limiting and recovery slow. Other **side-effects** include gastrointestinal disturbances, constipation, weight loss, polyuria and alopecia.

Vinblastine §

Brand name: Velbe §

Vinblastine has the actions and uses of vincristine, but is used mainly in the treatment of generalized Hodgkin's disease and lymphosarcoma. It is given by intravenous injection as an initial dose of 100 micrograms/kg, increasing at weekly intervals according to response up to a maximum dose of 500 micrograms/kg.

Vinblastine is less likely to cause neurotoxicity, but the bone marrow depression may be greater than with vincristine, and close haematological control is essential.

Vindesine §

Brand name: Eldesine §

Vindesine has the general properties of the vinca alkaloids, and is used mainly in acute lymphoblastic leukaemia in children, particularly that resistant to other resistant neoplasms.

Vindesine is given by intravenous injection in initial doses of 3 mg/m^2, increased at weekly intervals by increments of 0.5 mg/m^2 up to $4–5 \text{ mg/m}^2$, adjusted at all times according to granulocyte and platelet counts. **Side-effects** are similar to those of the other vinca alkaloids.

Etoposide §

Brand name: Vepesid §

Etoposide is a semi-synthetic derivative of the plant substance podophyllotoxin and inhibits DNA synthesis at the late S and G_2 phases. It is used in the treatment of lymphomas, small-cell carcinoma of the bronchi, and in some testicular carcinomas, sometimes in association with other cytotoxic drugs. Etoposide may be given initially by intravenous infusion in doses of $60–120 \text{ mg/m}^2$ daily for 5 days, repeated at intervals of 21 days.

The drug is irritant, and care must be taken to avoid extravasation. Etoposide may also be given orally in doses double those used intravenously.

Side-effects are myelodepression, requiring laboratory control, nausea, vomiting and alopecia.

Paclitaxel §▼

Brand name: Taxol §▼

Paclitaxel is a new and potent cytotoxic agent obtained from the bark of the Pacific yew. Its action differs from that of other anticancer drugs, as it acts by promoting and stabilizing the production of microtubules. Such stabilization disrupts mitosis and leads to cell death. At present, paclitaxel is used for the treatment of metastatic ovarian cancer where platinum therapy has failed, but careful premedication of the patient to avoid hypersensitivity reactions is necessary. Dexamethasone 20 mg is given 12 and 6 hours previously, and chlorpheniramine and cimetidine by intravenous injection an hour previous to treatment. Paclitaxel is given in doses of 175 mg/m^2 by intravenous infusion over 3 hours, followed by subsequent doses at 3-week intervals according to tolerance. The diluted infusion fluid should be used within 3 hours of preparation, and not be refrigerator stored.

Bone marrow suppression, mainly severe neutropenia, is the dose-limiting toxicity factor, and frequent monitoring of blood counts is necessary. Treatment should not be renewed until neutrophil and platelet counts have returned to satisfactory levels. The use of paclitaxel requires care under expert supervision, as hypersensitivity reactions may require treatment and withdrawal of therapy.

OTHER CYTOTOXIC DRUGS
Aminoglutethimide §

Brand name: Orimeton §

Aminoglutethimide is an enzyme inhibitor and blocks the production of steroids by the adrenal cortex. It also inhibits the conversion of androgens to oestrogens in the peripheral tissues. It functions as a hormone antagonist, and is used in the treatment of post-menopausal metastatic breast cancer in doses of 250 mg twice daily for 1 week, later increased to four times a day. It is also used in advanced prostatic carcinoma. Much larger doses are given in Cushing's syndrome associated with malignancy. Because of its general inhibitory action on the adrenal cortex, it is essential to give supportive corticosteroid therapy during aminoglutethimide therapy.

Side-effects include drowsiness, drug fever and skin reactions. Aminoglutethimide has an enzyme induction effect on the liver, and the doses of some other drugs such as the oral anticoagulants may have to be increased.

Amsacrine §

Brand name: Amsidine §

Amsacrine is a synthetic drug with the cytotoxic action of doxorubicin, but used mainly in the treatment of refractory acute leukaemia. It appears to act by inhibiting the synthesis of DNA by a binding mechanism. Amsacrine is given by slow intravenous infusion as a solution in 5% glucose (no other diluent is suitable) in doses of 90 mg/m^2 daily for 5 days initially to induce remission, and repeated at intervals of 2–4 weeks according to response. Subsequent maintenance doses of about one-third of the induction dose may be given at intervals of 3–4 weeks, based on the degree of recovery of the granulocyte and platelet counts. Close laboratory control is essential during amsacrine therapy.

   Side-effects apart from myelodepression, which may be dose-limiting include gastrointestinal disturbances, mucositis and occasional epileptiform episodes. Amsacrine may cause hypokalaemia and cardiac arrhythmias, and monitoring of electrolytes has been recommended. Care is necessary in renal and hepatic dysfunction.

Buserelin §

Brand name: Suprefact §

Buserelin is a synthetic analogue of gonadorelin, the gonado-trophin-releasing hormone of the hypothalamus (see p. 379). It is used in the treatment of metastatic prostatic carcinoma on the basis that it initially stimulates the release of the luteinizing hormone, and that stimulation results in a temporary increase in testosterone secretion by the testes. Following that initial stimula-tion, a secondary inhibition of luteinizing hormone occurs, with a subsequent inhibition of testosterone secretion, and relief of symptoms.

   Buserelin is given initially by subcutaneous injection in doses of 500 micrograms 8-hourly for 7 days, after which doses of 100 micrograms are given by intranasal spray up to six times a day. It is also used in the treatment of endometriosis (p. 454).

   A **side-effect** of buserelin is an increase of tumour growth during the first 2–3 weeks of treatment, which may have the undesirable effect of causing pain and spinal cord compression (p. 296).

Cisplatin §

Brand names: Neoplatin §, Platosin §

Cisplatin has an exceptional chemical structure, as it contains platinum bound up in an organic complex. It appears to have an action similar to that of the alkylating agents, and is used mainly in metastatic ovarian and testicular tumours, often as secondary therapy in association with other cytotoxic drugs in resistant conditions. It is given by intravenous injection in doses of 50–120 mg/m² body surface area every 3 or 4 weeks.

Cisplatin has a cumulative nephrotoxic action, as well as ototoxic and myelosuppressive effects. Its use requires care, with monitoring of the creatinine clearance rate. *Severe nausea and vomiting* almost invariably follow cisplatin therapy, and, if uncontrolled by anti-emetic drugs, may limit treatment.

Carboplatin (Paraplatin §) is a derivative of cisplatin, with which side-effects such as nausea and vomiting are less severe, and the ototoxic and nephrotoxic effects are also reduced. A second course of treatment should be delayed for some weeks.

Crisantaspase §

Brand name: Erwinase §

Some malignant cells are unable to synthesize asparagine, and so utilize exogenous sources of that essential amino acid. The development of such cells can be prevented by crisantaspase, which is an enzyme that breaks down asparagine, and is thought to act specifically at the G_1 stage of the cell cycle. It is used mainly to induce remission of acute lymphoblastic leukaemia in children, after pre-treatment with vincristine and prednisolone. It is given in doses of 1000 units/kg by slow intravenous injection daily for 10 days, or by intramuscular injection in doses of 6000 units/m² every third day for nine doses. Not more than 2 ml of the injection solution should be injected at any one site.

Side-effects include anaphylactic reactions and hyperglycaemia, and skin tests for sensitivity with 2 unit doses should be carried out before treatment, and before re-treatment after an interval.

Cyproterone §

Brand name: Cyprostat §

Cyproterone blocks androgen receptors, and so has an anti-androgen action. It also has some direct inhibitory action on the production of testicular androgens. Cyproterone is used for the symptomatic treatment of metastatic prostatic carcinoma, often in association with other drugs such as buserelin, and is given in doses of 100 mg three times a day after food. Care is necessary in hepatic disease.

Formestane §▼

Brand Name: Lentaron §▼

Formestane is a steroid derivative that specifically inhibits aromatase, the enzyme involved in the conversion of androgen to oestrogens. It has a prolonged action, as it binds irreversibly with the enzyme, and oestrogen production is suspended until new enzyme is biosynthesized. Its cytostatic action is a result of oestrogen deficiency. It is used in advanced breast cancer in post-menopausal women, and is given in doses of 250 mg by deep intragluteal injection at intervals of 2 weeks. Care should be taken to avoid intravascular injection. Side-effects include rash, pruritus, pain and irritation at the injection site (which should be varied). Headache, dizziness and vaginal bleeding may also occur. It has a more selective action than aminoglutethimide, and supplementary corticosteroid therapy is unnecessary.

Coombes R C et al 1992. A new treatment for post-menopausal patients with breast cancer. European Journal of Cancer 28: 1941–1945

Flutamide §

Brand name: Drogenil §

Flutamide is an androgen-blocking agent, and inhibits the uptake and binding of androgens by target organs. On that account it is used for the treatment of advanced prostatic carcinoma in patients who have not responded to, or cannot tolerate other forms of anti-androgen therapy. It is usually given in association with a LHRH agonist such as goserelin. Flutamide is given in doses of 250 mg three times a day, *preferably 3 days before* LHRH therapy is commenced, in order to reduce the initial 'flare' response.

A frequent **side-effect** of flutamide is gynaecomastia, which may occur less often with combined goserelin treatment. Gastrointestinal disturbances may occur, but liver dysfunction is a risk, and periodic hepatic tests should be carried out if treatment is prolonged. An increase in the prothrombin time may occur in patients receiving warfarin, and adjustment of the dose of anticoagulant may be necessary.

Goserilin §

Brand name: Zoladex §

Goserelin is a synthetic analogue of gonadorelin (LHRH), the gonadotrophin-releasing hormone of the hypothalamus and, like buserelin, it is used in the treatment of prostatic carcinoma. Goserelin is given in a dose of 3.6 mg by the subcutaneous injection of a special depot product from which the drug is slowly released at a rate that permits subsequent injections at intervals of 4 weeks.

Goserelin is also used in similar doses for the treatment of advanced breast cancer in pre-menopausal women, as it inhibits oestrogen production by the same mechanism as it inhibits androgen production, i.e., via depression of LH secretion. With extended treatment, oestrogen levels are similar to those of the menopause. It has no place in the treatment of post-menopausal breast cancer, as ovarian oestrogen production has already ceased.

Like buserelin, goserelin causes an initial rise in the plasma testosterone level, which may be associated with some increase in bone pain. Other **side-effects** are hot flushes and rash, but are usually mild and transient.

Leuprorelin § (dose: 3.75 mg monthly)

Brand name: Prostap SR §

Leuprorelin is a potent analogue of the gonadotrophic releasing hormones (GnRH) of the pituitary gland, which is ultimately concerned with the production of androgens (p. 364) and is used in the treatment of advanced prostatic cancer. Many such cancers are androgen-dependent, and medical treatment is with oestrogens that depress androgen activity. Oestrogen therapy has some undesirable **side-effects**, but a similar action can be achieved paradoxically by depressing GnRH activity with large doses of that hormone as leuprorelin. The initial effect of leuprorelin is to bring about a temporary rise in plasma testosterone levels which causes an exacerbation of symptoms (the 'flare' effect), but the sustained action of the drug inhibits subsequent testosterone production which results in a chemical castration. In prostatic cancer, treatment with leuprorelin brings about symptomatic relief, a reduction in bone pain, and in many cases a regression of the cancerous condition. Prostap SR is a sustained release product of leuprorelin, and is given as a dose of 3.75 mg by subcutaneous injection every 4 weeks, usually in the abdominal wall. Patients should be warned about the 'flare' effect, which may cause for a time an increase in bone pain and urinary difficulties, but such problems can be reduced by giving an anti-androgen before and during the first 2–3 weeks of treatment. Other side-effects are sweating, flushing, impotence, oedema and fatigue.

Pentostatin §▼

Brand name: Nipent §▼

Pentostatin was originally obtained as a fungal metabolite, and was found to have a cytotoxic action as a potent inhibitor of the enzyme adenosine deaminase, and could inhibit RNA synthesis and cause DNA damage. It is used in the treatment of hairy cell leukaemia, and may evoke a more rapid response as compared with the extended treatment necessary with interferon. It is given in doses of 4 mg/m^2 every other week by bolus intravenous injection or by intravenous infusion after dilution. Treatment should be discontinued if response has not occurred after 6 months. Frequent monitoring of the blood count is necessary, and treatment should be suspended if the neutrophil count falls below 200 cells/mm^3.

Procarbazine §

Brand name: Natulan §

Procarbazine is a methylhydrazine derivative of primary value in the treatment of Hodgkin's disease (lymphadenoma), as well as in other lymphomas, and in conditions resistant to other therapy, including small cell carcinoma of the bronchi. It is given orally in doses of 50 mg initially, rising by 50 mg daily up to 300 mg daily in divided doses. Maintenance doses of 50–150 mg daily may then be given up to a total dose of at least 6 g. Regular blood counts are essential during procarbazine therapy.

Side-effects are myelodepression, nausea and loss of appetite. The development of an allergic skin reaction is an indication of withdrawal of the drug. The taking of alcohol may cause a disulfiram like reaction (p. 9).

Tamoxifen §

Brand names: Nolvadex §, Tamofen §

Tamoxifen is a synthetic oestrogen antagonist, and acts as a cytotoxic agent by blocking receptor sites in oestrogen-dependent tumours. It is now regarded as a first-line drug in the treatment of all stages of breast cancer, and is given in doses of 10 mg twice a day, subsequently increased as required up to 20 mg twice a day. It was first used only in post-menopausal women with metastases, but it is now in use for pre-menopausal women with breast cancer. It may delay the development of metastases and prolong survival.

Side-effects are hot flushes, dizziness, vaginal bleeding and gastrointestinal disturbances. Amenorrhoea may occur with pre-menopausal patients receiving tamoxifen. The drug may also cause some hypercalcaemia at the initial stages of treatment, especially when metastases are present. An increase in bone pain may precede the initial response, and nurses can help by encouraging patients to continue treatment. Tamoxifen markedly increases the activity of warfarin and related anticoagulants, and close control is necessary when tamoxifen is given to or withdrawn from patients receiving oral anticoagulants.

 Furr B J A, Jordan V C 1984 The pharmacology and clinical use of tamoxifen. Pharmacology and Therapeutics 25: 127–205

Other cytotoxic drugs used less frequently include **dacarbazine** § (DTIC), **hydroxyurea** § (Hydrea §) and **mitozantrone** § (Novantrone §). The use of oestrogens in prostatic carcinoma is referred to on page 382.

IMMUNOSTIMULANTS

A few natural substances have an influence in stimulating or augmenting the immunological defence system of the body (see p. 557) and are useful in some forms of malignancy.

Interferon §

Brand names: Intron A §, Roferon A §, Wellferon §

The interferons (alfa, beta and gamma) are glycoproteins produced in mammalian cells, and are part of the natural defence system of the body, particularly against viral infections. They also have a modulating influence on the immune system, but the mode of action is not clear. Interferons are species specific, and only human interferon is of potential therapeutic value, of which supplies are extremely limited. The supply problem has been overcome by recombinant DNA technology, using human lymphoblastoid cells cultured with *Escherichia coli*. Recent studies have shown that human alfa-interferon has some antitumour properties, and it is used in the treatment of hairy-cell leukaemia, chronic myeloid leukaemia, some AIDS-associated Kaposi's sarcoma and genital warts (condylomata acuminata). A standard dose is 2 million units/m^2 by subcutaneous injection three times a week, but in chronic myeloid leukaemia doses of 4–5 million units daily until the white cell count returns to normal, followed by doses on alternate days, are continued indefinitely. Genital warts are treated with local injection of 1 million units three times a week for 3 weeks.

Side-effects of alfa-interferon include influenza-like symptoms, anorexia and lethargy. Myelodepression may also occur, and care is necessary in renal, hepatic or cardiovascular dysfunction.

It is of interest that beta-interferon is being investigated for possible use in multiple sclerosis (MS).

Interleukins

The interleukins, sometimes referred to as cytokines or lymphokines, are a group of polypeptides, some of which are involved in the complex hormonal control of the immune response.

Interleukin-2 is a lymphokinine which stimulates the production of both T-lymphocytes and interferon, and activates killer cells. Aldesleukin §▼ (Proleukin) is a recombinant form that may be useful in the treatment of metastatic renal cell carcinoma, but it is a highly toxic drug used only in specialist units.

RADIOPHARMACEUTICALS

As some radioactive drugs have been used to a limited extent in the treatment of malignancy, it is convenient to consider the group here.

Because of the potential dangers of radioactive substances, special precautions must be taken during storage and use. Storage must be in containers and in areas designed for the purpose, adequately shielded and under the control of a duly qualified individual. During the handling of radiopharmaceuticals, nurses and all others concerned must wear suitable protective clothing, and take other measures to prevent unnecessary exposure to radiation. Considerable care is also essential in disposing of the excreta of patients undergoing treatment with radiopharmaceuticals. Such disposal is under official control, but any local hospital regulations for the control of the use and disposal of radioactive substances must also be strictly observed.

Chromium-51

Chromium-51 is used as sodium chromate to label red cells in the circulation and to estimate gastrointestinal bleeding.

Cobalt-57 (^{57}Co) and Cobalt-58 (^{58}Co)

As the metal cobalt forms part of the structure of vitamin B_{12}, synthetic vitamin B_{12} containing cobalt-57, referred to as cyanocobalamin (^{57}Co) (which has a short half-life) is used to measure the absorption of cyanocobalamin in the diagnosis of pernicious anaemia, based on the radioactivity of the urine. A mixture of ^{57}Co and ^{58}Co is used to differentiate between failure of absorption because of the absence of the intrinsic factor (p. 496) and that due to poor ileal absorption.

Gallium-67

Gallium-67, as gallium citrate, is taken up and concentrated in some lymphatic tumours, and is used for tumour visualization by scanning techniques.

Gold-198

Gold-198 has been used as a colloidal suspension of metallic particles in the treatment of pleural and other malignant effusions, including those associated with rheumatoid arthritis.

Indium-111

Indium-111 as a complex with bleomycin and other substances has been used for tumour scanning, the investigation of the lymphatic system and in cerebrospinal fluid studies.

Indium-113

Indium-113 is an isotope with a short half-life. It is used as a complex with mannitol and other substances for the scanning of the lungs and other organs.

Iodine-131

Iodine-131 is used as sodium iodide in the diagnosis of thyroid functions and treatment of thyrotoxicosis. As it is taken up selectively by the gland, large doses are sometimes used in the treatment of thyroid carcinoma. As iodinated serum albumin it is used in the determination of plasma volume.

Iron-59

Iron-59 is used as the ferric citrate in the determination of iron absorption and utilization. The amount absorbed can be measured by whole body radiation tests.

Phosphorus-32

As sodium phosphate, this isotope is taken up by rapidly growing tissues such as the bone marrow. It reduces the production of red cells and has been used in the treatment of polycythaemia vera. It is also used in diagnosis and location of tumours of the eye and brain.

Technetium-99

This isotope is generated from the metal molybdenum. It has a half-life of about 6 hours, and can be given in relatively high doses, and is widely used. Following intravenous injection of the freshly prepared isotope, localization in tumours of the brain and many other tissues can be easily detected.

Xenon-133

This radioactive gas is used by intravenous injection as a solution in saline. It is rapidly excreted by the lungs, and is used to determine pulmonary function.

Yttrium-90

Yttrium is used as a suspension of colloidal yttrium silicate, in the treatment of malignant ascites.

Anticoagulants and haemostatics

Blood is a fluid that is as complex in the nature of its constituents as
it is in the scope of its functions. Those functions include the
maintenance and repair of body tissues, the transport of nutrients,
the maintenance of body temperature and the elimination of waste
products and foreign substances. The main constituents of blood
are the plasma, red and white blood cells and platelets. In addition,
the plasma contains various factors concerned with both the initiation and prevention of blood clotting. Some minor clotting occurs
as part of the natural repair process of the vascular system, and the
haemostasis or blood clotting that follows severe tissue damage is a
protective mechanism to reduce blood loss. Haemostasis is initiated by the aggregation of blood platelets at the damaged site
under the influence of thromboxane A_2 (p. 421). The platelets
adhere both to the damaged tissues and to each other, and form a
plug of platelets that reduces immediate blood loss. Such plug
formation in turn initiates a cascade of reactions that involves a
variety of blood factors and results in the formation of a stable clot
at the damaged site. The most important factors are fibrinogen
(Factor I), prothrombin (Factor II), thromboplastin (Factor III) and
calcium (Factor IV). Thromboplastin when released after tissue
damage forms a complex with calcium and prothrombin to form
thrombin, which in turn acts on fibrinogen, one of the soluble
proteins of the plasma, and leads to the formation of an insoluble
and stable fibrin clot. Subsidiary blood factors include Factor VIII,
which if absent causes haemophilia A, and Factor IX (the
Christmas factor) which is absent in haemophilia B, and vitamin
K. The process may be summarized very briefly thus:

$$\text{Prothrombin} + \text{thromboplastin} + \text{calcium} \longrightarrow \text{thrombin}$$
$$\text{Thrombin} + \text{fibrinogen} \longrightarrow \text{fibrin}$$

The fibrin forms a matrix upon which the blood clot is built up.

Normally the clotting of blood in the vascular system is prevented by heparin and other anticoagulating factors in the plasma, (such as antithrombin, which antagonizes any circulating thrombin), as well as by the inhibition of platelet aggregation by prostacyclin, but intravascular clotting may occur as a result of damage to, or alterations in the vascular epithelium especially under conditions associated with reduced blood flow. In such conditions, thrombosis may be initiated by the adhesion of blood platelets to a damaged site, with the liberation of thromboxane A_2 (TXA_2) (pp. 311 and 421), which stimulates platelet aggregation. Such aggregations act as a focal point for the deposition of fibrin and the development of an intravascular clot.

If this process takes place in one of the coronary arteries the supply of blood to the heart is restricted, the local concentration of thrombin may rise again and the dangerous condition of coronary thrombosis may result.

Thrombosis may also occur in the deep veins of the legs, especially during prolonged bed rest, and there is the added danger that the clot may become detached at a later stage, and may eventually cause a pulmonary embolism. A superficial thrombosis, as in varicose veins, is far less dangerous.

Much remains to be known about blood clot formation, and it is worth remembering that as with insulin and diabetes, the control of an abnormality may be possible long before the causes of the abnormality are fully understood.

Points about anticoagulants

(a) Two types: heparin products, given by injection and having a rapid action, and slow-acting oral anticoagulants.

(b) Standard heparin given intravenously; under laboratory control: some fractionated or low-molecular-weight heparins are injected subcutaneously and have a longer action that permits single daily doses.

(c) Effects of heparin can be neutralized rapidly by an injection of protamine; excessive response to oral anticoagulants controlled by phytomenadione (vitamin K_1).

Scott A K 1989 Prescribing anticoagulants. Prescribers' Journal
29: 24–30

Heparin § (dose: 10 000 units intravenously; 5000 units by subcutaneous injection)

Brand names: Monoparin §, Unihep § (intravenous), Calciparine §, Minihep §, Uniparin § (subcutaneous)

Heparin is the anticoagulant present in mammalian tissues, and for use it is extracted from animal lung and intestinal mucosa. It is an acidic polysaccharide, and its wide-ranging action is mediated via antithrombin III, which functions as a heparin co-factor. Antithrombin III is the major inhibitor of thrombin, activated Factor X(Xa) and other blood-clotting factors, and heparin increases the rate of such inhibition in a dose-dependent manner. Heparin, also referred to as standard or unfractionated heparin is a high molecular weight polysaccharide, but it can be depolymerized by enzymatic or chemical manipulation to yield fractions of low molecular weight. These fractions retain some of the properties of heparin although they have less effect on blood platelet aggregation, but they have a longer action than standard heparin, and have value in the prophylactic treatment of venous thrombosis. They are given by subcutaneous injection once a day for 5 days and, as is the case with subcutaneous injection of standard heparin, the usual laboratory monitoring is not required. The dose varies from 2500–3500 units according to the product used.

Heparin is widely used in the treatment of deep vein thrombosis, disseminated intravascular clotting, and the prophylaxis of postoperative thrombosis, and is given by intravenous injection in initial doses of 10 000 units or more, followed by maintenance doses of 5000–10 000 units every 4–6 hours.

Hirsh J 1991 Heparin. New England Journal of Medicine 324:
1565–1574

Alternatively, heparin may be given by continuous intravenous infusion in doses of 20 000–40 000 units over 24 hours. Maintenance doses are based on laboratory reports of the activated partial thromboplastin time. If a later change to oral anticoagulant therapy is intended, such treatment should be commenced at the same time as heparin therapy, and the latter withdrawn after 3 days, subject to laboratory control.

For the prophylaxis of postoperative deep-vein thrombosis and pulmonary embolism, especially in patients at risk, heparin, often as heparin calcium, is given by subcutaneous injection into the abdominal wall in doses 5000 units 2 hours before surgery, and repeated every 12 hours for 7 days, or until the patient is mobile. In such cases, the risk of heparin-induced haemorrhage is slight, and laboratory control of dose is not normally necessary. Such prophylactic use is not recommended in ophthalmic and neuro-surgery, because of the risks of ocular or cerebral haemorrhage. Heparin is contraindicated in severe liver disease and severe hypertension, in peptic ulcer and in any haemorrhagic disorders.

Heparin is also used to prevent the intravascular thrombosis that may occur during the extended drip infusion of intravenous fluids by the addition of 1 unit per ml of such fluid. Heparin also has a non-therapeutic use, as in small amounts of 50–200 units it is used to flush out and maintain the potency of catheters and cannulae (**Hep-Flush, Heplok, Hepsal**).

Side-effects of heparin include bruising, haemorrhage, transient alopecia, and hypersensitivity reactions. Osteoporosis has occurred after prolonged use.

Platelet counts should be measured in patients receiving heparin for more than 5 days, and treatment withdrawn if thrombocytopenia develops. Haemorrhage due to slight overdose can be controlled by withdrawal of the drug, but if severe, a rapid reversal of the anticoagulant action can be obtained by the intravenous injection of protamine sulphate, which is a specific antidote.

Protamine is a simple protein obtained from salmon sperm, and is given as a 1% solution in doses depending on the degree of heparin overdose, (as 1 mg will neutralize 80–100 units of heparin), up to a total dose of 50 mg, if given within 15 minutes of overdose. Lower doses are adequate after a longer interval, as heparin is rapidly excreted, and paradoxically, an overdose of protamine has an anticoagulant effect.

Some low-molecular-weight heparin fractions have a more selective action on certain stages of the coagulation process. They also have a longer action, and when used prophylactically by subcutaneous injection, the usual laboratory control of heparin administration are not necessary.

Prandoni P et al 1992 Subcutaneous low-molecular-weight heparin compared with intravenous standard heparin in the treatment of proximal vein thrombosis. Lancet 339: 441–445

Enoxaparin § (dose: 20–40 mg daily by subcutaneous injection)

Brand name: Clexane §

Enoxaparin is a low-molecular-weight heparin with a more specific and prolonged action than standard heparin that permits once-daily dosage. It has a higher ratio of anti-Factor Xa, but has little effect on platelet function or the bleeding time.

It is used for the prophylaxis of thromboembolic disorders associated with orthopaedic and general surgery, and in the prevention of clot formation during haemodialysis. Enoxaparin is given by *subcutaneous* injection in doses of 20–40 mg daily, the first dose being given 2–12 hours pre-operatively according to the degree of risk. During haemodialysis, a dose of 1 mg/kg is given through the arterial line at the beginning of the session. Overdose, as with heparin, can be neutralized by protamine. Care is necessary in patients with hepatic insufficiency, and with those taking platelet aggregation inhibitors, oral anticoagulants and NSAIDs.

Dalteparin (Fragmin), tinzaparin (Innohep▼, Longiparin▼) and danaparoid (Orgaran▼) are related products given by subcutaneous injection, and not requiring laboratory control when used prophylactically.

Ancrod § (dose: 2–3 units/kg by intravenous infusion)

Brand name: Arvin §

Ancrod is a glycoprotein with enzymatic properties, obtained from viper venom. It is used in the treatment of deep-vein and retinal thrombosis, and in the prophylaxis of postoperative thrombosis, as it brings about a breakdown of microparticles of fibrin in the blood, which are then removed by fibrinolysis.

Ancrod is given by intravenous infusion in doses of 2–3 units/kg in intravenous saline solution over 6–8 hours or more, followed by maintenance doses of 2 units/kg every 12 hours. Initial doses must be given very slowly to avoid an increase in blood viscosity, and the blood fibrinogen levels should be monitored daily. Ancrod is also given by subcutaneous injection for prophylaxis in doses of 2 units/kg initially, with doses of 1 unit/kg daily for 4 days or more. Alternatively, a single dose of 280 units may be given subcutaneously immediately after operation, followed by daily doses of 70 units for 4–7 days. Resistance may develop after a second course of ancrod.

Side-effects and contraindications of ancrod are similar to those of heparin. Severe haemorrhage requires the intravenous use of a specific antiserum (ancrod antidote) of which 1 ml will neutralize 70 units of ancrod. An initial dose of 0.2 ml of the antidote is given subcutaneously, and if there is no reaction after 30 minutes, a second dose of 0.8 ml is given by intramuscular injection, followed by a dose of 1 ml intravenously. In life-threatening haemorrhage, ancrod antidote should be given intravenously without a previous test dose, but as the antidote may cause an anaphylactic shock, adrenaline, an antihistamine and hydrocortisone must always be available whenever ancrod antidote is used. If the antidote is not available, fibrinogen or fresh whole blood or plasma should be given. Dextran should not be used during ancrod therapy.

ORAL ANTICOAGULANTS

Oral anticoagulants are synthetic substances that differ from heparin in both nature and mode of action, as they function as vitamin K antagonists. That vitamin is essential for the formation in the liver of prothrombin (Factor II) as well as Factors VII, IX and X. The oral anticoagulants act by interfering with the biosynthesis of those factors and they may also inhibit the further synthesis of vitamin K. They therefore have an indirect anticoagulant action that is slow in onset (36–48 hours), as the plasma level of circulating clotting factors has to fall by normal metabolism before the inhibition of prothrombin synthesis can exert its effects. They are not suitable for use in cerebral thrombosis or peripheral occlusion.

In practice, when an immediate anticoagulant action is required, therapy is commenced with both heparin and an orally active drug, and the former continued for 48 hours, after which heparin may be discontinued, as by that time the oral anticoagulant drug should have become effective. In all cases, laboratory control of dose in relation to the prothrombin time in terms of the International Normalized Ratio (INR) is essential throughout treatment. Omission of dose requires re-assessment of the prothrombin time. All patients receiving anticoagulant therapy should carry the official treatment card.

Warfarin § (dose: 3–10 mg daily)

Brand name: Marevan §

Warfarin is a coumarin derivative that is widely used as an orally active anticoagulant in the treatment and prevention of venous thrombosis and pulmonary embolism, in the treatment of transient cerebral ischaemia, and to prevent the formation of clots on prosthetic heart valves. It is also used prophylactically against deep-vein thrombosis in high-risk surgery.

Warfarin is usually given as an initial dose of 10 mg daily for 3 days, and subsequent doses are often designed to maintain the prothrombin time at about $2-2\frac{1}{2}$ times that of normal, with a higher ratio in deep-vein thrombosis and pulmonary embolism. Maintenance doses range from 3 to 9 mg daily, best taken at the same time every day. Warfarin is usually well tolerated, and is often regarded as a first-choice drug, but it should be used with care in hepatic and renal disease, and after surgery, and is contraindicated in pregnancy, severe hypertension, or any potentially haemorrhagic condition.

Side-effects include nausea, alopecia and skin reactions, but the most serious side-effect is haemorrhage from almost any organ of the body. Early signs of overdose are bleeding from the gums and the presence of erythrocytes in the urine, but severe haemorrhage requires withdrawal of the drug, and the administration by slow intravenous injection of phytomenadione (vitamin K_1) in doses of 2.5–20 mg, together with fresh plasma. In less severe overdose, phytomenadione may be given orally in doses of 2–20 mg.

Phytomenadione (also known as vitamin K_1) has a slow action that may take up to 12 hours to develop, and may persist for as long as 2 weeks or more.

The action of warfarin may be modified by many other drugs, including aspirin and anti-inflammatory drugs such as the NSAIDs. The anticoagulant action is reduced by rifampicin and griseofulvin, and potentiated by clofibrate and related drugs, by sulphonamides and some antibiotics, and combined treatment requires care.

(Note. *Vitamin K_1 is a modified form of vitamin K; standard forms of vitamin K such as menadiol are much less effective than K_1 in the treatment of overdose with oral anticoagulants.*)

Nicoumalone § (dose: 1–12 mg daily)

Brand name: Sinthrome §

Nicoumalone is a coumarin derivative with the actions, uses and side-effects of warfarin. Dosage depends, as with warfarin, on the prothrombin time, but a standard scheme of dose is a single dose of 8–12 mg on the first day of treatment, 4–8 mg on the second day, followed by maintenance doses of 1–8 mg or more daily, under laboratory control. Phytomenadione is indicated in haemorrhage due to nicoumalone overdose.

Phenindione § (dose: 25–200 mg daily)

Brand name: Dindevan §

Phenindione was once the most widely used of the oral anticoagulants, but it has now been largely replaced by warfarin. It is mainly used for patients who cannot tolerate coumarin derivatives. Treatment is commenced with a dose of 200 mg, followed by 100 mg on the second day, with maintenance doses of 50–150 mg according to laboratory reports of the prothrombin time.

It may colour the urine pink. Phenindione may cause hypersensitivity reactions, ulcerative colitis, renal and hepatic damage, and agranulocytosis. It may appear in breast milk, and should be avoided during breast-feeding.

PLATELET AGGREGATION INHIBITORS

Conventional anticoagulants are of value in the prophylaxis and treatment of venous thrombosis, but have little influence on thrombus formation on the arterial side of the circulation. Increasing attention has been turned towards drugs that can inhibit thrombus formation due to platelet aggregation in the arterial circulation by inhibiting platelet adhesion.

Platelet aggregation is normally controlled by a balance between thromboxane A_2 (TXA$_2$) (p. 422) which is present in the platelets, and is an inducer of aggregation, and prostacyclin, found mainly in the vascular endothelium, which has the reverse action. Platelets adhere to damaged areas of the endothelium and release TXA$_2$ and so start the chain of reactions that leads to the formation of a thrombus.

Aspirin has an antiplatelet action by irreversibly inhibiting platelet cyclo-oxygenase, and so preventing the synthesis of TXA$_2$, whereas the activity of prostacyclin is less affected. The inhibition lasts for the life-span of the platelet, so new platelets must be formed before the aggregation ability is restored.

Aspirin is being used for the secondary prophylaxis of myocardial infarction and cerebral vascular disease, but the dose likely to evoke the optimum response has yet to be determined. At present it is given in doses varying from 75–300 mg daily or on alternate days. It is also being used for the prevention of occlusion after by-pass surgery.

Dipyridamole § (dose: 300–600 mg daily)

Brand name: Persantin §

Dipyridamole is given in doses of 100–200 mg three times a day, and its antithrombotic action is mediated by inhibiting the enzyme phosphodiesterase, thus enhancing the action of prostacyclin. It is used, together with anticoagulants for the prevention of thrombosis in prosthetic heart valves. It has also been given in doses of 50 mg three times a day for the treatment of chronic angina. Dipyridamole is sometimes given intravenously as an adjunct in diagnosis by thallium-201 myocardial scanning.

Side-effects are nausea, diarrhoea, headache and rash.

Epoprostenol §

Brand name: Flolan §

Epoprostenol, also known as prostacyclin, is a prostaglandin produced in the intima of blood vessels. It has a powerful inhibitory action on platelet aggregation, as well as being a potent vasodilator. Epoprostenol has a very brief action, and is given only by continuous intravenous infusion.

It is used to prevent platelet aggregation in cardiopulmonary bypass, it may improve postoperative haemostasis, and is of value in charcoal haemoperfusion of patients with fulminating hepatic failure. In renal dialysis, it is used as an alternative to heparin. Epoprostenol is given by continuous intravenous infusion in doses of 2–16 nanograms/kg/minute, but the use of the drug requires close monitoring.

Side-effects include flushing, as it has a marked vasodilator action, headache, bradycardia and hypotension.

FIBRINOLYTIC AGENTS

In health, the small blood clots that are formed as part of the natural repair process of the vascular system are broken down by plasmin, a fibrinolytic agent derived from plasminogen by an activator present in the vascular endothelium. If clotting activity is excessive, deep-vein thrombosis and pulmonary embolism may occur, but fibrinolysis can be increased by treatment with plasminogen activators.

Streptokinase § (dose: 100 000–1 500 000 units by intravenous infusion)

Brand names: Kabikinase §, Streptase §

Streptokinase is a protein obtained from cultures of certain strains of haemolytic streptococci that combines with and activates plasminogen to form plasmin, which has a direct fibrinolytic action on intravascular blood clots. It is of value in severe thromboembolic disorders such as deep-vein thrombosis, myocardial infarction and pulmonary embolism, but early treatment is essential. It has also been used to clear thrombosed arteriovenous shunts.

Streptokinase is given by intravenous infusion in initial doses of 250 000 units, followed by hourly doses of 100 000 units for 24–72 hours under laboratory control of the clotting time. In myocardial infarction a single dose of 1 500 000 units over 1 hour is given, supported by extended oral treatment for some weeks with daily doses of 150 mg of aspirin. Hydrocortisone 100 mg is sometimes given with the first dose to reduce the risk of an allergic reaction, and adrenaline and an antihistamine should always be readily available for anaphylactic emergencies. When treatment is discontinued, anticoagulant therapy should be given to prevent a recurrence of the thrombosis. Streptokinase should not be used after recent haemorrhage or surgery, or in early pregnancy as it may cause placental separation. It should be avoided after strepto-coccal infection, as the blood may contain streptokinase-neutralizing antibodies. For the same reason, a second course of streptokinase should not be given within at least 3 months.

Side-effects include anaphylactic reactions, fever, rash and haemorrhage. The latter, if severe, can be controlled by injections of tranexamic acid.

Anistreplase § (dose: 30 units)

Brand name: Eminase §

Anistreplase is an inactive complex of plasminogen and strepto-kinase, used in myocardial infarction to break up coronary artery occlusion. Following intravenous injection, it binds firmly with fibrin, and is subsequently metabolized at a steady rate within the occlusion to release the fibrinolytic agent plasmin.

Anistreplase is given as a single dose of 30 units by slow intra-venous injection, as soon as possible after the infarction, and not later than 6 hours after.

Side-effects include haemoptysis, haematuria, allergic reactions and transient hypotension. Bleeding may occur at the injection site. The formation of antistreptokinase antibodies limits repeated treatment for at least 6 months.

Alteplase § (dose: 10–15 mg)

Brand name: Actilyse §

Alteplase is a form of human plasminogen activator obtained by recombinant DNA technology, and so has the advantage of being non-antigenic. It has a selective action on plasminogen bound to fibrin in a clot. Alteplase is used in the fibrinolytic treatment of acute thrombosis and coronary artery occlusion, and is given as an initial dose of 10 mg by slow intravenous injection, followed by a 90 mg dose over 3 hours by intravenous infusion. Early treatment is essential, if possible within 6 hours of the occlusion. Combined treatment with heparin may be necessary.

Side-effects include nausea and vomiting; bleeding may occur at the injection site and intracerebral haemorrhage has also occurred.

Urokinase § (dose: 5000–37 500 units)

Brand name: Ukidan §

Urokinase is an enzyme obtained from human urine or from cultures of human kidney cells. It acts directly on plasminogen to form plasmin, and so has fibrinolytic properties. It is used mainly in the dissolution of blood clots in the eye, and is given intra-ocularly in doses of 5000–7500 units in 2 ml of saline solution, and in vitreous haemorrhage doses up to 37 500 units are used. As urokinase is of human origin, it has the advantage of being non-antigenic. Urokinase is also effective in clearing thrombosed arteriovenous shunts by the instillation of a solution containing 5000–37 500 units.

Stanozolol § (dose: 5–10 mg daily)

Brand name: Stromba §

Stanozolol is an anabolic steroid (p. 390) that also has some fibrinolytic properties. It has been used in doses of 2.5–10 mg daily in the treatment of Behçet's disease and angio-oedema.

As it has some virilizing properties, it should not be used during pregnancy, or in prostatic carcinoma. Acne and hirsutism are occasional side-effects. Stanozolol may potentiate the action of oral anticoagulants.

HAEMOSTATICS

The haemostatics used clinically include certain products that can be applied locally to bleeding surfaces, and which in some cases may be left in place for subsequent absorption, and those used systemically for haemorrhagic states. Plasmin, derived from plasminogen by activating substances in the blood, has fibrinolytic properties, and haemorrhage may occur in conditions associated with excessive production of plasmin. Treatment is based mainly on drugs that reduce plasmin formation and fibrinolysis by the inhibition of fibrinogen activators.

Aprotinin § (dose: 500 000–1 000 000 units)

Brand name: Trasylol §

Aprotinin is a polypeptide obtained from bovine lung tissue that inhibits the action of plasmin, plasminogen activators and proteolytic enzymes. It is used in the treatment of haemorrhage due to hyperfibrinolysis and hyperplasminaemia. More recently it has been used to reduce blood loss during open heart surgery with extracorporeal circulation.

Aprotinin is given by an initial dose of 500 000 units by slow intravenous injection (to detect possible allergy), followed by doses of 200 000 units hourly by intravenous infusion until the haemorrhage is brought under control.

Occasional **side-effects** are hypersensitivity reactions and local thrombophlebitis.

Ethamsylate § (dose: 2 g daily)

Brand name: Dicynene §

Ethamsylate is a synthetic compound used as a systemic haemostatic. The mode of action is unknown, but may be linked with an increase in the number of circulating platelets or increasing their adhesion to the capillary walls. It is used in the control of bleeding due to damage and rupture of small blood vessels during surgery, as well as in haematesis, haematuria and menorrhagia.

Ethamsylate is given orally in doses of 500 mg four times a day, or in severe conditions by intramuscular or intravenous injection in doses of 500 mg every hour for 4–6 hours. Small doses of 12.5 mg/kg are given by injection to low-birth-weight infants for the prophylaxis and treatment of periventricular haemorrhage.

Blood plasma expanders should be given after ethamsylate, not before.

Occasional **side-effects** include nausea, headache and rash.

Tranexamic acid § (dose: 2–6 g daily)

Brand name: Cyklokapron §

Tranexamic acid is used to control the localized fibrinolysis and haemorrhage that may occur in prostatectomy, as well as in the generalized fibrinolysis associated with major surgery. It is also used in angio-oedema, in streptokinase overdose, and a 0.1% solution has been used for bladder irrigation. Tranexamic acid may be given orally in doses of 1 g four times a day, but in severe conditions it should be given by slow intravenous injection in doses of 1 g 8-hourly for up to 3 days before transfer to oral therapy.

The main **side-effects** are nausea, vomiting and diarrhoea, which may subside with a reduction in dose. Giddiness may occur if the injection is made too quickly. Care is necessary in thromboembolic disease, as the inhibition of fibrinolysis may affect the patency of blood vessels.

Some blood products used as haemostatics

The factors concerned in the formation of a blood clot have been referred to briefly on page 303 and certain blood fractions containing some of these factors have a limited use as haemostatics. They are mainly used to control capillary oozing.

Human Fibrin Foam, Thrombin and Factor VIII

The fibrin formed by mixing fibrinogen and thrombin can, by suitable manipulation, be prepared as a dry, spongy product. As such it is occasionally used as a haemostatic in surgery, and as it is of human origin, it is non-antigenic, and can be left in place, the foam is eventually absorbed. Thrombin, being the enzyme that converts fibrinogen into fibrin, is sometimes used by local application to control capillary bleeding. Alternatively, it may be used as fibrin glue by a twin-syringe device loaded with fibrinogen and thrombin. The method is used to control the oozing of blood from multiple pin points after surgery of delicate tissues.

A deficiency of the blood clotting agent Factor VIII is the cause of haemophilia A. Purified preparations of Factor VIII, obtained from pooled plasma, have been used as replacement therapy to prevent haemorrhage in patients with haemophilia A undergoing surgery. Such products may provoke allergic reactions, as they contain fibrinogen and other factors. A more highly purified preparation of Factor VIII is Monoclate P, with which the risk of allergic reactions, although not eliminated, has been markedly reduced. The dose is based on the degree of deficiency of Factor VIII, as some patients with haemophilia A may have plasma levels of Factor VIII as much as 95% below normal.

Recently, a recombinant form of human Factor VIII has become available as Kogenate §. It is essentially similar to Factor VIII derived from plasma, but avoids the risk of transmitting blood-borne viruses. It is indicated in haemophilia A (congenital Factor VIII deficiency), both for prophylaxis and treatment. Dosage is based on the degree of Factor VIII deficiency, the body-weight of the patient and the extent of bleeding. As a guide 1 unit of Kogenate/kg by intravenous injection will cause a rise of about 2% of Factor VIII activity. It is also effective in patients who have developed antibody inhibitors of Factor VIII, but dosage requires specialist supervision.

A deficiency of Factor IX is the cause of haemophilia B (Christmas disease). Plasma-derived products of Factor IX contain impurities, but a new preparation, obtained by mono-clonal antibody technique is Mononine §▼. It contains Factor IX in an exceptionally pure form, and is used as replacement treatment to prevent and control haemorrhage in Factor IX deficiency states. Mononine is given by intravenous injection, and the dosage varies according to the individual patient. Treatment carries the potential risks of allergic reaction, thrombosis and intravascular clotting, and the use of the drug requires great care.

Drugs acting on the gastrointestinal tract

Gastrointestinal disturbance of some kind afflicts most people at times from the cradle to the grave, and the variety of these disturbances is matched by the variety of preparations available to treat them. These preparations vary widely in nature and pharmacological properties, and will be considered under the headings of antacids, spasmolytics, ulcer-healing agents, anti-emetics, intestinal sedatives, adsorbents and laxatives. Figure 11.1 indicates the points of action of some gastric ulcer-healing agents.

ANTACIDS

Antacids are used to reduce gastric acidity and afford relief in gastritis, heartburn, dyspepsia, and other forms of hyperacidity. The ideal antacid would reduce but not neutralize gastric acid completely, otherwise a compensatory over-secretion of acid might occur. It should also have a prolonged action without significant side-effects. In practice, mixtures of antacids are used to obtain the best response, and many proprietary antacids, too numerous to list here, are available. In the past, antacids were widely used in the treatment of peptic ulcer, but for that purpose they have been superseded by the histamine H_2-receptor blocking agents (p. 322).

Points about antacids

(a) Used for the symptomatic relief of ulcer and non-ulcer dyspepsia and similar conditions.
(b) Often best taken between meals.
(c) Should not be taken with other drugs as they may reduce absorption or form insoluble complexes.
(d) May affect the special coating of some slow-absorption products.

Aluminium hydroxide

Brand names: Aludrox, Alu-cap

Aluminium hydroxide, usually used as aluminium hydroxide gel or mixture, but also available as capsules and tablets, has antacid properties that are useful in the treatment of dyspepsia. It has a slow and extended action with few side-effects, but unlike magnesium-based antacids, it may cause constipation. Magaldrate (Dynese) is a complex of aluminium and magnesium hydroxides and sulphates available as a suspension containing 800 mg per 5 ml. It is given in dyspepsia in doses of 5–10 ml after food, and at night.

Calcium carbonate (dose: 1–5 g)

Chalk is natural calcium carbonate, and has a useful and extended antacid action. It is often used in association with magnesium carbonate as Calcium Carbonate Compound Powder as, unlike most other antacids, it has a constipating effect.

Magnesium carbonate (dose: 250–500 mg)

Magnesium carbonate is a slow-acting antacid, and is a constituent of a wide range of proprietary products sold for dyspepsia and mild acidity. It is also used as Aromatic Magnesium Carbonate Mixture. Magnesium hydroxide (cream of magnesia) also has mild antacid action, but is used mainly as a laxative (p. 338).

Magnesium trisilicate (dose: 0.5–2 g)

Magnesium trisilicate has a slow and prolonged antacid action. It has been used extensively in the treatment of peptic ulcer, as in the stomach it forms a gel which has a local protective action, but it is now used mainly in dyspepsia. It is usually given in association with magnesium carbonate and sodium bicarbonate as Compound Magnesium Trisilicate Mixture (BP) (dose: 10 ml) or Compound Magnesium Trisilicate Oral Powder (dose: 1–5 g), as when given alone it has a laxative action.

Sodium bicarbonate (dose: 1–4 g)

Sodium bicarbonate is soluble in water and neutralizes gastric acid very quickly, with the evolution of carbon dioxide. Continued use may lead to alkalosis and rebound acid formation, and it is therefore seldom given alone except for the immediate relief of gastric pain. For such occasional use sodium bicarbonate is invaluable. The carbon dioxide liberated in the stomach by the reaction of gastric acid with the sodium bicarbonate may also relieve distension as the gas is eructed, and such eructation is useful as a proof to the patient of the efficacy of the antacid.

Other antacid products

Many proprietary products, too numerous to list here, are available containing standard or newer antacids, but all have a basically similar pharmacological action. In some, the antacid action is augmented by the use of auxiliary drugs to reduce spasm and inhibit the secretion of gastric acid (p. 329) or they may contain dimethicone to reduce flatulence, or assist in the breakdown of froth bubbles that may form as the result of the action of the antacid. The value of these products depends largely on individual need and response.

Gastrils contain an aluminium hydroxide-magnesium carbonate complex incorporated in a slow-dissolving pastille base. **Nulacin** tablets contain antacids and milk solids, and are intended to be sucked slowly at frequent intervals and thus provide the equivalent of a prolonged and continuous effect. **Mucaine** contains a local anaesthetic with aluminium hydroxide, and may be useful in oesophagitis and hiatus hernia.

Carminatives and bitters

Carminatives are survivors of older therapy. They produce a feeling of warmth in the stomach, and tend to relieve gastric distension by promoting the elimination of gas by belching. Oil of peppermint and tincture of ginger are carminatives, and are sometimes given with small doses of sodium bicarbonate, often with a bitter mixture. They have a useful but limited place in the treatment of abdominal colic and dyspepsia.

Interest in oil of peppermint has revived with its presentation as capsules containing 0.2 ml (**Colpermin, Mintec**).

Bitters are vegetable substances that, by their taste, promote a reflex secretion of gastric juice, and so stimulate the appetite. Gentian is a traditional bitter, and is still used as Alkaline Gentian Mixture or as Acid Gentian Mixture.

PEPTIC ULCER-HEALING DRUGS

Peptic ulcers are the result of autodigestion, which occurs when the natural defences such as the protective mucus lining of the stomach and duodenum break down. As ulcers do not occur in the absence of gastric acid, treatment was formerly based on the extended use of antacids such as magnesium trisilicate. Relapse after such treatment was common. It had long been known that histamine has a powerful influence on gastric acid secretion, but conventional antihistamines have no acid-inhibiting properties. It was then found that two types of histamine receptors exist, the histamine H_1-receptors associated with the systemic effects of histamine such as allergy, and the H_2-receptors found chiefly in the oxyntic cells, which are concerned with the secretion of gastric acid and pepsin. Conventional antihistamines block the H_1-receptors only, and a search for new drugs with a selective blocking action on the H_2-receptors resulted in the introduction of cimetidine, the first of the now many histamine H_2-receptor antagonists.

These drugs revolutionized the treatment of peptic ulcer, and are now widely used in the control of benign gastric and duodenal ulcer and related disorders, and the less common Zollinger–Ellison syndrome. They are also useful in the prophylaxis and treatment of gastric ulcers induced by non-steroidal anti-inflammatory agents (NSAIDs). Relapse after treatment

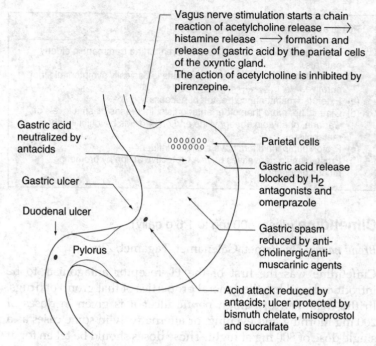

Figure 11.1 Points of action of ulcer healing-drugs.

with H_2-receptor antagonists may be due to the presence in the stomach of *Helicobacter pylori*. It was once thought that bacteria could not survive in gastric acid, but *H. pylori*, which is found in the gastric mucus, has developed an enzyme that protects it from acid attack by an alkalization of its immediate gastric environment. At present, eradication of *H. pylori* in peptic ulcer depends on multiple treatment with bismuth chelate, metronidazole and antibiotics. Some of these H_2-antagonists have an influence on drug-metabolizing enzymes in the liver, and the doses of drugs such as warfarin and phenytoin may need adjustment.

More recently, the therapeutic treatment of peptic ulcer has been widened by the introduction of omeprazole, which blocks the formation of gastric acid at a later stage than the H_2-receptor antagonists. In general the possibility of gastric carcinoma should be considered before treatment with a drug of this type is commenced with elderly patients.

Points about ulcer-healing drugs

(a) Malignancy should be excluded before starting treatment in elderly patients.
(b) Treatment with H_2-receptor antagonists is basically symptomatic, not curative.
(c) Extended maintenance treatment necessary.
(d) Cimetidine, more than other antagonists, increases plasma levels of warfarin, phenytoin, theophylline and other drugs by inhibiting their metabolism.
(e) Proton pump inhibitors have a similar influence.
(f) Prostaglandin derivatives have a protective action by promoting mucus production.

Cimetidine (dose: 800 mg to 1.6 g daily)

Brand names: Dyspamet, Galenamet, Tagamet, Zita

Cimetidine was the first of the H_2-receptor antagonists to be introduced, and has the general properties of that group of drugs. In the treatment of benign peptic ulcer it is given in doses of 200 mg morning and evening, or alternatively in some cases as a single dose of 800 mg at night. Those doses should be taken for at least 4 weeks, or longer in ulcers linked with NSAID therapy. In the latter, increased doses of 400 mg four times a day may be required. Subsequent maintenance doses vary from 400 mg once or twice a day. Cimetidine is given in similar doses for reflux oesophagitis, but doses up to 1.6 g daily or more may be required in the Zollinger–Ellison syndrome. In severe cases, cimetidine may be given by intramuscular or slow intravenous injection or intravenous infusion in doses of 200 mg at intervals of 4–6 hours. It is also used pre-operatively when a reduction in gastric acid secretion is required.

Cimetidine is usually well tolerated, but diarrhoea, dizziness and rash may occur. It may cause confusion in the elderly and severely ill patients, which rapidly subsides if the drug is withdrawn. Gynaecomastia has occasionally been reported as a result of cimetidine binding to the androgen receptors. It may increase the action of oral anticoagulants and theophylline, and modify the effects of some benzodiazepines, and care is necessary in hepatic and renal impairment. (Algitec is a mixed product containing cimetidine with alginic acid as a mucosal protectant.)

Famotidine (dose: 20–40 mg daily)

Brand name: Pepcid-PM

Famotidine has the actions, uses and side-effects of cimetidine, but it is effective in smaller doses and has a more prolonged action. In peptic ulcer it is given as a nightly dose of 40 mg for 4–8 weeks, followed by maintenance doses of 20 mg also at night. In the Z–E syndrome, larger doses of 20 mg every 6 hours are necessary. Unlike cimetidine, famotidine does not affect drug metabolism mediated by hepatic microsomal enzymes.

Nizatidine (dose: 150–300 mg daily)

Brand name: Axid

Nizatidine has the general properties and uses of the H_2-receptor antagonists, but has a more prolonged action. In the treatment of duodenal and benign gastric ulcer, it is given in doses of 300 mg at night, or 150 mg twice a day for at least 4 weeks. For the prevention of recurrence after ulcer healing, evening doses of 150 mg are given, and prolonged treatment for some months may be required. In short-term hospital treatment, nizatidine is given by continuous intravenous infusion in doses of 10 mg/hour.

Nizatidine is excreted mainly in the urine, and in renal impairment a reduction in dose to 150 mg daily or on alternate days may be necessary. Part of a dose is also excreted in breast milk, and its use during lactation should be avoided.

Reported **side-effects** include myalgia, chest pain, abnormal dreams and pruritus. Unlike cimetidine, androgen binding does not occur with nizatidine.

Ranitidine (dose: 150–300 mg daily)

Brand name: Zantac

Ranitidine resembles cimetidine in its general pattern of activity, and in the treatment of peptic ulcer it is given in doses of 150 mg twice a day or as a 300 mg dose at night for 4–8 weeks, with maintenance doses of 150 mg at night. In severe conditions, ranitidine may be given by intramuscular or slow intravenous injection in doses of 50 mg at intervals of 6–8 hours. It is also given by injection before surgery to prevent acid aspiration.

Large doses up to 6 g daily may be necessary to reduce the gastric acid secretion in the Zollinger–Ellison syndrome.

Ranitidine is well tolerated and has few **side-effects**, although it may cause confusion in some elderly patients, and care is necessary in renal impairment. It is less likely to cause gynaecomastia, or interfere with the metabolism of other drugs such as the oral anticoagulants. Gastric carcinoma should be eliminated before ranitidine treatment is considered.

Omeprazole § (dose: 20–40mg daily)

Brand name: Losec §

The final stage in the formation of gastric acid before it can be released from the parietal cells is the transfer of hydrogen ions (protons) across the cell membrane in exchange for potassium ions. That transfer is mediated by the enzyme H^+K^+-APTase, and the exchange system is referred to as the proton pump. A selective inhibitor of that enzyme could prevent gastric acid secretion at a different stage, and be of value in ulcer patients resistant to H_2-receptor antagonists. It could also be useful in reflux oesophagitis, where such antagonists are not always fully effective.

Omeprazole is a proton pump inhibitor of the required type. It is taken up selectively by the parietal cells, as only traces remain in the circulation after 24 hours, and brings about a more rapid rate of ulcer healing than the H_2-receptor antagonists. It is the preferred drug in the treatment of the Zollinger–Ellison syndrome. Omeprazole is used in the treatment of gastric and duodenal ulcers that have not responded to other drugs, including ulcers associated with NSAID therapy, and is given in doses of 20 mg daily for 4 weeks initially (8 weeks in gastric ulcer) with daily doses of 20 mg for maintenance treatment. Initial doses can be increased to 40 mg daily in severe conditions. Similar doses are given in erosive reflux oesophagitis. In the Z–E syndrome, initial doses of 60 mg daily are required, with subsequent maintenance doses varying from 20–120 mg daily according to need and response.

Omeprazole is well tolerated, and **side-effects** of headache and gastrointestinal disturbances are usually mild and transient. It is not recommended at present for maintenance treatment, because the prolonged achlorhydria induced may be undesirable. Adjustment of dose may be necessary in patients receiving warfarin, diazepam and phenytoin, as omeprazole also inhibits the action of the liver enzyme cytochrome P450, which is concerned with drug elimination. It has been suggested that omeprazole may assist in the elimination of *Campylobacter pylori* (now known as *Helicobacter pylori*), the organism linked with the relapse of gastric ulcer.

 Maton P M 1991 Omeprazole. New England Journal of Medicine 324: 965–975

Lansoprazole § (dose: 30 mg daily)

Brand name: Zoton §

Lansoprazole is a proton pump inhibitor of the omeprazole type. In duodenal ulcer it is given in doses of 30 mg daily for 4 weeks, but for 8 weeks in gastric ulcer. Similar doses are given in reflex oesophagitis. Side-effects are similar to those of omeprzole.

Misoprostol § (dose: 800 micrograms daily)

Brand name: Cytotec §

Misoprostol is a synthetic analogue of alphaprostadil (prostaglandin E_1, p. 421). Prostaglandins are mediators in the maintenance of the mucosal lining of the alimentary tract, and the biosynthesis of endogenous prostaglandins may be impaired in patients with peptic ulcer, and inhibited by non-steroidal anti-inflammatory agents (NSAIDs). Misoprostol both inhibits gastric acid secretion and promotes mucus production, and is used in the treatment of established peptic ulcer as well as in the prophylaxis of NSAID-induced ulceration, particularly in the elderly. It is given in doses of 800 micrograms daily in two or four divided doses, taken with meals and a last dose at night. Although early symptomatic relief may be obtained, treatment should be continued for at least 4 weeks, or longer up to 8 weeks if necessary. Doses of 200 micrograms two to four times a day are given for the prophylaxis of

NSAID-induced peptic ulcers. Misoprostol is not indicated in simple dyspepsia. Side-effects include diarrhoea (requiring a reduction in dose), nausea, abdominal pain and occasional abnormal vaginal bleeding. Care is necessary in cardiovascular disease, as misoprostol may cause hypotension.

Misoprostol preparations are contraindicated in pregnancy.

Arthrotec is a mixed product containing misoprostol 200 micrograms with diclofenac 50 mg.

Pirenzepine § (dose: 100–150 mg daily)

Brand name: Gastrozepin §

Pirenzepine is an anticholinergic/antimuscarinic drug with selective inhibitory effects on acid and pepsin secretion mediated by its action on the M_1-receptors in the gastrointestinal tract. It is used like the H_2-receptor antagonists in the initial and maintenance treatment of gastric and duodenal ulcers, and is given in doses of 50 mg two or three times a day before meals for at least 4 weeks, although therapy for 3 months may be required in some cases. Unlike most anticholinergic drugs, pirenzepine does not penetrate into the CSF, so central **side-effects** are uncommon. It is well tolerated but some transient dryness of the mouth and visual disturbances may occur.

Bismuth chelate (dose: 480 mg daily)

Brand name: DeNol

Bismuth chelate is a bismuth-potassium-citrate complex that appears to promote peptic ulcer healing by forming an insoluble protective coating over the ulcerated area. It is given in doses of 120 mg four times a day, increased to 240 mg six times a day if necessary. As the complex may coat food as well as an ulcer, it should be taken with plenty of water half an hour before meals. Milk, except in nominal amounts, should be avoided. Constipation is a side-effect.

Sucralfate § (Antepsin §) is a complex of aluminium hydroxide with sulphated sucrose, and has a similar ulcer-protective action, but little antacid activity. Dose 1–2 g four times a day before meals.

Carbenoxolone

Carbenoxolone is a derivative of an acid present in liquorice root, and it has some anti-inflammatory properties. It has been given in the treatment of peptic ulcer, but is now used in association with antacids as Pyrogastrone for the control of oesophageal ulceration as a tablet to be chewed after meals three times a day, with a double dose at night. Extended treatment for 6–12 weeks may be required. It is contraindicated in cardiac failure, hepatic or renal impairment, and in patients over 75 years of age.

Cisapride § (dose: 30–40 mg daily)

Brand names: Alimix §, Prepulsid §

Cisapride is used in the treatment of gastro-oesophageal reflux. At one time antacids were widely used, but the reflux may be due more to a delay in gastric emptying than to acidity. Treatment is now directed more towards stimulating gastric transit. Metoclopramide has centrally-mediated anti-emetic properties, and has been used in oesophageal reflux, but a drug with a more selective action on the gastrointestinal tract is cisapride. Its gastric stimulation action appears to be linked with a local release of acetylcholine in the gastrointestinal tract. It is given for the relief of the symptoms of reflux and non-ulcer dyspepsia in doses of 10 mg three or four times a day, continued for some weeks. It should be taken about 15–30 minutes before meals to obtain the optimum benefit, with a dose at night to prevent nocturnal reflux.

Some **side-effects** such as abdominal pain and diarrhoea are associated with the gastric stimulant action of the drug, but occasional headache, lightheadedness and convulsions have occurred. As cisapride is not a dopamine antagonist, the extrapyramidal side-effects of metoclopramide are unlikely to occur.

Spasmolytics

Spasmolytics are used as supplementary treatment in a variety of disturbances of the gastrointestinal tract, including non-ulcer dyspepsia and the irritable bowel syndrome. They are mainly antimuscarinic (anticholinergic) in action, and so have a relaxed effect on smooth muscle. Atropine is one of the oldest spasmolytics

(p. 251) but its side-effects such as dryness of the mouth limit its value.

Table 11.1 indicates some available products, but many others, not listed, contain auxiliary substances such as antacids.

Table 11.1 Intestinal antispasmodics

Approved name	Brand name	Daily dose
alverine	Spasmonal	180–360 mg
dicyclomine	Merbentyl	30–60 mg
hyoscine butylbromide	Buscopan	40–80 mg
mebeverine	Colofac	405 mg
mepenzolate	Cantil	75–200 mg
pipenzolate	Piptalin	15–25 mg
poldine	Nacton	8–16 mg
propantheline	Pro-Banthine	75 mg

ULCERATIVE COLITIS

Ulcerative colitis is a chronic inflammatory and ulcerative disease of the colon, manifested by attacks of bloody diarrhoea, interspersed with apparently capricious periods of asymptomatic remission. In severe conditions treatment with corticosteroids orally and by enema is necessary, but in milder ulcerative colitis reliance is largely placed on sulphasalazine and related drugs. With continued treatment they also reduce the risks of relapse. In resistant ulcerative colitis, azathioprine in doses of 2 mg/kg daily has been given.

Sulphasalazine §

Brand name: Salazopyrin §

Sulphasalazine is a sulphonamide derivative. It appears to be taken up selectively by the connective tissues of the intestinal tract with the release of 5-aminosalicylic acid (mesalazine), the active part of the molecule. It is used in the treatment of ulcerative colitis and regional enteritis (Crohn's disease) often in association with a corticosteroid, but the response is variable.

Sulphasalazine is given initially in doses of 1 g four times a day together with adequate fluids for 2–3 weeks for the control of acute attacks, reduced to maintenance doses of 500 mg four times a day when remission occurs. For children initial doses of 40–60 mg/kg daily are used, with maintenance doses of 20–30 mg/kg daily. Oral therapy can be supplemented by daily retention enemas of 3 g, or suppositories of 500 mg twice a day. Extended maintenance treatment should be given to avoid relapse.

Side-effects include nausea, headache, fever, rash, pruritus and neurotoxicity. Patients should be warned to report immediately if soreness of the throat, fever or malaise occurs, as blood disorders require prompt withdrawal of treatment. It is contraindicated in patients known to react to sulphonamides or salicylates.

Mesalazine § (dose: 1.2–2.4 g daily)

Brand names: Asacol §, Pentasa §

Mesalazine is the active metabolite of sulphasalazine, but it is absorbed too rapidly to be suitable for the treatment of ulcerative colitis. Absorption can be delayed by using the drug as a resin-bound complex (Asacol) from which the active constituent is released in the lower intestinal tract. It is given in doses of 400–800 mg three times a day when the side-effects of the parent drug are unacceptable. Mesalazine may cause nausea, diarrhoea and abdominal pain. Salicylate sensitivity is a contraindication. Suppositories of mesalazine (250 and 500 mg) are also available, and may be useful in patients with the distal form of the disease.

Osalazine § (dose: 1.5–3 g daily)

Brand name: Dipentum §

Osalazine represents an attempt to avoid the side-effects of sulphasalazine, which are mainly due to the splitting of the molecule, the release of the sulphonamide fragment, and the over-rapid absorption of the active derivative mesalazine. In osalazine, the sulphonamide has been eliminated, as the compound represents the combination of two molecules of mesalazine. The major part of a dose reaches the colon unchanged, where the compound is broken down by intestinal bacteria to release the active substance. In the treatment of ulcerative colitis, osalazine is given in doses of 500 mg–1 g three times a day, increased in severe conditions to 3 g daily. For maintenance, doses of 500 mg twice a day are given for long periods.

The main **side-effect** is a watery diarrhoea. Osalazine is contraindicated in patients sensitive to salicylates.

ANTI-EMETICS

Anti-emetics are drugs that prevent or modify nausea and vomiting. Vomiting is basically a protective mechanism to promote the rejection of ingested toxins, but it can be initiated by other stimuli, and then serves no useful purpose. The act of vomiting is governed by a complex system involving the vagus nerve, the chemoreceptor trigger zone (CTZ) and vomiting centre of the brain, and the release of serotonin and dopamine. It is initiated by the release of serotonin (5HT) from the enterochromaffin cells of the small intestine, which is followed by stimulation of the vague nerve, CTZ and vomiting centre of the brain. Impulses from the vomiting centre, mediated by dopamine, give rise to propulsive waves which may cause nausea and vomiting. Vomiting can also arise as a result of shock and injury; it may hinder post-operative recovery, and the loss of electrolytes caused by vomiting may result in serious metabolic disturbances. The control of vomiting has become more important with the introduction of some new platinum-containing cytotoxic agents, which cause intense nausea and vomiting to the point where some patients have refused further treatment.

In view of the complex nature of the vomiting process, it is not surprising that anti-emetic activity is found in a wide range of substances, many of which have some degree of central depressant activity. Hyoscine is the active constituent of some travel sickness remedies, and the newer and much more powerful anti-emetics are the serotonin and dopamine blocking agents represented by ondansetron and domperidone.

Many of the phenothiazine-derived tranquillizers also have anti-emetic properties mediated by blocking the action of dopamine on the chemoreceptor trigger zone. **Thiethylperazine** § (Torecan), **prochlorperazine** § (Stemetil §) and **trifluoperazine** § (Stelazine) are representative compounds. **Methotrimeprazine** (Nozinan), the phenothiazine antipsychotic, is also used by subcutaneous infusion as an anti-emetic and anxiolytic in the supportive treatment of advanced cancer.

Certain antihistamines such as **cyclizine** (Valoid) and **dimenhydrinate** (Dramamine) are also useful as anti-emetics. Promethazine theoclate (Avomine) is useful in travel sickness. **Betahistine** § (dose: 8–16 mg) (Serc) and **cinnarizine** (dose: 15–30 mg) (Stugeron), represent drugs that are of value in Meniere's disease, vertigo, and other labyrinthine disturbances. The use of anti-emetics to control the vomiting of pregnancy requires great care, and if possible should be avoided during the first trimester because of the risks of drug-associated fetal damage.

Points about anti-emetics

(a) Hyoscine and antihistamines are useful in motion sickness.
(b) Some phenothiazines, but not thioridazine, are effective in more severe vomiting.
(c) In very severe nausea and vomiting secondary to disease and cytotoxic therapy, domperidone and nabilone are effective.
(d) The selective serotonin antagonists are valuable in severe cytotoxic drug-induced vomiting not controlled by other anti-emetics.

Domperidone § (dose: 30–120 mg daily)

Brand name: Motilium §

Domperidone is a potent dopamine antagonist, and by preventing the access of dopamine to receptors in the chemoreceptor trigger zone (CTZ), the activation of that zone by emesis-provoking stimuli is inhibited. It also binds selectively with dopamine D_2-receptors in the stomach, and so inhibits the dopamine-mediated propulsive waves in the stomach that can result in vomiting. Domperidone does not cross the blood–brain barrier very easily, and is less likely to cause sedation, extrapyramidal symptoms and other central side-effects than anti-emetics of the pheno-thiazine type. It is given orally in doses of 10–20 mg every 4–8 hours, or by suppositories of 30 mg. It is not intended for routine use in postoperative vomiting. Domperidone also increases gastrointestinal mobility and has been used in functional dyspepsia, and to expedite the transit of barium sulphate in gastrointestinal radiological investigations.

Metoclopramide § (dose: 15–30 mg daily)

Brand names: Maxolon §, Primperan §; Parmid §

Metoclopramide is a dopamine antagonist, and differs from most other anti-emetics by its multiple action. It has a central effect by depressing the threshold of activity of the vomiting centre, and by its weak serotonin antagonist properties, it also reduces the sensitivity of nerves linking that centre with the pylorus and duodenum. It also increases gastric peristalsis.

Metoclopramide is given in doses of 10 mg, orally or by injection, up to three times a day, and is useful in many conditions associated with nausea and vomiting. Gastrobid Continus, Gastromax and Maxolon SR are slow-release products and are not suitable for patients under 20 years of age.

In the control of the nausea due to cytotoxic therapy, metoclopramide is given in large doses (2–4 mg/kg) every 2 hours by intravenous infusion up to a maximum of 10 mg/kg over 24 hours, the initial dose being given before cytotoxic therapy is commenced. In standard doses, the stimulating effects of metoclopramide on the gastrointestinal tract are useful in facilitating barium meal examinations.

Side-effects include extrapyramidal reactions, especially in children and young adults, and careful dosing may be necessary. Hyperprolactinaemia has been reported.

Nabilone § (dose: 4–6 mg daily)

Brand name: Cesamet §

Nabilone is a synthetic cannabinoid with anti-emetic properties of value in the nausea and vomiting associated with cytotoxic therapy. It is not a dopamine antagonist, and appears to act on certain opiate receptors. It is given in oral doses of 1–2 mg twice a day during each period of treatment (commencing before such therapy) and continued for 24 hours after the end of the course.

Side-effects include drowsiness, confusion, hallucinations, depression and hypotension. Nabilone should be used with care in patients with a history of psychosis, and if renal impairment is present.

Prochlorperazine § (dose: 10–30 mg daily)

Brand names: Buccastem §, Stemetil §

Prochlorperazine is a chlorpromazine-like drug with similar

actions and uses. It blocks the access of dopamine to the CTZ, and so has valuable anti-emetic properties. It is used in the control of severe nausea and vomiting, as well as in labyrinthine disorders. In prophylaxis, doses of 5–10 mg are given two or three times a day, but for the treatment of nausea and vomiting the initial dose is 20 mg, followed by doses of 10 mg as required. Alternatively, an initial dose of 25 mg may be given by suppository. In severe conditions, prochlorperazine can be given in doses of 12.5 mg by deep intramuscular injection, followed by oral therapy. Buccastem is a product designed for buccal administration to provide a longer action from a 3 mg dose of prochlorperazine. In labyrinthine disorders, initial doses of 5 mg three times a day may be increased slowly up to 30 mg daily, and extended treatment may be required.

Side-effects such as sedation, dryness of the mouth and drowsiness are usually mild with anti-emetic doses of prochlorperazine but extrapyramidal reactions may occur with higher doses, especially in children and the elderly.

Serotonin (5HT₃)-receptor antagonists

Cytotoxic chemotherapeutic agents and radiotherapy can cause very severe nausea and vomiting, considered to be due to the release of serotonin (5HT) from the enterochromaffin cells in the intestinal mucosa, which contain most of the body stores of serotonin. Such released serotonin acts on a specific subgroup of receptors in the gut, identified as the 5HT₃-receptors, which in turn leads to stimulation of the vagus nerve and activation of central 5HT₃-receptors in the chemoreceptor trigger zone (CTZ), and subsequent initiation of the vomiting reflex.

When the anti-emetic properties of metoclopramide were found to be linked with its weak serotonin antagonist action, attention was turned to the development of more selective 5HT₃-receptor antagonists, represented by granisetron, ondansetron and tropisetron. These drugs act on the 5HT₃-receptors in the gut and CTZ, and have no action on other types of serotonin receptors. They have no dopamine antagonist properties, and so are unlikely to cause the extrapyramidal side-effectss of metoclopramide. To obtain the best anti-emetic response, these 5HT₃-receptor antagonists should be given before chemotherapy or radiotherapy is commenced.

Granisetron §▼ (dose: 2 mg daily)

Brand name: Kytril §▼

Granisetron is a $5HT_3$-receptor antagonist with the general properties of that group of drugs. It is given for the prophylaxis and treatment of nausea and vomiting induced by cytotoxic therapy in doses of 1 mg orally, preferably an hour before treatment, followed by a second dose of 1 mg 12 hours later. Alternatively, granisetron may be given as a 3 mg dose by intravenous infusion, repeated at intervals if necessary up to a total dose of 9 mg in 24 hours. **Side-effects** include headache and constipation.

Ondansetron §▼ (dose: 24 mg daily)

Brand name: Zofran §▼

Ondansetron is another $5HT_3$-receptor antagonist used like granisetron and tropisetron for drug-induced nausea and vomiting. When severe vomiting is anticipated it is given before chemotherapy in a dose of 8 mg by intravenous injection, followed by two more doses of 8 mg at 4-hourly intervals. Alternatively, an intravenous dose of 1 mg hourly for up to 24 hours may be given. A dose of 20 mg of dexamethasone, given intravenously before chemotherapy may enhance the anti-emetic response. In less severe vomiting, the initial intravenous dose of 8 mg can be followed by oral therapy in doses of 8 mg 8-hourly. Maintenance treatment is with doses of 8 mg 8-hourly for up to 5 days. Ondansetron is well tolerated, but **side-effects** include constipation, headache and a sensation of flushing or warmth.

Tropisetron §▼ (dose: 5 mg daily)

Brand name: Navoban §▼

Tropisetron is a $5HT_3$-receptor antagonist that differs from others by its extended action which permits single daily dosage. It is used as a 6-day treatment for the prevention of cancer chemotherapy-induced nausea and vomiting, and is given initially as a single dose of 5 mg by intravenous infusion. Over the next 5 days it is given orally in a dose of 5 mg, to be taken before food. Tropisetron is generally well tolerated, but **side-effects** such as

headache, constipation, dizziness and gastrointestinal disturbances may occur.

ADSORBENTS

Adsorbents are solids that have the ability to bind with gases and
other substances, including bacterial toxins, and so prevent their
absorption. They are used mainly in the treatment of mild
diarrhoea. Activated charcoal is also used in the treatment of
poisoning by some toxic drugs (p. 575).

Kaolin (dose: 15–60 g)

Kaolin, or china clay, is a purified silicate of aluminium. It is used
in the treatment of food poisoning, enteritis, dysentery and
diarrhoea. Mixture of Kaolin and Morphine BP, BNF is widely
employed in the treatment of mild gastrointestinal disturbances
as the kaolin adsorbs any toxins, and the morphine constituent
reduces gastrointestinal motility.

Charcoal (dose: 4–8 g)

Activated charcoal has adsorbent properties similar to those of
kaolin, and is sometimes used in the treatment of flatulence and
distention, and in poisoning by alkaloids and related drugs. It is
also used by the charcoal perfusion technique in cases of
poisoning by methyl alcohol, lithium salts and salicylates.

ANTIDIARRHOEAL DRUGS

Co-phenotrope (Lomotil, Tropergen) contains the antimotility
agent diphenoxylate 2.5 mg with atropine 25 micrograms and is
useful in both acute and chronic diarrhoea. Loperamide (Imodium,
Loperagen) is of value in acute diarrhoea, given as an initial dose
of 4 mg, followed by subsequent doses of 2 mg.

Codeine phosphate, dose 15–30 mg, is also useful in acute
diarrhoea, and is present in the proprietary products Diarrest and
Kaodene. Kaolin and Morphine Mixture B.P., dose 10 ml
4-hourly, is also used in mild diarrhoea.

In simple acute diarrhoea, particularly in children and the
elderly, it is essential to replace fluid and electrolyte loss, and this

should precede drug therapy. Compound Sodium Chloride and Glucose Powder, or Oral Rehydration Salts (ORS) is a suitable product for that purpose, or alternatively, for short periods, a solution of glucose or sugar with a small amount of salt may be used. Proprietary products for oral rehydration therapy include Diocalm, Diorylate, Electrolade, Gluco-lyte, Rapolyte and Rehidrat. Infective diarrhoeas are usually self-limiting as they are caused by viruses, and antibacterial drugs are seldom required.

In more severe and extended diarrhoeas, the cause, such as ulcerative colitis, should be sought, as more specific drugs may be required (p. 330).

LAXATIVES

Sometimes termed aperients, laxatives are substances which stimulate peristalsis, promote evacuation and relieve constipation. At one time they were used extensively regardless of need, but their routine use has declined. Their use is primarily indicated for the treatment of constipation in (1) illness and pregnancy, (2) elderly patients with inadequate diets and poor abdominal muscle tone, (3) when intestinal activity has been reduced by medication, and (4) preparation for surgery or diagnosis. They can be classified as stimulant, osmotic, bulk forming and softening laxatives. The following products are in use:

Osmotic laxatives

Substances such as the well-known magnesium sulphate (Epsom salts) are not absorbed when given orally, and in the intestines they increase the bulk and fluidity of the faeces and function as osmotic laxatives. When given in doses of 5–15 g, well diluted, in the morning on an empty stomach, the action is rapid and effective.

Magnesium hyroxide, although an antacid, is converted by stomach acid to magnesium chloride, and has a laxative action similar to that of magnesium sulphate. Citromag is a preparation of magnesium citrate, used mainly for bowel evacuation before radiology or surgery. Patients should be advised that Citromag is an effervescent powder, and hot water should be used to prepare the solution.

Klean-Prep is a bowel cleansing product containing sodium sulphate as the laxative constituent. It is used before colonic surgery, and before radiology so that the bowel is free from any solid matter. In use, the contents of four sachets, dissolved in 4 litres of water, are given in doses of 250 ml every 10–15 minutes until all the solution has been taken or the desired response obtained.

Stimulant vegetable laxatives

These drugs contain anthraquinones, which are thought to stimulate Auerbach's plexus in the large intestine and so increase the rate of peristaltic movement, but may cause abdominal cramp. They are slow in action and are best taken at night. They are now used less extensively, but still have a limited place in therapeutics. The chronic use of stimulant laxatives is not recommended, as they may then exacerbate the problem of constipation by inducing an atonic colon. It is worth remembering that enough of the drug may be excreted in the milk of nursing mothers to have an effect on the infant.

Cascara

Cascara bark is a useful purgative that has a mild slow action that results in the passage of a soft stool. Cascara is now used mainly as standardized tablets, dose, 1 or 2 at night.

Senna (dose: 0.5–2 g)

Both the leaves and the seed pods of senna have laxative properties, and have long been used domestically as 'senna tea'. Senna is very effective but may cause some griping. Senokot is a proprietary product containing a standardized extract of senna, which is more consistent in action and better tolerated.

Castor oil (dose: 5–20 ml)

The oil expressed from castor seeds contains a derivative of ricinoleic acid, and following oral administration it is split up in the intestine, like other fats, by the enzyme lipase. The liberated ricinoleic acid has a stimulant action on the small intestine, and castor oil is a useful purgative in diarrhoea and food poisoning and in preparation for radiological examination of the intestinal tract. The action is self-limiting, as evacuation is followed by a quiescent period and subsequent constipation.

Cathartics

The drastic purgatives are represented by vegetable drugs such as aloes, colocynth and jalap, but are now rarely used.

SYNTHETIC LAXATIVES

Bisacodyl (dose: 5–10 mg)

Brand name: Dulcolax

Bisacodyl is not absorbed when given orally but has a stimulant action on the walls of the colon. It is sometimes described as a contact laxative, and is useful not only as a general laxative, but also to secure evacuation of the colon before X-ray examination. Tablets containing 5 mg and suppositories of 10 mg are available.

Docusate sodium (dose: 50–500 mg)

Brand name: Dioctyl

Docusate sodium, also known as dioctyl sodium sulphosuccinate, is a surface-active agent, and acts as a faecal softener by increasing the amount of water that remains in or penetrates into the faeces. It is present in the mixed laxative product Danthron.

Lactulose (dose: 50% solution, 15–50 ml)

Brand names: Duphalac, Lactugal, Osmolax, Regulose

Lactulose is an artificial sugar that escapes digestion as there is no enzyme in the gut capable of metabolizing such sugars. Lactulose reaches the colon unchanged, and so functions as a slow-acting osmotic laxative. It is then rapidly broken down by bacteria to form lactic and other acids, and promotes the formation of softer faeces of low pH.

Lactulose solution is given to relieve constipation in doses of 15 ml twice a day. It is also of value in doses of 30–50 ml three times a day in hepatic encephalopathy, as it limits the formation and absorption of nitrogenous breakdown products in the intestinal tract. Such breakdown products are normally converted in the liver to urea, and could accumulate when liver damage has occured. The **side-effects** of lactulose are flatulence, abdominal cramp and intestinal discomfort.

Lactitol is a semisynthetic sugar similar in actions and uses to lactulose. For constipation it is given as a single daily dose of 10–20 g, mixed with food, and taken with adequate fluid. In hepatic encephalopathy, it is given in doses of 500–700 mg/kg three times a day.

Phenolphthalein (dose: 50–300 mg)

Phenolphthalein has a mild irritant action on the intestines, and is used in habitual constipation. It is absorbed in part by the entero-hepatic circulation and excreted later in the bile, so that the action may extend over several days. It may cause rash and albumin-uria, and its use has now declined. It is present in some propri-etary laxative products.

Sodium picosulphate (dose: 5–15 mg)

Brand names: Laxoberal, Picolax

Sodium picosulphate is a synthetic laxative of the bisacodyl type, and is used for similar purposes. It is slow acting (10–12 hours), and is useful for bowel evacuation before surgery. Sodium Picolate Elixir is the official product (dose, 5–15 ml at night). Products of this type are not suitable for prolonged use.

BULK AND LUBRICANT LAXATIVES

Bulk laxatives are vegetable substances of a mucilaginous nature that are not digested, but excreted unchanged. During this process they absorb water and increase the bulk of the faeces, and so act as mechanical laxatives. They are therefore useful in the treatment of constipation where the faeces are dry and hard, but they may not be suitable when the intake of fluid is inadequate or in cases of faecal impaction.

Typical products are bran, ispaghula and psyllium seeds, and mucilaginous products from various plants from the basis of proprietary bulk laxatives such as Fybogel, Isogel, Metamucil, Normacol and Regulan. Bran products are Proctifibe and Trifyba. Celevac contains methylcellulose. All these bulk laxatives should be taken with an adequate amount of water to reduce the risk of intestinal obstruction.

Liquid paraffin (dose: 8–30 ml)

Liquid paraffin is a mineral oil that passes through the alimentary tract unchanged, and therefore acts as a simple lubricant laxative. It is particularly valuable in producing a soft stool after intestinal and rectal operations or in cases of haemorrhoids. It is now used mainly as Liquid Paraffin Oral Emulsion. Some proprietary emulsions may contain added phenolphthalein.

The oil-soluble vitamins of the diet may dissolve in liquid paraffin, and its extended use as a laxative may cause some vitamin deficiency. It is contraindicated for children under 3 years of age. Some absorption of the oil may occur after prolonged use, and paraffinomas have developed after prolonged self-medication, which should be discouraged. The Committee on Safety of Medicines has recommended that preparations containing liquid paraffin should no longer be directly available to the public, and restrictions should be placed on its sale through pharmacies.

LAXATIVE ENEMAS

Locally acting laxatives are sometimes useful in softening impacted faeces and facilitating evacuation. Those used as enemas may contain oils, osmotic laxatives, surface-active faecal-softening agents, and the following are some representative products: arachis oil retention enema, magnesium sulphate enema, phosphates enema, Micralax, Relaxit and Veripaque.

MISCELLANEOUS DRUGS

It is convenient to refer here to a few drugs that have some exceptional influence on secretory or excretory functions.

Penicillamine § (dose: 1.5 g daily)

Brand names: Distamine §, Pendramine §

Penicillamine, also referred to on page 423, is used in the treatment of Wilson's disease, a hepatolenticular degeneration brought about by the excessive retention of copper in the body. Penicillamine binds with and mobilizes the excess copper as a soluble chelate, which is excreted in the urine. It is given in doses of 500 mg three times a day before food, but treatment must be continued indefinitely with maintenance doses of 750 mg daily once a negative copper balance has been achieved. Hypersensitivity reactions may limit prolonged treatment.

It is also used in the treatment of cystinuria, as it combines with cystine to form a more soluble complex. It is given initially in divided doses of 1–3 g daily before food, aimed at reducing urinary cystine excretion to 200 mg/litre. Subsequent maintenance doses are 0.5–1 g, together with a fluid intake of at least three litres daily.

Penicillamine is also used in the treatment of poisoning by lead, mercury, copper and gold.

Trientine §

Trientine is also a copper chelating agent used in the treatment of Wilson's disease, but it is usually reserved for patients unable to tolerate penicillamine. It is given in doses of 300–600 mg four times a day before food. Trientine may cause nausea, and interfere with the absorption of iron.

Cholelitholytic drugs

Cholelitholytic drugs are those that are used orally for the dissolution of cholesterol-containing gall stones present in a functioning gall bladder. They appear to act by inhibiting the hepatic synthesis of cholesterol, and as the bile becomes less saturated with cholesterol, so steroid-containing gall stones tend to dissolve, but stones larger than 15 mm are less likely to dissolve completely. They are suitable for the treatment of radiolucent stones only, as calcium-containing or bile-pigment stones are unlikely to dissolve. Chenodeoxycholic acid (**Chendol** §, **Chendecon** §, **Chenofalk** §), is given in doses of 750–1250 mg daily; ursodeoxycholic acid (**Destolit** §, **Ursofalk** §), is given in doses of 450–600 mg daily. Combidol contains both acids, and is given in doses of 500–750 mg daily. They are used only when surgery or other biliary techniques are inadvisable, as very prolonged treatment is required, and recurrence is common within a year after treatment is discontinued. Oestrogen-containing oral contraceptives, and drugs of the clofibrate type, which increase bile cholesterol, should be avoided.

Glutamic acid hydrochloride (dose: 1.5–3 g daily)

Brand name: Muripsin

Glutamic acid hydrochloride yields hydrochloric acid in solution, and is given in doses of 500 mg–1 g with meals in conditions of reduced or absent gastric acid secretion, as in hypochlorhydria and achlorhydria.

Pancreatin

Pancreatin is a preparation of mammalian pancreas, and contains a mixture of the enzymes protease, amylase and lipase, necessary for the digestion of proteins, carbohydrates and fats. It is given orally in the treatment of cystic fibrosis and other conditions of pancreatic deficiency, but its use requires care, as pancreatin is inactivated by heat and gastric acid. It is used as a powder or granules, and may be taken mixed with food or fluids, which should not be too hot, and not allowed to stand before being taken.

Inactivation by gastric acid can be reduced by taking pancreatin with an antacid or an acid-inhibiting agent of the cimetidine type. Some preparations of pancreatin are supplied as enteric coated granules, by which means larger amounts of lipase and other enzymes escape inactivation and reach the duodenum unchanged. Nurses should advise patients that these enteric coated granules should be swallowed whole, and not chewed, otherwise the benefits of the enteric coating will be lost. The standard dose of pancreatin is up to 8 g daily, but requires individual adjustment according to need and the nature and frequency of the stools. **Side-effects** include nausea, vomiting and abdominal discomfort; anal irritation may also occur. Some very high strength pancreatin preparations have been used in cystic fibrosis, but recent reports indicate that with these high potency products, there is a risk that fibrotic strictures of the colon may develop with extended treatment, and require major surgery. Until the extent of the risk becomes known, the Committee on Safety of Medicines has recommended that the treatment of patients receiving these high potency products should be reviewed, and unless there are special reasons, a change should be made for the time being to other pancreatin preparations. If symptoms indicative of gastrointestinal obstruction occur with any pancreatin preparation, the possibility of bowel stricture should be reported without delay.

Pancreatin preparations

Creon; Nutrizym GR; Nutrizym 10; Pancrease; Pancrex; Pancrex V.

High potency pancreatin products ▼

Creon 25000; Nutrizym 22; Pancrease HL; Panzytrat.

(A new product for the treatment of cystic fibrosis is dornase alfa (p. 446).)

Drugs acting on the urinary system

DIURETICS

Diuretics are drugs that increase the excretion of urine. They are used extensively in heart failure, where they are regarded as first-line treatment, as by increasing urinary output they decrease plasma volume, lower the venous return and so reduce the cardiac pre-load. They are also used in renal, hepatic and pulmonary disease associated with fluid retention. The mode of action varies, as the renal system is complex, and different diuretics may act at a different or more than one point.

Anatomically, each kidney is made up of about a million nephrons, each consisting of a glomerulus and two tubules connected by the loop of Henle. Each nephron functions as a filtering unit and can be represented diagrammatically (Fig. 12.1).

The glomerulus consists of a group of fine blood vessels, in which the blood circulates under pressure (about 1200 ml of blood pass through the glomeruli of the kidneys every minute). The glomerulus is enclosed in a cup-like structure (Bowman's capsule), connected with an extended tubular system consisting of the proximal convoluted tubule, which ends in the collecting duct. It functions as a filter, for a large amount of water and dissolved salts is separated from the protein and lipid constituents of the blood passing through the glomerulus.

This protein-free filtrate passes on to the tubules, where much of the water, glucose, sodium chloride, sodium bicarbonate,

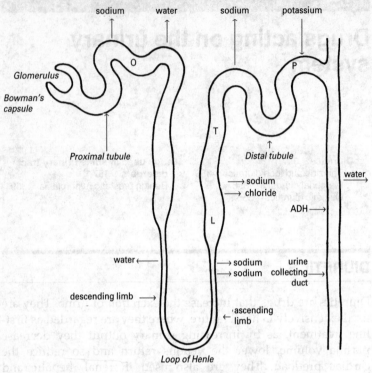

Figure 12.1 Diagram of nephron unit and some points of electrolyte exchange and diuretic action.

potassium chloride and other substances are selectively re-absorbed and pass back into the circulation, leaving the excess water, urea and other unwanted substances to be excreted as urine. About 70% of the sodium, all the potassium, and much of the water are re-absorbed by the proximal tubule, and a further 20% of sodium is absorbed in the loop of Henle. About 20 ml of the original filtrate leaves the loop to enter the distal tubule. Here, the urine is further concentrated, and according to the electrolyte balance more sodium is absorbed in exchange for potassium.

In the collecting duct, under the influence of the antidiuretic hormone, water passes into the interstitial tissues and then back into the general circulation.

Electrolyte balance

Thus the kidney is an organ of considerable complexity, and in health it is capable of maintaining the composition of the blood within narrow limits in spite of varying fluid intake or extremes of climatic conditions. The antidiuretic hormone of the pituitary gland present as vasopressin plays an important part in this control of the electrolyte balance of the body, but disease can upset this delicate balance, and heart failure and liver disease are among the most important causes of kidney dysfunction.

If the blood supply to the glomerulus is reduced as a consequence of an impaired circulation, or excessive drug-induced lowering of blood pressure, the filtration rate is slowed down. Yet tubular re-absorption continues unchecked, so that excess water and salts which are normally excreted, soon begin to accumulate in the body tissues.

In conditions such as congestive heart failure, or renal, hepatic or pulmonary disease, where salt and water retention have resulted in oedema or ascites, diuretics can afford relief by checking tubular re-absorption, and so increasing the elimination of water and the dissolved salts.

Some diuretics have a limited antihypertensive action, and are useful in supplementing the response to more specific blood pressure lowering agents. They are also useful in the treatment of drug overdose by increasing the rate of renal elimination.

Mode of action of diuretics

Because of the complex structure of the kidney, different diuretics may produce the same final effect by different modes of action. Thus diuresis may be achieved by drugs which dilate the renal blood vessels and so increase the glomerular filtration rate, or by those that prevent the re-absorption of salts and water by the tubules or the loop of Henle.

Some drugs have a general action at several points, others, such as frusemide and ethacrynic acid, act largely on the loop, whereas spironolactone has a selective action on the distal tubule. Diuretics that act mainly on the distal tubule alter the sodium–potassium balance, and permit a larger amount of potassium to be excreted. Occasionally this loss of potassium may result in hypokalaemia, with muscle weakness and cardiac arrhythmias especially in patients with heart failure who are receiving digoxin. The supplementary administration of potassium chloride may be necessary, often as effervescent potassium tablets (Kloref, Sando-K) or as a slow-release product (Slow-K). Such products should always be taken with water, and while the patient is in a standing or sitting position to prevent oesophageal damage.

Available diuretics fall into three main groups, the thiazide diuretics, the loop or high ceiling diuretics, represented by frusemide, and the potassium-sparing diuretics. (See amiloride and osmotic diuretics on p. 356). It should be obvious that potassium supplements, referred to above, should not be given with potassium-sparing diuretics.

Points about diuretics

(a) Thiazides are used mainly to reduce oedema due to heart failure, and in hypertension.
(b) Loop diuretics are of value in pulmonary oedema caused by left ventricular failure, and when response to thiazides is inadequate.
(c) Hypokalaemia is potentially dangerous in patients with coronary heart disease receiving digoxin and those on anti-arrhythmics.
(d) Best taken in the morning to reduce nocturia.
(e) May cause postural hypotension, especially after sleep.
(f) Lethargy, weakness and anorexia may indicate electrolyte disturbance and hypokalaemia.

THIAZIDE AND LOOP DIURETICS

Some of the early sulphonamides had a certain degree of diuretic activity, and further research led to the introduction of the thiazide class of diuretics, followed by the discovery of the loop diuretics. The thiazides act mainly on the distal tubule and are of value in congestive heart failure, whereas the loop diuretics, which influence re-absorption in the loop of Henle, are also used in pulmonary oedema. The thiazides are also useful in reduced doses as supplementary drugs in the treatment of hypertension (p. 188).

Chlorothiazide (Saluric, dose: 0.5–2 g) was the first thiazide diuretic, but it has been largely replaced by more potent drugs. Table 12.1 indicates the range of diuretics in use. When possible, these diuretics should be given at times when the subsequent diuresis is less likely to interfere with sleep.

Although in general these potent diuretics are well tolerated, the **side-effects** are numerous and include gastrointestinal distur-

Table 12.1 Diuretics

Approved name	Brand name	Products
amiloride	Midamor	Tablets, 5 mg
bendrofluazide	Aprinox	Tablets, 2.5 mg; 5 mg
	Centyl	Tablets, 2.5 mg; 5 mg
	Neo-Naclex	Tablets, 2.5 mg; 5 mg
bumetanide[a]	Burinex	Tablets, 1 mg; 5 mg
chlorothiazide	Saluric	Tablets, 500 mg
chlorthalidone	Hygroton	Tablets, 50 mg; 100 mg
cyclopenthiazide	Navidrex	Tablets, 0.5 mg
ethacrynic acid[a]	Edecrin	Tablets, 50 mg
frusemide[a]	Lasix	Tablets, 20 mg; 40 mg
	Dryptal	Tablets, 40 mg
hydrochlorothiazide	Esidrex	Tablets, 25 mg; 50 mg
	HydroSaluric	Tablets, 25 mg, 50 mg
hydroflumethiazide	Hydrenox	Tablets, 50 mg
indapamide	Natrilix	Tablets, 2.5 mg
mefruside	Baycaron	Tablets, 25 mg
methylclothiazide	Enduron	Tablets, 5 mg
metolazone	Metenix; Xuret	Tablets, 5 mg
piretanide	Arelix	Capsules, 6 mg
polythiazide	Nephril	Tablets, 1 mg
torasemide	Torem	Tablets 2.5, 5 and 10 mg
triamterene	Dytac	Capsules, 50 mg
xipamide	Diurexan	Tablets, 20 mg

[a] 'Loop diuretics'.
Note. The suffix 'K' is added to the brand name of several of the above products when a compound tablet containing both potassium chloride and diuretic is available. It should not be assumed that these products contain the same amount of diuretic as the plain tablet, as in some cases they contain less. In some mixed tablets potassium chloride is contained in an enteric-coated core of the tablet, and the release of the potassium chloride in the small intestine may cause small bowel ulceration and obstruction. Patients taking such tablets should be advised to report any gastrointestinal disturbances.

bances, hyperglycaemia, hyperuricaemia, gout, rash and thrombocytopenia. Photosensitivity has been reported. The loop diuretics may also cause tinnitus and deafness. Care is necessary in renal and hepatic impairment.

Bendrofluazide § (dose: 2.5–10 mg daily)

Brand names: Aprinox §, Berkozide §, NeoNaclex §

Bendrofluazide is a representative of the thiazide diuretics generally in its actions and uses. It is rapidly absorbed orally, and has an action that lasts 10–12 hours or more, so the standard dose of

2.5–5 mg should be taken in the morning so that the diuresis does not disturb sleep.

Bendrofluazide acts mainly on the descending loop of Henle and the distal tubule, and produces diuresis by preventing the reabsorption of salts and water. It is widely used in the treatment of congestive heart failure and many other oedematous conditions, including pre-menstrual tension.

Frusemide § (dose: 40 mg–2 g daily)

Brand names: Lasix §, Dryptal §, Diuresal §

Frusemide is classed as a 'loop' diuretic, as it acts on the loop of Henle as well as the proximal and distal tubules.

It is a powerful diuretic, and is frequently effective in oedema and the oliguria of renal failure when other diuretics fail to evoke an adequate response. Frusemide is given in doses of 40 mg or more daily, and the onset of diuresis is rapid, and may extend over 6 hours. Maintenance doses may vary from 20–80 mg daily according to need and response.

If a very rapid diuresis is required, as in pulmonary oedema, frusemide may be given by intramuscular or intravenous injection in doses of 20–50 mg, and the response may be dramatic both in its rapidity and in the magnitude of the diuresis. Nausea and weakness may follow the copious diuresis, and some hypotension may occur. In severe oliguria associated with renal failure, much larger doses are given, ranging from 250 mg 4–6 hourly up to a maximum single dose of 2 g. Alternatively, treatment may be commenced with a dose of 250 mg by intravenous infusion, increased if necessary to 500 mg followed by oral treatment on the basis that 500 mg orally is equivalent to 250 mg intravenously.

Side-effects include rash, tinnitus and occasional deafness. Frusemide may cause hypokalaemia, and care is necessary in diabetes and gout. It is contraindicated in cirrhosis of the liver.

Bumetanide § (dose: 1–5 mg daily)

Brand name: Burinex §

Bumetanide is a 'loop' diuretic with a rapid but brief action, and is often effective in a dose as low as 1 mg daily but a second dose may be given after 6–8 hours if required. Larger doses of 5 mg or more daily have been given in oliguria. In severe conditions such as pulmonary oedema, bumetanide may be given by intravenous or intramuscular injection in doses of 1 or 2 mg, repeated if required after 20 minutes or later. Doses of 2–5 mg may be given by slow intravenous infusion. The action of bumetanide is similar to that of frusemide, and electrolyte disturbances and loss of potassium may occur as with other diuretics. Some muscle pain and damage has been reported after high doses. In the elderly, the rapid relief of oedema may cause sudden disturbances of the circulation with hypotension and collapse.

Piretanide (Arelix §), is a loop diuretic with similar properties to those of frusemide and bumetanide, but it is used mainly in the treatment of hypertension (p. 186).

Amiloride § (dose: 5–20 mg daily)

Brand name: Midamor §

Amiloride is a potassium-sparing diuretic which acts mainly on the distal tubules. The diuresis is slow in onset, but the effects may persist for 48 hours. It is useful in patients receiving digitalis, as such patients are sensitive to lowered potassium levels.

The dose of amiloride when given alone is 10–20 mg daily. Reduced doses are given in association with other diuretics, as the action is then potentiated, and the loss of sodium (natriuresis) is increased, but the loss of potassium is decreased.

Side-effects of amiloride are rash, anorexia, pruritus, dizziness and confusion. It is contraindicated in renal failure and hyperkalaemia.

Moduretic § is a mixed product, and contains amiloride 5 mg and hydrochlorothiazide 50 mg.

Ethacrynic acid § (dose: 50–400 mg daily)

Brand name: Edecrin §

Ethacrynic acid is a 'loop' diuretic with an action similar to that of frusemide and may evoke a prompt and copious diuresis in patients who are resistant to, or who have failed to respond to other diuretics. It is given in doses of 50 mg daily after food initially, with subsequent maintenance doses of 50 mg two or three times a day, or up to a maximum daily dose of 400 mg in cases of refractory oedema. In severe conditions, ethacrynic acid may be given in doses of 50 mg by slow i.v. injection but care is necessary, as a too marked response may cause an acute hypotensive episode.

Side-effects include gastrointestinal disturbances, occasionally with a watery diarrhoea. Deafness has been reported as a side-effect after intravenous use, especially with high doses and in reduced renal efficiency. Potassium supplements may be required with continued therapy, as potassium loss, although less with ethacrynic acid, may still occur.

Spironolactone § (dose: 50–400 mg daily)

Brand names: Aldactone §, Spiroctan §

Spironolactone is a synthetic steroid that is converted in the liver to the active metabolite canrenone, which blocks the action of aldosterone on the kidney. Aldosterone is one of the steroid hormones of the adrenal cortex, and is concerned with the electrolyte balance of the body by its influence on the re-absorption of sodium and excretion of potassium by the distal tubules.

Some patients with cirrhotic oedema, ascites or the nephrotic syndrome do not always respond fully to standard diuretics, possibly because they secrete excessive amounts of aldosterone. When that occurs, the effects of a diuretic are largely nullified by the increased re-absorption of sodium in the distal tubules brought about by the action of aldosterone.

In such resistant conditions spironolactone may promote a diuresis by its aldosterone-blocking action and so reducing the re-absorption of sodium. It is also used in congestive heart failure. It is given in doses of 25–50 mg four times a day, together with a thiazide diuretic. The initial response is slow in onset, and if the diuresis is still inadequate after 5 days, the higher dose of 400 mg daily should be given.

These high doses may cause headache and drowsiness, and impotence and gynaecomastia have been reported as side-effects. The drug should be used with care in hepatic disease.

Potassium canrenoate (Spiroctan-M §) has a similar action, as it is also metabolized in the body to canrenone. It has the advantage of being soluble, and is given by slow intravenous infusion in doses of 200–400 mg daily.

Torasemide § (dose: 5–40 mg daily)

Brand name: Torem §

Torasemide is a diuretic that in low doses resembles the thiazides, and in high doses promotes a loop-diuretic type of diuresis. In hypertension it is given in morning doses of 2.5 mg, with water, but in oedema larger doses of 5–20 mg or more daily may be necessary. In congestive heart failure or hepatic oedema, torasemide may be given by slow intravenous infusion in doses of 10 mg daily initially, slowly increased if required up to a maximum of 40 mg daily. Torasemide has the general **side-effects** of the potent diuretics. It may potentiate the action of antihypertensive drugs and curare-like muscle relaxants, but the effects of NSAIDs and antidiabetic drugs may be reduced.

Triamterene § (dose: 100–250 mg daily)

Brand name: Dytac §

Triamterene is a potassium-sparing diuretic similar to amiloride and functions mainly by inhibiting the re-absorption of salts and water by the distal tubules of the kidney. Triamterene is given in initial doses of 50 mg three to five times a day, adjusted after 1 week according to need, and given on alternate days.

If given with a thiazide diuretic, the potassium loss may be reduced, and the overall diuretic effect increased, and such combined treatment may be useful in resistant oedema.

Side-effects are nausea, dry mouth and rash. Patients should be advised that, in some lights, the urine may appear bluish. Potassium supplements should not be given with triamterene, or with any other potassium-sparing diuretic.

Metyrapone § (dose: 3–4.5 g daily)

Brand name: Metopirone §

Metyrapone inhibits the formation of aldosterone by the adrenal cortex, and so has an indirect diuretic action (see spironolactone). It is occasionally used in oedema resistant to other therapy in doses of 2.5–4.5 g daily in divided doses. Metyrapone is also used in the treatment of Cushing's syndrome and other **side-effects** of corticosteroid therapy. The dose is based on the degree of disturbance of cortisol production, and may vary from 250 micrograms to 6 g daily. Nausea and vomiting are **side-effects**. Metyrapone is also used as a test for pituitary function (p. 376).

MERCURIAL DIURETICS

The mercurial diuretic Mersalyl, once widely employed, is now virtually obsolete. It is still used very occasionally in oedema resistant to other drugs, and is given *solely* by deep intramuscular injection in doses of 0.5–2 ml. Intravenous injection of mersalyl has caused severe hypotension and sudden death.

OSMOTIC DIURETICS

Osmotic diuretics are pharmacologically inert substances that are not metabolized in the body, but have the ability to attract water from the tissues. If given by injection, they bring about a transient increase in blood volume by this transfer of water, but the increase is soon compensated for by an increased urinary output. Substances that bring about this indirect diuresis are referred to as osmotic diuretics, and of chief therapeutic interest are mannitol and urea.

Mannitol (dose: 50–200 g)

Mannitol, sometimes termed manna sugar, is a carbohydrate that largely escapes metabolism, and is excreted unchanged in the urine, and so functions as an osmotic diuretic. It is mainly used intravenously to reduce the intracerebral pressure in cerebral oedema, for forced diuresis in the treatment of poisoning, and in the treatment of oliguria associated with acute renal failure.

Mannitol is given by intravenous infusion of a 10–20% solution in doses of 50–100 g over 24 hours, after an intravenous sensitivity test dose of 200 mg/kg. Careful control of the fluid balance and plasma electrolytes is necessary to prevent circulatory overload.

Side-effects of mannitol are chills, fever, nausea and tachycardia. Care is necessary to avoid extravasation, as necrosis may occur. It is contraindicated in congestive heart failure and pulmonary oedema.

Urea (dose: 40–80 g)

Urea is one of the end products of protein metabolism, and has been used orally as a non-toxic diuretic, but the large dose required limits its value. When given intravenously it functions as an osmotic diuretic, and it has been used to treat the acute rise in intracranial pressure in cerebral oedema, although mannitol is now preferred. Urea is given in doses of 40–80 g by intravenous infusion as a 30% solution in 5 or 10% glucose injection. It is now used less frequently.

DRUGS USED IN SOME URINARY TRACT DISORDERS AND IN BENIGN PROSTATIC HYPERPLASIA

Many of the anticholinergic drugs of the propantheline type are useful in the treatment of urinary frequency and incontinence, and other drugs with anticholinergic side-effects, such as amitriptyline and other tricyclic antidepressants, are also given in enuresis and similar conditions.

They act mainly by reducing the contractile activity of the detrusor muscle, but they have the disadvantages of most anticholinergic agents of causing dryness of the mouth and blurred vision. Care is also necessary in the elderly, as they may precipitate glaucoma, and in males, may add to the problems of prostatic hypertrophy. Some other drugs used in the treatment of urinary frequency and other bladder disorders are represented by the following:

Desmopressin § (dose: 10–40 micrograms intranasally)

Brand names: Desmospray §, DDAVP §

Desmopressin is an analogue of vasopressin (p. 365) and is used in the control of primary nocturnal enuresis in children and adults. It is given by nasal spray at bedtime in doses of 10–20 micrograms, increased to a maximum of 40 micrograms if necessary. It is not recommended for children under 5 years of age. The response should be checked at monthly intervals by suspending treatment for a week. Although desmopressin has little pressor activity, care should be taken in hypertension and cardiovascular disorders. Its use in diabetes insipidus is referred to on page 365.

Ephedrine § (dose: 30–60 mg daily)

Ephedrine is a sympathomimetic amine (p. 243) that is sometimes useful in nocturnal enuresis. It appears to act by influencing bladder neck closure, and possibly contraction of the distal sphincter. It is given in doses of 30–60 mg at night according to age.

Side-effects include restlessness and insomnia. Ephedrine is contraindicated in prostatic hypertrophy as it may cause urinary retention.

Flavoxate § (dose: 600 mg daily)

Brand name: Urispas §

Flavoxate has some smooth muscle relaxant properties, and is indicated in the control of spasm of the urinary tract, and in the symptomatic relief of dysuria, urgency and cystitis. It is given in doses of 200 mg three times a day.

Side-effects may include headache, nausea and blurred vision. Like related drugs, it should be used with care if glaucoma is present.

Oxybutynin § (dose: 10–20 mg daily)

Brand names: Cystrin §, Ditropan §

Oxybutynin resembles flavoxate in having antispasmodic properties, and is useful in relieving the symptoms of neurogenic bladder instability, such as frequency and urgency. It is given in doses of 5 mg two to four times a day according to need. The elderly may be more susceptible to the atropine-like **side-effects** of oxybutynin, and should be given half-doses.

Pseudoephedrine (dose: 30–60 mg)

Brand name: Sudafed

Pseudoephedrine is an isomer of ephedrine that has been used in nocturnal enuresis in doses of 30–60 mg at night. Pseudoephedrine also has some decongestive properties, and is present in some expectorant preparations.

Side-effects. Visual hallucinations have sometimes occurred in children given such pseudoephedrine-containing products (p. 444).

BENIGN PROSTATIC HYPERPLASIA

Benign prostatic hyperplasia (BPH) is common in men over 50 years of age, and causes a varying degree of bladder outlet obstruction. The associated incomplete emptying of the bladder may promote infection and secondary inflammation of the bladder which may also involve the upper urinary tract with progressive urinary frequency and nocturia. Surgery is the radical treatment, but when surgery is contraindicated or postponed, symptomatic treatment is with certain anticholinergic agents, alpha receptor-blocking agents, or an enzyme inhibitor.

Points about drugs used in BPH

(a) Useful when surgery is contraindicated or postponed.
(b) Usually given to elderly patients, some may cause postural
    hypotension especially with first dose.
(c) Low doses initially and in renal impairment.
(d) Some are also used in hypertension — extra care needed.

Alfuzosin §▼ (dose: 7.5 mg daily)

Brand name: Xatral §

Alfuzosin is a selective antagonist of post-synaptic alpha$_1$-adrenoceptors, and lowers the tone of bladder and prostatic smooth muscle. It is used for the symptomatic relief of benign prostatic hyperplasia, and is also of value when surgery has to be delayed. Alfuzosin is given as an initial dose of 2.5 mg at bedtime, as it may cause hypotension, afterwards three times a day. Reduced doses should be given to the elderly, and patients with renal and hepatic insufficiency. **Side-effects** include dizziness, vertigo and gastrointestinal disturbances. Combined treatment with anti-hypertensive agents should be avoided because of additive effects and treatment should be withdrawn before general anaesthesia.

Jardin A et al 1991 Alfuzosin for the treatment of benign prostatic hypertrophy. Lancet 337: 1457–1461

Finasteride § (dose: 5 mg daily)

Brand name: Proscar §

The development of the prostate gland and any prostatic enlargement in later life is linked with the conversion of testosterone to dihydrotestosterone in the gland by the enzyme 5-alpha reductase. The inhibition of that enzyme in BPH should lead to a regression of the hyperplasia, and finasteride is a synthetic steroid with the required highly specific inhibitory action. It is given in doses of 5 mg daily, but prolonged administration is necessary to obtain a shrinkage in size of the prostate gland and symptomatic relief. Finasteride has no androgenic properties or affinity for androgen receptors in other tissues. It is well tolerated, and the mild **side-effects** are due to its anti-androgenic properties.

Gormley G J et al 1992 The effect of finasteride in men with benign prostatic hyperplasia. New England Journal of Medicine 327: 1185–1191

Indoramin § (dose: 50–100 mg daily)

Brand name: Doralese §

Indoramin is an alpha receptor blocking agent with a relatively selective action on the alpha receptors of the sympathetic nerves that control bladder muscle tone. By blocking those receptors, the tone of the bladder neck muscle is relaxed, and the degree of bladder outlet obstruction is relieved to some extent. Indoramin is given in doses of 20 mg twice daily initially, slowly increased if required up to a maximum of 100 mg daily. In elderly patients with reduced renal clearance, a single nightly dose of 20 mg may be adequate. **Side-effects** are dry mouth, drowsiness and nasal congestion. The use of indoramin in hypertension is referred to on page 194.

Prazosin § (dose: 2–4 mg daily)

Brand name: Hypovase §

Prazosin is an alpha-adrenoceptor blocking agent used mainly in hypertension (p. 196) but it is also useful for the symptomatic treatment of benign prostatic hyperplasia. It is given in doses of 1–2 mg twice a day, and with extended treatment it reduces urinary frequency and nocturia, as well as reducing the volume of residual urine. The initial dose of prazosin should be small, and taken at night, on account of its hypotensive action. **Side-effects** are dizziness, dry mouth and blurred vision.

Hormones and the endocrine system

Hormones are chemical substances released into the blood stream by the endocrine glands. These glands, sometimes referred to as ductless glands, are small pockets of highly specialized tissues situated in various parts of the body, and they play a fundamental part in growth and development and in the maintenance of the health of the body.

The hormones of the endocrine system are released according to physiological needs, but the hormones of one gland may influence the activity of another, others may be affected by impulses from the central nervous system, and the whole mechanism of production and release of hormones is so complex that the final response is due to the interaction of many factors.

Many of these hormones have been extracted from the glands concerned and adrenaline and insulin are familiar examples of hormones used therapeutically. In some cases it has been possible to make hormones synthetically, and some derivatives are more powerful and selective in action than the natural hormones. These advances in biological chemistry have led to a wider understanding of the action and importance of hormones, and their value, as well as their limitations, as therapeutic agents.

THE PITUITARY GLAND

The pituitary or hypophysis is a small gland about the size of a pea, situated in the base of the skull and it is attached by a stalk to the hypothalamus. It consists of two parts, the anterior and posterior lobes, and secretes a number of hormones which affect other endocrine glands as well as various physiological processes. These secretions are themselves stimulated or inhibited by the action of the regulatory hormones of the hypothalamus, a 'feed-back' system that plays an important part in the control of hormonal activity. The relationship between the pituitary gland and the hormones which it ultimately controls is indicated in Figure 13.1.

POSTERIOR LOBE

This part of the pituitary gland is a store for two hormones,

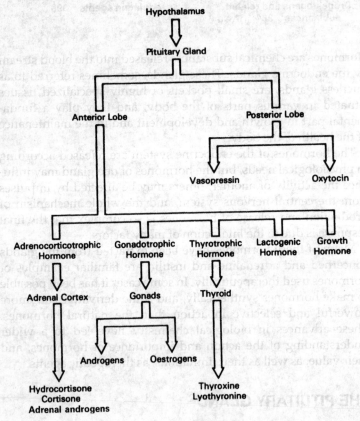

Figure 13.1 The relationship between the pituitary gland and hormones.

vasopressin and oxytocin, derived from the hypothalamus. Vasopressin is the antidiuretic hormone, and plays an essential part in maintaining the water balance of the body. Oxytocin stimulates contractions of uterine smooth muscle, particularly at the end of pregnancy.

Vasopressin, now obtained by recombinant technology, increases the re-absorption of water by the renal tubules when the fluid intake is low, and so reduces the urinary output, whereas with a high intake of fluid it decreases absorption and preserves the fluid balance by increasing urinary excretion. Vasopressin is used mainly in the treatment of diabetes insipidus which is caused by pituitary dysfunction. It is a deficiency condition that may occur abruptly at almost any age, or it may follow injury, and is characterized by thirst and a high output of very dilute urine. A correspondingly high fluid intake is required that may amount to several litres a day. Two forms of the disease are recognized, pituitary diabetes insipidus (PDI), and nephrogenic or partial diabetes insipidus (NDI). Vasopressin is replacement therapy, as the symptoms of PDI can be relieved by injections of vasopressin. In practice, vasopressin is used mainly for the diagnosis of PDI, and its differentiation from NDI, as for prolonged-treatment longer-acting derivatives, some of which can be given by nasal spray (see desmopressin, lypressin and terlipressin) are preferred. In nephrogenic diabetes insipidus the kidneys are resistant to exogenous ADH and treatment is with chlorpropamide, chlorthalidone and carbamazepine. Those drugs appear to sensitize the renal tubules to respond to any remaining endogenous vasopressin.

Vasopressin § (dose: 5–20 units)

Brand name: Pitressin §

Vasopressin is used in the diagnosis and treatment of pituitary diabetes insipidus and is given in doses of 5–20 units by subcutaneous or intramuscular injection every 4 hours. When the diabetes insipidus is due to injury, only short-term treatment may be necessary. For long-term use treatment with alternative drugs such as desmopressin, lypressin and terlipressin is usually preferred, which in some cases can be given by nasal spray. Vasopressin is also used for the control of variceal bleeding, and is then given in doses of 20 units by intravenous infusion. **Side-effects** of vasopressin are nausea and intestinal disturbances, cramp and occasionally angina.

Desmopressin § (dose: 10–40 micrograms)

Brand names: DDAVP §, Desmospray §

Desmopressin is a synthetic analogue of vasopressin with a much longer antidiuretic action and reduced pressor side-effects. It is used in pituitary diabetes insipidus as nasal drops or spray once or twice a day in doses of 10–20 micrograms (one to two puffs). It may also be given by intramuscular or intravenous injection in doses of 1–4 micrograms daily. Liquid intake must be adjusted during desmopressin treatment to avoid fluid retention and hyponatria. **Side-effects** of desmopressin are similar to those of vasopressin. Desmopressin is sometimes useful in nocturnal enuresis when endogenous vasopressin may be deficient. In doses of 20–40 micrograms at night it may control the eneuresis without affecting day-time kidney function. It may also be of value in nocturia associated with multiple sclerosis. Withdrawal of such treatment should be carried out after 3 months to permit an assessment of renal function.

Lypressin § (dose: 2.5–10 units as required)

Brand name: Syntopressin §

Lypressin resembles desmopressin in action, and in pituitary diabetes insipidus it is given as a nasal spray in doses of 2.5–10 units (one to four puffs) up to seven times a day. Local **side-effects** are nasal congestion and ulceration; it may also cause nausea and abdominal pain.

Terlipressin § (dose: 1–2 mg by injection)

Brand name: Glypressin §

Terlipressin is a vasopressin analogue for the treatment of bleeding from oesophageal varices. It is given by intravenous injection as an initial dose of 2 mg, followed by doses of 1–2 mg 4- to 6-hourly until bleeding is controlled up to a maximum of

12 doses. The **side-effects** of terlipressin are similar to those of vasopressin, but less marked.

Oxytocin § (dose: 1–5 units)

Brand name: Syntocinon §

Oxytocin has a selective stimulating action on uterine muscle, but it has no pressor or antidiuretic properties. The degree of activity is related to the physiological state of the uterus, and is greatest during the late stages of pregnancy. In practice oxytocin is used mainly in uterine inertia and for the induction of labour. It is given by intravenous drip infusion in dextrose solution, in small doses of 1–3 milliunits per minute, as the rapid response requires careful control of the dose.

Oxytocin is also used to control post-partum haemorrhage, and is given in doses of 5–10 units by slow intravenous infusion. Doses of 2–5 units may also be given by intramuscular injection, often together with 500 micrograms of the longer-acting ergometrine, as Syntometrine (p. 450). Oxytocin is also used by intravenous infusion in the management of missed abortion.

ANTERIOR LOBE

The anterior lobe of the pituitary gland is one of the most important glands of the body. It secretes at least six hormones, including the adrenocorticotrophic, the gonadotrophic, the thyrotrophic, the lactogenic, and the growth hormone. Some are used therapeutically, others in diagnosis, but as they are protein in nature they are not effective orally, and must be given by injection.

With a few exceptions their therapeutic use is disappointing. Their action is basically that of stimulating the related endocrine gland, i.e. the thyrotrophic hormone controls the activity of the thyroid gland, and in therapy the use of the hormones of the gland concerned is preferred.

Corticotrophin §

Corticotrophin is the adrenocorticotrophic hormone, sometimes referred to as ACTH, and was originally obtained from animal

368 DRUGS AND PHARMACOLOGY FOR NURSES

pituitary gland. It has a direct action on the cortex of the adrenal gland, and stimulates the production of hydrocortisone, cortisone and other steroids. The final action of the hormone is basically that of hydrocortisone, and direct treatment with that drug or related steroids is usually preferred.

Corticotrophin exerts its effects through the medium of the adrenal gland, and in health there is a balance between the activity of the gland and the level of corticosteroids in circulation. The balance is achieved by a 'feed-back' mechanism, as a rise in the blood corticosteroid level causes a fall in corticotrophin secretion. That fall results in a reduction in the release of the steroids from the adrenal cortex, which then stimulates the anterior pituitary gland to produce more ACTH. As more ACTH is released, the level of corticosteroids again rises, and this 'see-saw' rise and fall in hormone production is an essential part of the physiological balance of the body (Fig. 13.2).

When the cortex is damaged, as in Addison's disease, corticotrophin is of no value, and corticosteroid replacement therapy is necessary. Corticotrophin has been used in the treatment of chronic asthma and many other disorders but its use has declined.

It is now used as tetracosactrin to test the efficiency of adrenocortical function.

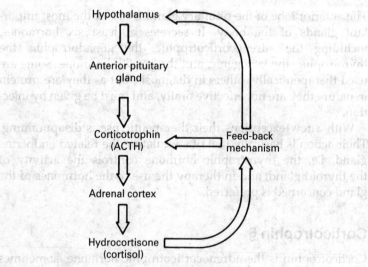

Figure 13.2 Feed-back control of adrenal cortex activity.

Tetracosactrin § (dose: 250 micrograms by injection)

Brand names: Synacthen §, Synacthen Depot §

Tetracosactrin is used mainly in the 30-minute diagnostic test of adrenocorticol insufficiency. It is given in a dose of 250 micrograms by intramuscular or intravenous injection, and the plasma cortisol levels are measured immediately before and exactly 30 minutes after the injection. Normally a rise to at least 200 mmol/litre of cortisol should occur.

Tetracosactrin–zinc phosphate complex (Synacthen Depot) is a longer-acting form used for short-term treatment of conditions requiring corticosteroid therapy, particularly in patients unable to tolerate such treatment orally, or when the oral response is ineffective. The complex is given by intramuscular injection as an initial daily dose of 1 mg, reduced to 0.5 mg twice a week. It should be given under medical supervision, as serious anaphylactic reactions have occurred, and immediate treatment must be available (p. 233).

ADRENAL CORTEX

When the cortex of the adrenal gland is stimulated by corticotrophin, it forms two types of hormones biosynthesized from cholesterol, the corticosteroids and the adrenal androgens.

The natural corticosteroid hormones can be divided into two main groups, the glucocorticoid hormones exemplified by hydrocortisone (cortisol), which control carbohydrate and protein metabolism, and the mineraloid hormones, represented by aldosterone, which influence the salt and water balance of the body. This distinction is useful, but not exact, as the glucocorticoid hormones also influence the electrolyte balance to some extent, and some synthetic corticosteroids have a more selective action.

Corticosteroids

Hydrocortisone (cortisol) and cortisone are well-known examples of glucocorticoid hormones, and are closely related as cortisone is converted in the liver to hydrocortisone.

These steroids have a number of important actions, and are closely concerned with the metabolism of fats, proteins and carbohydrates. They promote the formation of glycogen by the liver, affect the excretion of salts and water, reduce capillary permeability, have a marked anti-allergic action, and increase the resistance of the body to stress and shock.

Therapeutic uses

The corticosteroids have a wide range of therapeutic applications, apart from their use in deficiency states. Dosage varies accordingly, and in principle the lowest dose that evokes the desired response should be given. In view of their numerous **side-effects**, they should not be used unless the benefits are likely to outweigh the disadvantages of treatment.

The corticosteroids are used mainly in deficiency states and in the suppression of various inflammatory disease processes, including rheumatoid arthritis, and the nephrotic syndrome.

In deficiency states, such as Addison's disease, the secretion of corticosteroids by the adrenal cortex is diminished or absent, and for replacement therapy, reliance is largely placed on hydrocortisone supplemented by fludrocortisone. The latter has an increased mineralocorticoid activity that provides the balance for complete replacement therapy.

The corticosteroids are also used in various inflammatory diseases such as rheumatoid condition, as they suppress inflammation indirectly by depressing the release of phospholipids from plasma cell membranes. Such lipids are necessary for the formation of prostaglandins, which play an important part in the inflammatory process (p. 416). Corticosteroids are also of value in allergic reactions and asthma, shock and stress.

The corticosteroids are also used with cytotoxic drugs in the control of malignant disease, and in association with drugs such as azathioprine, to reduce immune responses after organ transplantation. They are also used locally in various inflammatory conditions of the skin and eyes.

The potency of the corticosteroids is such that they should be used with great care, and in principle they should be used in the lowest effective dose for the shortest period of time. Patients should carry a card stating that they are receiving the drugs, so that in cases of emergency, treatment can be adapted to the patient concerned, as continuity of treatment is important, and higher doses may be necessary in illness. Table 13.1 shows the

Table 13.1 Comparable doses of some corticosteroids

Corticosteroid	Dose
Cortisone	25.0 mg
Hydrocortisone	20.0 mg
Prednisone	5.0 mg
Prednisolone	5.0 mg
Methylprednisolone	4.0 mg
Triamcinolone	4.0 mg
Dexamethasone	0.75 mg
Betamethasone	0.75 mg

anti-inflammatory doses of some corticosteroids, although larger doses may be required in allergic conditions (p. 372).

Points about corticosteroid therapy

(a) Potent drugs; lowest effective dose should be given and response balanced against the potential dangers.

(b) In long-term treatment, the side-effects may be worse than the disabilities caused by the illness being treated.

(c) In chronic conditions, treatment should be withdrawn very slowly to permit the return of normal adrenocortical function.

(d) Corticosteroids best taken in the morning to reduce suppressive effects on pituitary-adrenal function.

(e) All patients should carry a steroid warning card.

(f) Great care is necessary in anaesthesia, and measures must be taken to avoid a potentially precipitous fall in blood pressure due to corticosteroid therapy.

Side-effects. The profound influence of the corticosteroids on the physiological activities of the body is reflected in their side-effects. They delay tissue repair, increase gastric acidity, and may cause or exacerbate peptic ulcer, of which the symptoms may be disguised by the anti-inflammatory action. The influence of the corticosteroids on tissue reactions is also a potential danger in infection, as they may temporarily suppress signs of infection until the illness has become well established.

The salt and water balance of the body is also disturbed, and muscle wasting, loss of calcium and osteoporosis may occur, especially after long treatment. The retention of normally excreted fluid may lead to oedema and hypertension. Moonface and other signs of Cushing's syndrome may also occur, due to changes in the deposition of fat. The prolonged use of corticosteroids in high doses may cause a 'steroid cataract'.

In children, the corticosteroids may bring about a suppression of normal growth, and if given during pregnancy, may affect the fetal development of the adrenal glands.

Care is also necessary when corticosteroids are applied locally, as their action is suppressive, and the condition may return when treatment is discontinued. Systemic absorption with side-effects may occur if topical preparations of some corticosteroids are applied over large areas, especially if occlusive dressings are used. Small children are particularly susceptible to such side-effects, and for such patients a product containing a low potency corticosteroid should be used (p. 533).

Potassium loss, causing muscle weakness and cardiac irregularities are other side-effects of corticosteroids, and potassium supplements should be given if treatment is prolonged. Both euphoria and depression may occur, and the latter may be serious in patients with a history of mental disturbances. With the newer synthetic steroids the disturbances in the electrolyte balance have been reduced, and are less frequent and severe.

Hydrocortisone § (dose: 12.5–30 mg daily)

Brand names: Efcortelan §, Efcortesol §, Hydrocortistab §, Hydrocortone §, Solu-Cortef §

Hydrocortisone is the main glucocorticosteroid hormone of the adrenal cortex. It is used orally for replacement therapy in Addison's disease and other conditions of adrenal cortex deficiency in doses of 20 mg in the morning and 10 mg at night, adjusted to need, and supplemented by fludrocortisone, which has an increased mineralocorticoid activity. In severe deficiency states, and in the crises of Addison's disease hydrocortisone is given by intravenous injection in doses of 100 mg every 6–8 hours, followed by oral therapy as the condition is controlled.

Large doses of hydrocortisone intravenously are also used in the emergency treatment of severe acute asthma, and to supplement adrenaline injections in acute hypersensitivity reactions. It is also given intravenously for the treatment of septic shock in doses up to 300 mg, although the value of such therapy has been questioned. Large doses have been given orally in conditions such as pemphigus and exfoliative dermatitis.

Hydrocortisone is also highly effective when applied locally, and it is widely used as a 0.1–1% cream, ointment or lotion in the treatment of many inflamed and itching skin conditions. Some preparations of hydrocortisone for local use may contain an antibiotic such as neomycin to control or prevent any associated infection, as hydrocortisone has no antibacterial properties. A retention enema containing hydrocortisone 100 mg is sometimes used in ulcerative colitis to supplement other therapy. It should be noted that hydrocortisone is of no value in urticaria.

Cortisone § (dose: 25–37.5 mg daily)

Brand names: Cortistab §, Cortisyl §

Cortisone is a glucocorticoid with the actions and side-effects of hydrocortisone, to which it is converted in the liver. Hydrocortisone is now the preferred drug, as cortisone as such is inactive, and in liver disease the conversion of cortisone to hydrocortisone may not be complete.

Cortisone has distinct mineralocorticosteroid properties, and is still used for replacement therapy in Addison's disease and other conditions of adrenocortical deficiency, in divided doses of 25–37.5 mg daily. It has been used in many other inflammatory and allergic conditions, but prednisolone or other compounds with a reduced action on the sodium balance and fewer side-effects are now preferred. Cortisone is ineffective both locally and by injection into joints.

Prednisolone § and prednisone § (dose: 10–100 mg daily)

Prednisolone brand names: Deltastab §, Precortisyl §, Prednesol §, Sintisone §

Prednisone brand name: Decortisyl §

Prednisolone and prednisone are derivatives of hydrocortisone and cortisone respectively, but are about five times more potent. They have the same general action and uses of the parent drugs, but the increased glucocorticoid action is accompanied by a decrease in mineralocorticoid potency, with a reduction in some side-effects. Prednisone is itself inactive, and is converted in the liver to prednisolone, and the latter is now the preferred drug, particularly for extended treatment.

Prednisolone is used in a wide range of conditions requiring systemic corticosteroid therapy, including the suppression of the inflammatory reactions of rheumatoid arthritis, in allergic states, systemic lupus erythematosus and pemphigus, to name but a few. It is given orally in doses that may range from 5–60 mg daily in divided doses, but for the extended treatment of rheumatoid conditions doses above 10 mg daily are seldom required. In such long-term treatment, alternate-day, early-morning dosage may reduce side-effects by causing less depression of the pituitary-adrenal axis. For serious conditions such as acute lymphoblastic leukaemia and pemphigus, large doses are given, as the need to control the condition outweighs the risks of side-effects. In other cases, it may be given by intramuscular injection as prednisolone acetate in doses of 25–100 mg once or twice a week.

One of the chief disadvantages of corticosteroid therapy generally is the disturbance caused in the salt and water balance of the body. Although these disturbances are less with prednisolone, prednisone and other derivatives in all cases, and especially with long-term treatment, the maintenance doses should be the lowest dose that evokes a satisfactory response. Intermittent rather than daily doses have been recommended as pituitary-adrenal suppression may occur if treatment is prolonged. When treatment is to be discontinued, slow withdrawal of a corticosteroid over a period of weeks may be required to permit the natural production of corticosteroids to rise to a normal level.

The reduced tendency of some derivatives to cause salt and water retention is of advantage when long term therapy is needed, but conversely, they are less suitable for the treatment of Addison's disease, and in such cases a salt-retaining corticosteroid such as cortisone or fludrocortisone is required.

Corticosteroids such as prednisolone are given in high doses of 30–40 mg for the control of acute asthma, but for long-term use their systemic side-effects may cause complications. The difficulty has been solved to some extent by the introduction of some corticosteroids that are effective in asthma when given by oral inhalation. **Beclomethasone** (Becotide §, Becloforte §), **betamethasone** (Bextasol §) and **budesonide** (Pulmicort §) are available products, supplied in metered dose aerosols, and given in doses of 50–200 micrograms up to four doses daily. Fluticasone (Flixotide §)

is a new derivative effective in doses of 25–120 micrograms. They are used in conditions of chronic airway obstruction not responding adequately to drugs of the salbutamol type, and regular use is necessary to obtain the maximum response.

Patients should be given detailed instructions in the use of these aerosol products to obtain the maximum penetration of the drug, (p. 23). It has been recommended that a preparatory inhalation of a bronchodilator drug such as salbutamol should be given before inhalation of the corticosteroid to promote such penetration.

In some cases, the use of corticosteroid inhalations may permit a transfer from oral therapy, with a consequent reduction in side-effects, but such transfer must be made very slowly.

Dexamethasone § (dose: 0.5–9 mg daily)

Brand name: Decadron §

Dexamethasone has the general properties and uses of the corticosteroids, but it has little, if any, mineralocorticoid potency. It is given orally in doses of 0.5–9 mg daily, although larger doses up to 15 mg daily in divided doses may be required in severe conditions. Doses by intravenous injection range from 1–20 mg, but in the treatment of shock, doses of 2–6 mg/kg by intravenous infusion or injection have been given.

Dexamethasone is also of great value in the treatment of raised intracranial pressure, as in cerebral oedema, which can result from trauma or oxygen deprivation, and is then given intravenously as an initial dose of 10 mg, followed by intramuscular doses of 4 mg 6-hourly, continued if required for some days. The more selective action of dexamethasone on the hypothalamus-pituitary-adrenal axis is made use of in the dexamethasone suppression test for the diagnosis of Cushing's syndrome, in which a single dose of 1 mg is given at night. The degree of suppression of corticotrophin secretion is measured by the urinary excretion of certain hydroxycorticosteroids. **Betamethasone** is a related compound with similar actions and uses.

Mineralocorticosteroids

Hydrocortisone and analogous compounds are known as glucocorticosteroids because their main effect is on carbohydrate metabolism. Other hormones of the adrenal cortex, represented by aldosterone, are concerned with the maintenance of the electrolyte balance of the body, and are referred to as mineralocorticosteroids. One synthetic compound, however, fludrocortisone, has both glucocorticosteroid and a marked mineralocorticoid activity.

Fludrocortisone acetate § (dose: 0.1–2 mg)

Brand name: Florinef §

Fludrocortisone is a synthetic fluorine-containing derivative of hydrocortisone, and is characterized by a marked increase in potency and salt-retaining properties, of value in Addison's disease. In that disease the adrenal glands have been damaged or destroyed by tubercular infection, or have atrophied from other causes, and in consequence there is deficiency of adrenal corticosteroids.

As a result of the absence of those sodium and water-retaining factors, large amounts of salt and fluid are excreted. Fludrocortisone can restore the electrolyte and fluid balance but doses of fludrocortisone that just maintain the electrolyte balance may not evoke an adequate glucocorticoid response. Therapeutically it is used only for partial replacement treatment of adrenocortical insufficiency in Addison's disease to supplement hydrocortisone therapy. Fludrocortisone is given in doses of 50–300 micrograms daily, together with hydrocortisone 20–30 mg daily, carefully adjusted to individual need and response. Both salt and fluid intake should be controlled to avoid the development of oedema, hypertension and weight gain. Occasionally, potassium supplements may be required.

Inhibitors of corticosteroid synthesis

These are considered here because of their biochemical association with hydrocortisone.

Metyrapone §

Brand name: Metopirone §

Metyrapone inhibits the action of an enzyme concerned with the synthesis of the precursors of hydrocortisone and cortisone, and is used as a test of anterior pituitary gland function. It is given in doses of 750 mg 4-hourly for six doses, and the consequent reduction in the level of glucocorticoids in the plasma stimulates the anterior pituitary to secrete more corticotrophin. That increase stimulates the production of more precursors, but as further conversion to hydrocortisone is inhibited by metyrapone these precursors are excreted in the urine, and can be measured as an assessment of activity of the gland.

Metyrapone has also been used in the treatment of Cushing's syndrome, in doses based on hydrocortisone production, under specialist supervision.

Trilostane § (dose: 120–480 mg daily)

Brand name: Modrenal §

Trilostane is a steroid antagonist that inhibits one stage in the biosynthesis of corticosteroids by the adrenal cortex. It is used in the treatment of Cushing's syndrome, primary aldosteronism, and other conditions of adrenal cortex hyperfunction. The standard dose is 60 mg four times a day for 3 days, afterwards adjusted to need. Much larger doses have been given, and prolonged treatment is usually required, with monitoring of the blood corticosteroid and electrolyte levels.

Trilostane has a secondary use in the treatment of breast cancer when oestrogen antagonists such as aminoglutethimide (p. 291) are no longer effective. It is then given in doses of 240 mg daily, doubled every third day up to 960 mg daily. Such doses require supplementary replacement therapy with a corticosteroid such as prednisolone.

Caution is necessary in liver and kidney dysfunction.

GONADOTROPHIC HORMONES

These hormones stimulate the gonads in both sexes. Two separate hormones are known, the follicle-stimulating hormone (FSH) and the luteinizing hormone (LH). They are produced in the anterior lobe of the pituitary gland and released under the influence of gonadorelin, the gonadotrophin releasing hormone (GnRH) of the hypothalamus. Their function is complex, as in the female the follicle-stimulating hormone (FSH) controls the development of the ovarian follicles and the production of oestrogens. The luteinizing hormone (LH) is concerned with the development in the ovary of the corpus luteum and the formation of progesterone, whereas in the male the LH controls the production of androgens.

It has not proved possible to extract these hormones from anterior pituitary glands except in very small amounts, but large quantities of hormones with very similar actions are obtainable from other sources. The urine of pregnant women contains a hormone derived from the placenta, and referred to as chorionic gonadotrophin, which resembles the luteinizing hormone. It is the presence of this gonadotrophin in urine that forms the basis of some pregnancy tests. Human follicle-stimulating hormone is obtained from the urine of postmenopausal women. Some semi-synthetic hormone products are also available.

Chorionic gonadotrophin §

Brand names: Gonadotrophon LH §, Pregnyl §, Profasi §

Human chorionic gonadotrophin (HCG) is used in infertility due to inadequate levels of natural gonadotrophins. It is given to induce ovulation after follicle development has been stimulated by injections of follicle-stimulating hormone, in doses based on individual need, and a course of treatment may require a total dose of 5000–10 000 units. The use of HCG requires care to avoid hyperstimulation and multiple pregnancy. In males, HCG has been given in doses of 500 units or more to stimulate the production of testosterone in delayed puberty.

Side-effects include headache, mood changes and oedema.

Human gonadotrophins

Intramuscular injections of FSH, followed by injections of HCG are used in anovulatory sterility due to low gonadotrophin secretion, particularly in patients who have not responded to clomiphene.

Humegon and Normegon are preparations of human menopausal gonadotrophin (HMG) containing the follicle-stimulating hormone (FSH) and the luteinizing hormone (LH). They are used in the treatment of female fertility disorders associated with hypopituitarism. Dose is based on the individual response. Metrodin is a preparation of the follicle-stimulating hormone.

Gonadorelin § (LHRH)

Brand names: Fertiral §, Relefact §, HRF §

Gonadorelin is a synthetic form of the hypothalamic hormone that controls the formation and release of the follicle-stimulating and luteinizing hormones of the anterior pituitary gland. It is used as a diagnostic agent to assess pituitary function, and is then given as a single intravenous dose of 100 micrograms, after which the level of circulating luteinizing hormone is assayed.

It is also used in the treatment of amenorrhoea and infertility due to a deficiency of endogenous gonadorelin. In such cases, gonadorelin is given by subcutaneous or intravenous pulsatile pump injections in initial doses of 10–20 micrograms, repeated every 90 minutes under careful control. Treatment is continued for 6 months unless conception occurs earlier.

Frazer H M, Waxman J 1989 Gonadotrophin releasing hormone analogues for gynaecological disorders and infertility. British Medical Journal 298: 475–476

Analogues of gonadorelin have an initial stimulating action on the production of gonadotrophin, followed by a secondary inhibition of ovarian and testicular activity. They have applications in the treatment of endometriosis and metastatic prostatic cancer. See buserelin (p. 454), goserelin (p. 455), leucoprorelin (p. 455) and nafarelin (p. 455).

Clomiphene citrate § (dose: 50–200 mg daily)

Brand names: Clomid §, Serophene §

Clomiphene is not a gonadotrophin, but is considered here because of its selective influence on ovulation. It is a synthetic compound that blocks the actions of oestrogens on receptor sites in the hypothalamus, and by disturbing the normal hormone balance, indirectly increases the release of pituitary gonadotrophins, and stimulates the maturation of the ovarian follicles. It can be regarded as an anti-oestrogen.

Clomiphene is used in the treatment of infertility provided that the patient is still capable of responding to an ovulatory stimulus. It is given in doses of 50 mg daily for 5 days, commencing about the 5th day of the menstrual cycle, or at any time if amenorrhoea is present, and such treatment may induce ovulation and produce an endometrium favourable to the establishment of pregnancy. The dose may be increased, if ovulation does not occur, up to 100 mg daily for 5 days as the cycle of treatment is continued, but if pregnancy is not achieved after three cycles, further treatment is unlikely to be successful.

Side-effects include visual disturbances, hot flushes, weight gain, dizziness and occasional hair loss. Care must be taken to avoid hyperstimulation, as multiple births have occurred. Clomiphene is contraindicated in conditions of abnormal uterine bleeding, or if ovarian cysts are present.

Cyclofenil § (dose: 400 mg daily)

Brand name: Rehibin §

Cyclofenil has the actions of clomiphene, and is used in the treatment of anovulatory infertility. It is given in doses of 200 mg twice a day for 10 days, starting on the 3rd day of the normal cycle, and the course should be repeated for at least 3 months.

Side-effects include hot flushes, nausea and abdominal discomfort.

Bromocriptine § (dose: 2.5–7.5 mg daily)

Brand name: Parlodel §

Bromocriptine is not a hormone, but a derivative of ergotoxine, one of the alkaloids of ergot, and is a stimulant of the dopamine receptors in the brain. The hypothalamus both stimulates and inhibits the secretion of prolactin by the anterior pituitary gland, and the inhibitory factor is thought to be dopamine.

The administration of bromocriptine has the effect of inhibiting prolactin release, and is used for the suppression of lactation and the relief of galactorrhoea. It is given in doses of 2.5 mg initially, followed by doses of 2.5 mg twice a day for 14 days. In galactorrhoea, an initial daily dose is increased to 7.5 mg daily up to a maximum of 30 mg daily. Doses of 2.5 mg twice daily are also used in some types of infertility. As bromocriptine also inhibits the release of growth hormone, it has been used in the treatment of acromegaly in doses of 20 mg daily.

Side-effects are numerous and include nausea, dizziness, postural hypotension, confusion and dyskinesia. Pleural effusions with high doses may require withdrawal.

The use of bromocriptine in the treatment of parkinsonism is referred to on page 259.

Cabergoline §▼ (dose: 1 mg)

Brand name: Dostinex §▼

Cabergoline, like bromocriptine, is a dopamine agonist and has similar actions and uses, but with the advantages of a longer duration of action and fewer side-effects. For the inhibition of lactation cabergoline is given as a single dose of 1 mg during the first post-partum day. For the suppression of established lactation it is given in doses of 0.25 mg every 12 hours for 2 days. In the treatment of hyperprolactinaemia, cabergoline is given in doses of 0.25 mg twice a week initially, gradually increased by 0.5 mg at monthly intervals. Subsequently doses range from 0.25–2 mg weekly. Serum prolactin levels tend to return to normal within 2–4 weeks, and monthly determinations of such levels should be carried out. Slow recurrence of the hyperprolactinaemia usually occurs when treatment is withdrawn. Cabergoline is better tolerated than bromocriptine, but dizziness, vertigo, headache, dyspepsia and depression are some of the many **side-effects**. Care is necessary if antihypertensive or antipsychotic therapy is also given. Pregnancy should be excluded before commencing cabergoline therapy. It should not be given with macrolide antibiotics or any dopamine antagonist.

Danazol § (dose: 200–800 mg daily)

Brand name: Danol §

Danazol is a synthetic compound with a selective inhibitory action on pituitary gonadotrophin secretion. It is used mainly in endometriosis, but it has been used in menorrhagia, gynaecomastia, precocious puberty and hereditary angio-oedema. The dose varies from 100 to 200 mg four times a day starting on the 1st day of the menstrual cycle, after excluding pregnancy.

Side-effects are those associated with its androgenic activity and include nausea, weight gain, oedema, voice changes and hirsutism.

OESTROGENS

Following the development of the ovarian follicles under the influence of the gonadotrophic hormone (FSH), oestrogens are formed and released according to physiological needs. These hormones are concerned with the general development and maintenance of the female genital system, and with the marked changes in the uterine mucosa that occur during the first half of the menstrual cycle. Together with progestogens, they are widely used in oral contraceptive products (p. 387).

Oestrogens are used therapeutically in a variety of conditions, including menopausal symptoms associated with the decline in the natural secretion of oestrogen. The aim of treatment, often referred to as hormone replacement therapy (HRT), is to relieve the flushes, palpitations and psychological disturbances of the menopause with the lowest effective dose of oestrogen, thus allowing the body to adjust itself to a lower hormone level more slowly. (*Note.* A non-hormonal treatment of menopausal flushing is **clonidine** (Dixarit) in doses of 50–75 micrograms twice daily (p. 106).) Oestrogens are also useful in relieving postmenopausal conditions such as senile vaginitis and pruritus vulvae.

Oestrogens are given in other conditions such as genital hypoplasia, primary amenorrhoea and delayed puberty, and in certain menstrual disturbances associated with ovarian deficiency. They are also used in the palliative treatment of postmenopausal mammary carcinoma and to relieve the pain associated with bony metastases. Oestrogens have also been used for the suppression of lactation, but as such use is associated with thrombo-embolism, **bromocriptine** is now preferred.

Oestrogens are also valuable in the treatment of carcinoma of the prostate gland and may give considerable symptomatic relief, although side-effects may be troublesome (p. 383). Oestradiol is the most important natural oestrogen, but synthetic oestrogens such as ethinyloestradiol and stilboestrol are available.

Ethinyloestradiol § (dose: 10–50 micrograms daily)

Ethinyloestradiol has the action of the natural hormone, but is some 20 times more potent, and has fewer side-effects. It is active in controlling menopausal symptoms in doses as low as 10 micrograms daily, and it is also used in primary amenorrhoea, functional uterine bleeding, sometimes in association with a progestogen. In general, long-term treatment should be avoided. Large doses up to 3 mg daily have been given in postmenopausal mammary carcinoma, and in prostatic carcinoma.

Side-effects include nausea, breast enlargement, weight gain and disturbances of liver function. Care is necessary in hypertension, and cardiac disease. Other oestrogens are represented by **oestriol** (Ovestin), **conjugated oestrogens** (Premarin), **piperazine-oestrone** (Harmogen) and **polyoestradiol** (Estradurin).

Stilboestrol § (dose: 100 micrograms–20 mg daily)

Stilboestrol, also known as diethylstilboestrol, is a synthetic compound that is unrelated to the natural oestrogens, yet it has powerful oestrogenic properties. It is effective orally and has been used in all conditions requiring oestrogen therapy, but nausea and vomiting are more common with stilboestrol than with associated drugs, and it is now used much less extensively.

Stilboestrol is effective in the palliative treatment of prostatic carcinoma and is given in doses of 1–3 mg daily, although much larger doses have been given. In males, it may have side-effects such as gynaecomastia and impotence.

An alternative is **fosfesterol** (Honvan §), which is given in doses of 100–200 mg three times a day, or in doses of about 550–1100 mg daily by intravenous injection, with weekly maintenance doses of 276 mg. Fosfesterol is broken down in the prostate gland by the enzyme acid phosphatase to give a high local concentration of stilboestrol in the prostatic tissues. It brings about a reduction in tumour size with symptomatic relief, although some perineal pain may follow the intravenous use of fosfesterol.

Hormone replacement therapy (HRT)

The vasomotor disturbances of the menopause are due to the

natural decline in oestrogen production, and can be relieved by suitable replacement therapy. Such treatment also relieves any associated menopausal vaginitis, and the long-term administration of low-dose oestrogens also reduces the risks of postmenopausal osteoporosis. Cyclical oestrogen/progestogen therapy is usually given to prevent endometrial hyperplasia, but oestrogen-only treatment is adequate in women who have had a hysterectomy.

Oestrogens can be given orally or as skin patches, less frequently as implants. Skin patches have the advantage of dermal absorption of the oestrogen, and so avoid the first-pass liver loss that follows oral administration. Oestrogen-containing skin patches should be applied to a clean, unbroken and dry skin area below the waistline, and detached after 3–4 days. Fresh patches should be applied to a different area.

The following products are available:

Oestrogen/progestogen
Climagest, Cyclo-Progynova, Menophase, Nuvelle, Prempak, Trisequens

Oestrogen only
Climaval, Progynova, Premarin, Harmogen, Hormonin, Zumenon

Patches
Estraderm, Evorel, Estracombi, Estrapak.

Tibolone §▼ (dose: 2.5 mg daily)

Brand name: Livial §▼

Tibolone is a synthetic steroid with progestogen and oestrogen activity. It is used mainly to control the flushing and other vasomotor disturbances of the menopause, and the daily dose of 2.5 mg should be continued for at least 3 months without interruption. The **side-effects** are those of related compounds. It is contraindicated in cardiovascular disease and in hormone-dependent neoplasm. Vaginal bleeding is an occasional side-effect of tibolone, and it should not be used within one year of the last natural menstrual period.

PROGESTOGENS AND RELATED SUBSTANCES

Progesterone and other hormones secreted by the corpus luteum are concerned with the maintenance of pregnancy and the development of lactation. Towards the end of pregnancy the secretion of the progestogens wanes. This influence on the maintenance of pregnancy led to the use of progestogens in the treatment of threatened abortion, but they are now chiefly employed in dysfunctional uterine bleeding and other menstrual disorders for their action on the development of the endometrium. They are also used as secondary drugs in the treatment of breast cancer.

Progesterone § (dose: 20–60 mg daily by injection)

Brand name: Gestone §

Progesterone is the natural hormone, and is given by deep intramuscular injection as an oily solution. In dysfunctional uterine bleeding doses of 5–10 mg may be given for a week before menstruation is expected, and in the premenstrual syndrome, doses of 50–100 mg are given on the 12th day of the cycle, and continued until menstruation commences. Alternatively, it may be given as a pessary or suppository (Cyclogest) of 200–400 mg twice daily.

Proluton Depot § (hydroxyprogesterone hexanoate) is a long-acting derivative. In habitual abortion it is given in doses of 250–500 mg by intramuscular injection at weekly intervals during the first half of pregnancy, but its value has been questioned.

Side-effects of progesterone include acne, urticaria and weight gain. It should be used with care in cardiac and renal disease, epilepsy, asthma, or conditions associated with fluid retention. (Progesterone should not be used during pregnancy because of the risk of virilization of a female fetus.)

Medroxyprogesterone § (dose: 2.5–30 mg daily)

Brand names: Farlutal §, Provera §

Medroxyprogesterone has the general properties of the progestogens, and is given in doses of 2.5–10 mg daily for 5–10 days in dysfunctional uterine bleeding. In endometriosis doses of 10 mg three times a day are given continuously for 3 months, or as doses of 50 mg weekly by deep intramuscular injection. It is also used in large doses in the treatment of breast, endometrial and prostatic cancer.

In breast cancer it is given orally in doses that may range widely according to need from 400 milligrams to as much as 1.5 g daily, or by deep intramuscular injection in doses varying from 250 mg weekly to 1 g daily. Lower doses are given in other conditions, and in prostatic cancer doses of 100–500 mg daily may be effective.

Side-effects are similar to those of progesterone.

Gestronol § (Depostat §), dose 200–400 mg weekly by intramuscular injection, and **megestrol** (Megace §), dose 40–320 mg daily, are other progestogens used in large doses in the treatment of breast cancer.

Norethisterone (dose: 10–30 mg daily)

Brand names: Menzol §, Primolut N §, Utovlan §

Norethisterone is an orally active progestogen, which is used mainly in the treatment of amenorrhoea, functional uterine bleeding and endometriosis. It has also been used in dysmenorrhoea and the premenstrual syndrome. Doses vary from 5–10 mg three times a day, at different stages of the menstrual cycle according to the condition under treatment.

It has been used to postpone menstruation in doses of 5 mg three times a day. It is also used as a second-line drug in the treatment of breast cancer in doses of 40 mg or more daily.

It is also a constituent of many oral contraceptive products (see p. 387). Norethisterone has the general side-effects of progesterone, but it has a more virilizing potency and in doses over 15 mg daily the incidence of liver disturbances may increase.

Dydrogesterone § (dose: 5–30 mg daily)

Brand name: Duphaston §

Dydrogesterone is a potent, orally active progestogen, and it is used in the treatment of endogenous progesterone deficiency. It is exceptional as it does not inhibit ovulation, yet it is capable of relieving the pain of dysmenorrhoea. It is given in doses of 10 mg twice daily for 3 weeks, followed by a break of 7 days before treatment is recommenced. It is also useful in some forms of endometriosis, dysfunctional uterine bleeding, infertility and abortion, and in control of the premenstrual syndrome.

Allyloestrenol (Gestanin), dose, 5–10 mg daily is used mainly in habitual abortion.

FERTILITY CONTROL

The explosive rise in population in recent years, particularly in underdeveloped countries, has led to the development of drugs for controlling fertility and birthrates.

It has long been recognized that the inhibition of ovulation by oestrogens would be effective, and later it was found that lower doses could be used if a progestogen was also given. Following the production of synthetic and highly active progestogens, oestrogen–progestogen preparations that can inhibit ovulation for long periods, apparently without influencing subsequent fertility, are now used as oral contraceptives (see Table 13.2). These products are in general well tolerated, but some nausea, acne, gain in weight, liver damage, and thrombosis may occur.

The possible relationship between thrombo-embolism and the

Table 13.2   Oral contraceptives

	Brand name	Progestogen dose of product
Mixed products containing 50 micrograms of mestranol	Norinyl-I Ortho-Novin 1/50	norethisterone 1 mg
Mixed products containing 50 micrograms of ethinyloestradiol	Minilyn Ovran	lynoestrenol 2.5 mg levonorgestrel 250 micrograms
Mixed products containing 35 micrograms of ethinyloestradiol	Brevinor Cilest Neocon 1/35 Norimin Ovysmen	norethisterone 500 micrograms norgestimate 250 micrograms norethisterone 1 mg norethisterone 1 mg norethisterone 500 micrograms
Mixed products containing 30 micrograms of ethinyloestradiol	Conova 30 Eugynon 30 Femodene Loestrin 30 Marvelon Microgynon 30 Minulet Ovran 30 Ovranette	ethynodiol 2 mg levonorgestrel 250 micrograms gestodene 75 micrograms norethisterone 1.5 mg desogestrel 10 micrograms levonorgestrel 150 micrograms gestodene 75 micrograms levonorgestrel 250 micrograms levonorgestrel 150 micrograms
Mixed products containing 20 micrograms of ethinyloestradiol	Loestrin 20 Mercilon	norethisterone 1 mg desogestrel 150 micrograms

Table 13.2   *(cont'd)*

	Brand name	Progestogen dose of product
Progestogen-only products	Femulen	ethynodiol 500 micrograms
	Micronor	norethisterone 350 micrograms
	Microval	levonorgestrel 30 micrograms
	Neogest	norgestrel 75 micrograms
	Norgeston	levonorgestrel 30 micrograms
	Noriday	norethisterone 350 micrograms

Logynon, Logynon ED, BiNovum, Synphase, Tri–Minulet, Triadene, Trinordiol and Trinovum are mixed products containing tablets of different strengths of ethinyloestradiol and norethisterone or levonorgestrel, and are designed to produce a phased hormonal response that mimics the natural hormone cycle more closely than is possible with fixed dose packs.

The progestogen-only products appear to act by increasing the viscosity of cervical mucus, and so reduce sperm penetration. Unlike mixed products, they are given continuously as single daily doses, to be taken at the same time every day. Additional protection is necessary for the first 14 days, or if any dose is omitted. In general, they are considered less reliable than the mixed products. Depo-Provera (medroxyprogesterone) is an injectable contraceptive, and is given as a single dose of 150 mg by deep intramuscular injection between the third and fifth day of the cycle, repeated after 3 months for long-term protection. Similarly, norethisterone enanthate (Noristerat) may be given in a dose of 200 mg by deep intramuscular injection, repeated after 8 weeks.

Post-coital contraception has been obtained by the use of mixed products containing levonorgestrel 250 micrograms and ethinyloestradiol 50 micrograms (Ovran and PC4). Treatment should be commenced within 72 hours of intercourse with a dose of two tablets, followed by a second dose 12 hours later. The risk of drug-induced vomiting can be reduced by an anti-emetic such as prochlorperazine.

Levonorgestrel is a progestogen widely used in oral contraceptives, but it is now available as implants (Norplant) claimed to have an action extending over 5 years. The product consists of six capsular implants each containing 38 mg of the drug, for subcutaneous insertion. The drug is slowly released from the capsules, and binds with progesterone receptors, and acts by thickening the cervical mucus so that it is impenetrable by spermatozoa. Suppression of ovulation may also occur. Should it be necessary to remove the implants, levonorgestrel plasma levels become undetectable within a few days.

use of oral contraceptives has caused some concern. The magnitude of the risk is difficult to assess, as thrombosis and pulmonary embolism may occur in a woman of child-bearing age who is not taking oral contraceptives. This risk appears to be associated with the oestrogen content, and many products now have a reduced dose of oestrogen. Some progestogen-only oral contraceptives are also available, but menstrual irregularities are more likely with these products.

It has also been suggested that there may be a possible link between breast cancer in women up to the age of 45 years and the prolonged use of oral contraceptives before a first pregnancy. An oral contraceptive containing the lowest suitable doses of both oestrogen and progestogen is recommended. The use of any oral contraceptive product should be discontinued if side-effects such as migraine-like headaches, visual disturbances, or any signs of thrombo-embolism or jaundice occur.

It should be noted that some drugs that induce hepatic enzyme activity, such as phenytoin, griseofulvin and carbamazepine, and some antibiotics, particularly rifampicin, may reduce the efficacy of oral contraceptives, and others such as ampicillin may hinder their absorption.

ANDROGENS

The androgens are the male sex hormones secreted by the testes, under the control of the anterior pituitary gland and are responsible for the development and maintenance of the male sexual system. They also have powerful anabolic or tissue building properties, and the rapid physical development of the male at puberty is associated with increased androgen activity.

Therapeutically, the androgens are used mainly in testicular deficiency in the male, and in carcinoma of the breast in females. Their anabolic effects are useful in osteoporosis and wasting diseases, but their virilizing action is a limiting factor when attempting to use the anabolic properties of androgens in the treatment of female patients. These two properties of the androgens can be separated to some extent by chemical modification of the hormones, and some modified androgens with a reduced virilizing action are described later under 'Anabolic steroids'.

Testosterone § (dose: 5–25 mg)

Brand names of testosterone esters: Primoteston §, Restandol §, Sustanon §, Virormone §

Testosterone is the most important natural androgen, originally obtained from the interstitial cells of the testes, but now prepared synthetically. In testicular deficiency or hypogonadism it is given as long-acting esters such as testosterone propionate by intramuscular injection in doses varying from 25–250 mg at intervals of

2–3 weeks. An alternative method is the subcutaneous implantation of sterile pellets. A pellet dose of 200–600 mg will provide a slow release of testosterone over a period of more than 6 months. Recently, a testosterone skin patch has been introduced as Testotop TTS 15, for daily application to the scrotal skin.

Testosterone undecanoate (Restandol) is given orally in doses of 120–160 mg daily initially, with subsequent maintenance doses varying from 40–120 mg daily. Doses of 100 mg or more have been given in the palliative treatment of carcinoma of the breast, but may have virilizing side-effects.

Mesterolone § (dose: 50–100 mg daily)

Brand name: Pro-Viron §

Mesterolone is an orally active androgen used in the treatment of hypogonadism and male infertility due to oligospermia. It is given in doses of 25 mg three or four times a day, but prolonged treatment for some months is required. Mesterolone is less likely to cause hepatic disturbances and other toxic effects.

Methyltestosterone § (dose: 20–50 mg daily)

Testosterone is inactivated by the liver when given orally, but methyltestosterone largely escapes hepatic inactivation. It has been given orally to maintain or supplement the effects of testosterone injections.

A side-effect is a dose-related cholestatic jaundice.

Anabolic steroids or non-virilizing androgens

Attempts have been made to exploit the protein-building properties of androgens in the treatment of wasting disease, but their side-effects limited their value. Some modified derivatives with reduced virilizing effects were subsequently introduced, but the results were largely disappointing. Such modified androgens are still used to a limited extent in the treatment of post-menopausal osteoporosis, and also in some aplastic and resistant anaemias, as steroids have some stimulating action on erythropoiesis. The response is highly variable. They should not be given to children to stimulate growth, as premature closing of the epiphyses may occur. Representative compounds include **nandrolone** (Decadurabolin §), given by deep intramuscular injection in doses of 25–50 mg at intervals varying from 1–3 weeks, and **stanozolol** (Stromba §), given orally in doses of 50 mg daily or by deep intramuscular injection in doses of 50 mg every 2 or 3 weeks.

Oxymetholone (Anapolon §) is given orally in doses of 2–3 mg/kg daily in aplastic and refractory anaemia, but prolonged treatment for some months is required. **Nandrolone** (as Decadurabolin §) is also used in aplastic anaemia in doses of 50–150 mg weekly by intramuscular injection.

Although these anabolic steroids have a reduced androgenic potency, some virilizing **side-effects** must be anticipated with the high doses used in the refractory anaemias, especially in children, and they are contraindicated in prostatic carcinoma and pregnancy. Another side-effect is cholestatic jaundice, which may occur more frequently with stanozolol. It is of interest that these anabolic steroids tend to reduce the itching associated with chronic biliary obstruction, yet paradoxically may make the jaundice worse.

Cyproterone § (dose: 100–300 mg daily)

Brand name: Androcur §

Cyproterone is referred to here as it has anti-androgenic properties, and is used in the treatment of hypersexuality in the male. It is given in doses of 50 mg twice daily.

On the basis that sebum secretion is linked with androgen activity, cyproterone is used in the treatment of severe acne in women not responding to other treatment, as **Dianette** § (cyproterone 2 mg with 35 micrograms of ethinyloestradiol), once daily for 21 days a month for several months. The use of cyproterone in the treatment of prostatic carcinoma is referred to on page 294.

Side-effects of cyproterone in full doses are fatigue, and weight gain; care is necessary in hepatic dysfunction, and blood counts should be made at regular intervals.

THYROID HORMONES

The thyroid gland is situated in the neck, on either side and in front of the trachea, and is one of the largest endocrine glands of the body. Its main physiological function is the control of the basal metabolic rate, which is mediated by the production of the thyroid hormones. A high output results in hyperthyroidism; a low output and consequent slowing down of the metabolic processes causes a condition which in adults is termed myxoedema, and in children is known as cretinism.

The thyroid gland selectively absorbs iodine circulating in the blood, derived from the diet, and forms two iodine-containing hormones, thyroxine and liothyronine. These hormones are stored in the gland as thyroglobulin, and subsequently released into the blood stream as required. Calcitonin, which is formed in another part of the thyroid gland, has a different function, and is described on page 397.

Points about thyroid drugs

(a) Early diagnosis and treatment are essential in cretinism.
(b) In hypothyroidism, maintenance doses should be taken before breakfast.
(c) Liothyronine is used in severe conditions when a rapid action is required, and is given by intravenous injection in hypothyroid coma.

Thyroxine § thyroxine sodium § (dose: 25–200 micrograms daily)

Thyroxine is used mainly in the control of thyroid deficiency states (hypothyroidism or myxoedema), and in neonatal hypothyroidism or cretinism. In myxoedema, treatment is commenced with small doses of 25–50 micrograms daily, slowly increased until a metabolic balance has again been achieved. Maintenance doses are 100–200 micrograms daily. The reason for these small initial doses is that the myocardium is often affected in myxoedema. Large initial doses of thyroxine may increase the heart rate, and add to the cardiac burden before the myocardium has had time to recover.

In cretinism early diagnosis and prompt treatment is essential, as if delayed, mental damage may occur which cannot be reversed by subsequent thyroid treatment. The initial dose for a cretinous infant is about 10 micrograms/kg daily, rising to 100 micrograms daily by about 5 years of age, and controlled by laboratory reports on plasma thyroxine levels. Maintenance doses in adults range from 100–200 micrograms daily, and treatment must be continued for life.

Side-effects, which may be associated with over-rapid therapy, include tachycardia, diarrhoea, restlessness, anginal pain and weight loss. Many such side-effects disappear with an adjustment of dose.

Liothyronine § (dose: 5–60 micrograms daily)

Brand names: Tertroxin §, Triiodothyronine §

The latent period of 10 days or so that elapses before thyroxine exerts a full effect is considered to be due to a slow conversion of the drug into liothyronine, which is the form of the hormone which finally affects the metabolism.

Liothyronine is used when a rapid action is required, as it is effective within a few hours, but the action is correspondingly short, and the drug is not suitable for maintenance treatment. It is given in initial doses of 5 micrograms three times a day, slowly increased to 60 micrograms daily according to need. In severe myxoedema, when coma may be imminent or present, liothyronine may be given by intravenous injection in initial doses of 50 micrograms, gradually reduced to 25 micrograms twice daily. Alternatively, doses of 5–20 micrograms may be given intravenously 12-hourly or more frequently as required.

Side-effects are similar to those of thyroxine, and care is necessary in hypertension and cardiovascular disease.

THYROID INHIBITORS[1]

Excessive activity of the thyroid gland, referred to as hyperthyroidism or thyrotoxicosis, is characterized by rapid pulse, loss of weight, raised metabolic rate, and enlargement of the thyroid. At one time surgical removal of much of the gland was the only effective treatment, but since the introduction of certain antithyroid substances, oral therapy has become an established method of control.

---

[1]These are not hormones, but are considered here because of their therapeutic connection with the thyroid.

Points about thyroid inhibitors
(a) Bone marrow suppression may occur.
(b) Withdraw treatment if any evidence of neutropenia.
(c) Advise patients to report sore throat or other indications of possible infection.
(d) White cell counts if any evidence of infection.

Carbimazole § (dose: 5–60 mg daily)

Brand name: Neo-Mercazole §

Carbimazole is the most effective and least toxic of the antithyroid drugs. These compounds reduce the formation of thyroxine and liothyronine in the thyroid gland by combining with the iodine absorbed from the blood. By this means the iodine necessary for the biosynthesis of thyroxine is made unavailable, and carbimazole brings about an indirect lowering of the basal metabolic rate by this interference with hormone synthesis.

Carbimazole is active orally, and the dose depends on the degree of thyrotoxicosis. An average initial dose is 30 mg daily, and the patient may feel better within 10–14 days, but the full response is slow as the thyroxine already formed and stored in the gland must first be metabolized, and the raised basal metabolic rate may not return to normal until after 3–5 weeks. The dose of carbimazole can then be slowly reduced to a maintenance dose of 5–15 mg daily, and prolonged treatment for months is usually required. Resistance to carbimazole is uncommon, and a poor response may indicate that the patient is not complying with treatment. Occasionally, carbimazole and thyroxine are given together in the so-called 'blocking-replacement regimen'.

Side-effects are most common in the early stages of treatment, and include gastrointestinal disturbances, pruritus, nausea and headache. Macropapular rash may also occur. Severe reactions such as agranulocytosis and aplastic anaemia have also been reported. It should be noted that carbimazole and related drugs may appear in breast milk, and may depress the thyroid activity of a breast-fed infant.

Propylthiouracil § (dose: 300–600 mg daily) also has an antithyroid action, but is more liable to cause toxic effects than carbimazole. It is useful occasionally when the rash caused by carbimazole is severe, and not controlled by antihistamines.

Iodine

Although iodine in very small amounts is necessary for normal thyroid activity, larger doses can depress thyroid function for short periods, and temporarily relieve the symptoms of thyrotoxicosis. This action appears to be a blocking effect on the release of thyroxine from the gland. The effect of large doses is at a maximum after about 2 weeks, and iodine is often given to reduce the basal metabolic rate during the preparation of patients for thyroidectomy. It also reduces the hyperplasia and vascularity of the gland, making it smaller and firmer, and so making subsequent surgery easier. It is usually given as Lugol's Solution (Aqueous Solution of Iodine) in doses of 0.1 to 0.3 ml well diluted, three times a day for 2 weeks before operation. **Potassium iodide** in doses of 60 mg three times a day is also effective. Lugol's Iodine Solution has been given in doses of 2 ml (after dilution with saline) by slow intravenous injection in thyrotoxic crisis.

Beta-adrenergic blocking agents are also used in thyrotoxicosis as they inhibit the adrenergic-mediated action of thyroxine, and so reduce tachycardia and tremor. They do not alter the levels of circulating thyroid hormones, and are used for short-term treatment in association with other antithyroid drugs. Propranolol is often used, in doses of 10–50 mg 6-hourly for a few days before thyroidectomy, and nadolol and sotalol are other beta-blockers used for the symptomatic treatment of thyrotoxicosis.

Propranolol is also used in association with other antithyroid drugs in the emergency treatment of thyrotoxic crisis, and is given by intravenous injection in doses of 5 mg every 6 hours, together with hydrocortisone 100 mg 6-hourly. **Radioactive iodine** (p. 301) is occasionally used in the diagnosis of thyroid dysfunction, in the treatment of thyrotoxicosis resistant to other drugs, and in cancer of the thyroid.

OTHER HORMONES

Lactogenic hormone (Prolactin)

Prolactin is concerned with milk formation. During pregnancy, premature lactation is suppressed by the relatively large amounts of oestrogen in the blood, but following delivery there is a sharp fall in the oestrogen level, and release of prolactin. In the breast prepared during pregnancy, prolactin stimulates milk production at term, and sustains subsequent lactation.

Oestrogens can suppress the action of the hormone, and stilboestrol and bromocriptine have been used to inhibit lactation. It should be noted that some drugs, such as methyldopa and the phenothiazines, may cause galactorrhoea as a side-effect via stimulation of prolactin release.

Growth hormone (somatotrophin)
Somatropin §

Brand names: Humatrope §, Norditropin §, Saizen, Genotropin §

Somatotrophin, or human growth hormone, is present in the anterior pituitary gland, and is released as required by controlling factors in the hypothalamus. One of its main actions is to increase the production of cartilage and so extend the length of the long bones. It has been used to stimulate growth in children with a deficiency of somatotrophin, but the hormone obtained by recombinant or enzyme-modified DNA technology, and known as somatropin, is now preferred. The dose must be individually determined, but is about 0.07 unit/kg weekly by subcutaneous or intramuscular injection. Growth hormone is contraindicated if epiphyseal closure has already taken place.

Octreotide § (dose: 50–600 micrograms daily by injection)

Brand name: Sandostatin §

Octreotide is a synthetic analogue of the natural regulatory hormone somatostatin. That hormone inhibits the release from the anterior pituitary gland of the growth hormone somatotrophin, as well as other pituitary hormones such as the thyroid stimulating hormone, corticotrophin and prolactin. It also acts on the pancreas and inhibits the release of insulin, glucagon, gastrin and the vasodilator intestinal peptide (VIP), and so blocks their action on the target tissues. Somatotrophin has too short a plasma life to be of therapeutic value, but octreotide is a derivative with a much longer action. It is used for the symptomatic relief of the flushing and severe diarrhoea of the carcinoid syndrome, which is associated with tumours that secrete excessive amounts of vasoactive substances such as VIP into the circulation.

Octreotide is given in doses of 50 micrograms by subcutaneous injection twice daily, increasing to 200 micrograms three times a day according to need. In most cases a complete remission of symptoms may be achieved, but the drug should be withdrawn in the absence of a response after 1 week's treatment. It may also be given by intravenous injection under ECG control when a rapid response is required. It should be noted that octreotide has no antitumour action, and has no effect on the underlying cause of the carcinoid syndrome. Similar doses have been given in the treatment of acromegaly.

PARATHYROID GLAND AND CALCIUM-REGULATING AGENTS

The parathyroid glands have no relationship with the thyroid glands other than that of position. They are situated in the neck, near the thyroid, and their function is the control of calcium and phosphate metabolism. A deficiency of parathyroid activity, or an accidental removal of the glands during thyroidectomy results in a lowering of blood calcium and an increase in the phosphate level. The former, if unchecked, leads to severe tetany.

Tetany due to low blood calcium can be relieved by the administration of calcium salts. For the acute attack, calcium gluconate solution (10%) can be injected intravenously or intramuscularly in doses of 10–20 ml, and treatment may be maintained by the oral administration of calcium gluconate or calcium lactate (dose: 1–5 g). **Vitamin D (calciferol)** and related drugs may also be given in the long-term control of calcium deficiency (p. 484).

Calcitonin § Salcatonin §

Brand names: Calcitare § (pork), Calsynar § (salmon)

Calcitonin is present in the thyroid and parathyroid glands, as well as in thymus tissue. It appears to complement the action of the parathyroid hormone in maintaining the calcium balance.

It lowers blood calcium by inhibiting bone metabolism, and it also brings about an increase in the urinary excretion of phosphates. It is used in the treatment of hypercalcaemia states, in osteoporosis, and in the severe hypercalcaemia that may occur in neoplastic disease. Calcitonin is also useful in relieving the pain and neurological complications of Paget's disease, including deafness. It also has applications in the treatment of postmenopausal osteoporosis.

Calcitonin can be obtained from pig thyroid, but a synthetic form is salcatonin (salmon calcitonin). Salcatonin is more potent than calcitonin, and is suitable for long-term treatment, as it is less likely to produce antibodies.

In Paget's disease, salcatonin is given in doses of 50 units (= calcitonin 80 units) three times a week by subcutaneous or intramuscular injection. In hypercalcaemia, doses up to 10 units/kg are given, based on need and biochemical response, but in the short-term treatment of the severe bone pain of malignancy, doses by injection of 200 units 6-hourly for 48 hours are given. In postmenopausal osteoporosis 100 units of salcatonin are injected daily, with vitamin D and calcium supplements orally.

Side-effects are nausea, flushing and tingling. Skin tests should be carried out before treatment in patients with a history of allergy.

Bisphosphonates

It is convenient to refer here to some phosphorus compounds, the bisphosphonates, that are used in disturbances of calcium metabolism. (The use of plicamycin in hypercalcaemia is referred to on p. 288.)

Etidronate disodium § (dose: 5 mg/kg daily)

Brand name: Didronel §

Etidronate disodium is a phosphorus-containing compound that has no relationship to calcitonin, but is considered here as it is used in the treatment of the pain of Paget's disease. It is adsorbed onto the hydroxyapatite (calcium-containing) crystals of bone, and reduces both their rate of growth as well as their subsequent dissolution. The rapid turnover of bone associated with Paget's disease is correspondingly reduced, and as a result the pain as well as the further development of the disease are reduced.

Etidronate disodium is given orally as a single daily dose of 5 mg/kg, preferably 2 hours before or 2 hours after food. Prolonged treatment for up to 6 months may be required, and calcium-containing food products should be avoided. Larger doses up to 10 mg/kg daily have been given when a more rapid response over a shorter period is required, but in all cases an interval of 3 months at least should be allowed before giving a second course of treatment. Didronel PMO is a mixture of etidronate disodium and calcium carbonate for use in vertebral osteoporosis.

Points about bisphosphonates

(a) Used in Paget's disease and the hypercalcaemia of malignancy.
(b) Should be given between meals; no food 2 hours before or 2 hours after a dose.
(c) Avoid milk and other calcium-containing products as well as iron and mineral supplements.

Ralston S H et al 1990 Use of bisphosphonates in hypercalcaemia due to malignancy. Lancet 335: 737

Etidronate is also used to control the hypercalcaemia of malignancy in doses of 7.5 mg/kg daily for 3 days by intravenous infusion, repeated after a rest period of at least 7 days. Subsequent oral doses of 20 mg/kg daily as a single dose are usually given for 30 days. Calcium levels should be monitored during treatment. (The hypercalcaemia of hyperparathyroidism seldom responds to etidronate therapy.)

Nausea and diarrhoea are **side-effects**, and an increase in bone pain with risks of fracture may occur with higher doses. Much of the drug is excreted in the urine, and severe renal impairment is a contraindication. Although disodium etidronate appears to have some effect on the activity of osteoclasts, it has little influence on normal turnover of bone.

Pamidronate disodium § (dose: 15–60 mg daily by intravenous infusion)

Brand name: Aredia §

The response to etidronate disodium is sometimes variable, and alternative drugs are pamidronate disodium and sodium clodronate. Pamidronate is used mainly in the control of tumour-induced hypercalcaemia, and it acts by blocking the transformation of osteoclast precursors into functioning osteoclasts. It is given by intravenous infusion in doses of 15–60 mg daily, according to the degree of hypercalcaemia. A fall in the plasma calcium level may occur within 24–48 hours, with a maximum response after 4–5 days. It may also cause some disturbance of the electrolyte balance of the body, and care is necessary in marked renal impairment.

Sodium clodronate § (dose: 1600 mg daily; 300 mg daily by intravenous infusion)

Brand name: Loron § Bonefos §▼

Sodium clodronate has actions and uses similar to those of disodium etidronate and pamidronate. It has a high affinity for bone, and suppresses osteoclast-mediated bone resorption, and increases the urinary excretion of calcium without adversely affecting mineralization. Sodium clodronate is given initially in doses of 300 mg daily by intravenous infusion over 2 hours, after dilution with 0.9% saline solution.

Beex L et al 1989 Pamidronate and hypercalcaemia of malignancy. Lancet ii: 617

The duration of treatment varies from 3–5 days, according to response, after which maintenance therapy with oral doses of 1600–3200 mg daily, in divided doses, may be given if required. The oral dose should be taken 1 hour before or 1 hour after food, with water or other fluid, but not milk. Extended treatment is required to achieve the maximum response, but should not exceed 6 months.

Side-effects include nausea and diarrhoea, and care is necessary in severe renal impairment.

The serum calcium and phosphate levels should be checked periodically.

Sodium cellulose phosphate (dose: 15 g daily)

Brand name: Calcisorb

Sodium cellulose phosphate functions in the intestinal tract as an ion-exchange substance, and binds with dietary calcium, thus preventing its absorption. It is used in the treatment of hypercalcaemia, and is given in doses of 5 g three times a day in association with a low-calcium diet.

Diarrhoea is an occasional side-effect, and renal impairment and congestive heart failure are considered to be contraindications.

Insulin and other hypoglycaemic agents

Insulin is the primary treatment for the symptomatic control of the chronic hypoglycaemic disease known as diabetes mellitus which affects nearly one million people in the UK alone. It is an insulin-deficiency disease, in which genetic and immunological factors may be involved. Two main types have been distinguished: type 1 or insulin-dependent diabetes mellitus (IDDM), and type 2, or non-insulin-dependent (NIDDM). Type 1 may occur at any age, but is most common in the young, and as such patients produce little or no endogenous insulin, life-long insulin replacement therapy is required. Patients with NIDDM, which is sometimes referred to as maturity-onset diabetes, produce some endogenous insulin, but it is not released according to need, and in such cases treatment with an oral hypoglycaemic agent coupled with a suitable diet is usually effective. Auxilliary drugs such as guar gum and acarbose may also be useful, as they modify the absorption of dietary carbohydrates. Insulin is one of the many hormones of the pancreas. That large gland secretes trypsin and other protein digestive hormones which enter the duodenum as pancreatic juice, but insulin is formed in the beta cells of the islets of Langerhans which are small pockets of specialized tissues found in the pancreas. It is of historical interest that it was demonstrated in 1890 that the pancreas was involved in some way with carbohydrate metabolism, yet insulin was not extracted from the gland in a form suitable for clinical use until 1922. In diabetes mellitus the beta cells no longer function, possibly because they are broken down by an autoimmune process, which may in turn be triggered by some environmental agent such as a virus.

Insulin controls the normal uptake and use of glucose by the tissues, as well as glucose storage in the liver as glycogen. In diabetes mellitus, the amount of available insulin is inadequate for glucose metabolism, and as a result excess glucose soon accumulates in the blood. Part of this excess is excreted in the urine, and acts as an osmotic diuretic, and increased amounts of water and electrolytes are excreted. The polyuria thus set up results in severe thirst, and if untreated, dehydration and coma result.

Because of the deficiency of insulin, proteins and fats are used as alternative sources of energy, leading to tissue breakdown and wasting. In health, fats are metabolized in the liver to simple substances, but in diabetes, this process is incomplete, and the so-called acetone- or ketone-bodies are formed.

Although these ketone bodies are excreted in part in the urine, they also accumulate in the body, leading to diabetic acidosis and coma. Insulin therefore plays an essential role in the control of glucose, protein and fat metabolism, and most of the symptoms of diabetes mellitus can be controlled by a suitable dose of one of the many insulin products available, provided the necessary dietary adjustments are made and adhered to. Insulin has a polypeptide structure, and is useless orally as it is inactivated by digestive enzymes, and it is usually given by subcutaneous injection.

For many years, insulin was extracted from beef or pork pancreas. These animal insulins differ slightly from human insulin in the arrangement of certain amino acids in the insulin molecule, but it is now possible to obtain human-type insulin from enzyme-modified pork insulin (H-emp), or by recombinant DNA technology in *Escherichia coli* (H-prb) or via yeast cells (H-pyr).

These human-type insulins are being used to an increasing extent, and although they are considered to have a potency comparable with that of standard insulins, some care should be taken when transferring a patient from an animal insulin to a human type insulin. Hypoglycaemia may occur during the changeover period, without the patient experiencing the normal warning symptoms of giddiness, tremor and palpitation, although some authorities consider that the risks have been exaggerated.

In all cases, the type and dose of insulin must be adjusted to the needs of the individual patients with modifications of diet and life-style to achieve the maximum degree of control. Blood or urine tests to determine glucose levels should be carried out regularly, for which reagent test strips are available for visual or meter measurement. Such tests may show variations throughout the day, and patients should be warned about such fluctuations, but levels between 4 and 10 mmol/litre of blood glucose for most of the time should reduce the risks of diabetic complications. Car drivers should be very careful to avoid hypoglycaemia and its consequences, and on long journeys should carry out a blood glucose test every 2 hours.

MAIN TYPES OF INSULIN

Three main types of insulin products are recognized, the short-acting, intermediate and long-acting preparations (Table 14.1, p. 406).

Soluble Insulin Injection (Neutral Insulin)

Soluble insulin is the standard form of insulin, and is the product to be used when Insulin Injection or Neutral Insulin is prescribed. Following subcutaneous injection it is rapidly absorbed, and a peak effect is reached in about 3 hours. With a suitable dose, the high blood-sugar level falls rapidly, the depleted glycogen reserves are restored, ketone bodies are oxidized, and as glucose is no longer excreted in the urine, the characteristic thirst and polyuria of diabetes are relieved.

Soluble insulin is used in the initial treatment of severe diabetes, in doses dependent on the degree of insulin deficiency and the condition of the patient. Soluble insulin is also the product of choice for the treatment of diabetic emergencies, and for increased control during operation. If required, it may be given by intramuscular or intravenous injection when the subcutaneous route is not indicated.

An advance in the administration of insulin is the introduction of the **Autopen**, **B-D Pen**, **Pur-In Pen**, **NovoPen** and **Penject** injection devices. These are used in conjunction with an insulin-containing cartridge or syringe, and permit the self-injection of a metered dose of soluble insulin as required, and offer the advantages over conventional syringes of portability and increased freedom.

Another refinement is the administration of soluble insulin by continuous subcutaneous infusion by an infusion pump. Such a device provides a basal insulin level and pre-meal supplementary

Table 14.1 Insulin products

Product	Brand or other name	Origin	Approximate duration of action in hours
Short-acting insulins			
soluble insulin	Soluble	Beef	6–8
	Human Actrapid	H-pyr	6–8
	Human Velosulin	H-emp	6–8
	Humulin S	H-prb	6–8
	Hypurin Neutral	Beef	6–8
	Pur-in Neutral	H-emp	6–8
	Velosulin	Pork	6–8
Intermediate-acting insulins			
insulin zinc (amorphous)	Semitard MC	Pork	12–16
biphasic insulin	Rapitard MC	Beef and pork	18–22
biphasic isophane insulin	Human Actraphane	H-pyr	18–22
	Human Initard 50/50	H-emp	18–22
	Human Mixtard 30/70	H-emp	18–22
	Humulin M1–4	H-prb	14–16
	Initard 50/50	Pork	14–16
	Mixtard 30/70	Pork	18–22
	PenMix 10/90–50/50 Pur-In Mix 15/85–50/50	H-pyr H-emp	18–22 18–22
isophane insulins	Isophane	Beef	18–22
	Hypurin Isophane	Beef	18–22
	Human Insulatard	H-emp	18–22
	Human Protophane	H-emp	18–22
	Humulin I	H-prb	18–22
	Insulatard	Pork	18–22
	Pur-In Isophane	H-emp	18–22
insulin zinc suspension (mixed)	Human Monotard	H-pyr	18–22
	Humulin Lente	H-prb	18–22
	Hypurin Lente	Beef	18–22
	Lente MC	Beef and pork	18–22
Long-acting insulins			
insulin zinc suspension (Crystalline)	Human Ultratard	H-pyr	22–30
	Humulin Zn	H-prb	18–22
protamine zinc insulin	Hypurin Protamine Zinc	Beef	24–30

doses, but is only suitable for use by well motivated and competent patients who are aware of the risks as well as the advantages of continuous insulin infusion. For such patients, the method offers a considerable improvement in the quality of life.

Modified insulins

The frequency with which injections of soluble insulin must be given has led to the development of a number of modified insulins with varying durations of effect to obtain a smoother control of the diabetic state. Some, such as isophane insulin and biphasic insulin can be given twice daily, others such as protamine zinc insulin and insulin zinc suspension permit once-daily administration. Table 14.1 indicates the range of products available and their approximate duration of activity.

Points about insulins
(a) Usually injected subcutaneously. (b) Soluble insulin has a rapid action and so is given 15–30 minutes before food. (c) They are injected intravenously in emergencies, but action disappears after about 30 minutes. (d) Soluble insulin may be mixed in the syringe with most other forms of insulin of the same type (bovine, porcine, human), but the soluble form should be drawn up first. (e) Vials of insulin suspension should be rotated and inverted to ensure even mixing; shaking will cause froth. (f) Date vial when first withdrawal is made. (g) Rotate injection site to reduce risk of local fat hypertrophy.

Protamine zinc insulin (PZ insulin)

Protamine zinc insulin is a suspension of insulin combined with protamine, a simple protein obtained from fish sperm, and a trace of zinc chloride. This modified insulin is not soluble in water, and a single daily dose may be sufficient to control the symptoms of diabetes when suitable dietary adjustments are made.

For patients who require a product with a more rapid initial action, yet with a sustained effect, a mixed injection of suitable doses of soluble and PZ insulin, prepared at the time of use may be given. With such mixtures in the same syringe, part of the soluble insulin becomes bound to the PZ insulin, thus modifying the effect, and the use of PZ insulin has declined.

Isophane (NPH) and biphasic insulins

These are modifications of insulin that have an action midway between those of soluble and PZ insulins. Isophane insulin is a neutral suspension of an insulin-protamine-zinc complex, and when given twice daily evokes a smooth response. It is a useful product for use in pregnancy, where adjustment of dose may be necessary. It can, if required, be mixed with soluble insulin, and **Actrapane**, **Initard** and **Mixtard** are such proprietary mixed products.

Biphasic isophane insulins are mixtures of soluble insulin and isophane insulin, and the rapidity of action depends on the proportion of soluble insulin present in a particular product.

INSULIN ZINC SUSPENSIONS

These preparations have also been known as the lente insulins. They are protamine-free suspensions of zinc insulin but the rate of absorption of these modified insulins is markedly influenced by the size of the insulin particles present in the suspension. When the particles are extremely small (amorphous zinc insulin) absorption is rapid; with larger crystalline particles the absorption is slower, but the action more prolonged. For many diabetics, the use of a form of insulin zinc suspension may permit control with a single daily injection.

These insulin modifications are basically for the maintenance control of stabilized diabetics. They are not suitable for emergency use, neither should they be mixed with any other form of insulin. Three forms of these insulins are in use:

Insulin zinc suspension (amorphous)

This product has slower but longer action than that of soluble insulin.

Insulin zinc suspension (crystalline)

The form with a duration of action that may extend over 24 hours.

Insulin zinc suspension (mixed)

This preparation contains both the amorphous and crystalline forms of zinc insulin. It has a peak effect about 6 hours after injection with a duration of activity of about 24 hours. It is often given twice a day, although with some patients a single daily dose may be adequate. Human as well as bovine and porcine preparations of insulin zinc suspension are available, but human forms have a shorter duration of activity.

Adverse reactions

Insulin overdose may cause hypoglycaemia, with faintness, giddiness and weakness, and if untreated, may lead to coma, convulsions and death. The immediate treatment is sugar or glucose, as a highly sweetened cup of tea if the patient is still able to swallow, but in severe hypoglycaemia, intravenous glucose will be required.

All diabetic patients should carry some glucose sweets for immediate use should they feel faint, as well as a warning card indicating that they are diabetics. Hypoglycaemic coma must be distinguished from diabetic coma, where the blood sugar is high, with marked acidosis, and treatment is the administration of repeated small doses of soluble insulin, if necessary by careful intravenous injection.

Minor reactions to insulin include local irritation, and a lipoma may occur at a repeatedly used injection site. Such lipomas are of little importance except from the cosmetic point of view. A long-term adverse effect is a diabetic nephropathy, with proteinuria, a decline in glomerular filtration and a rise in blood pressure. ACE-inhibitors (p. 197) may reduce the glomerular pressure by dilating the arteries, and may slow down the process of renal damage.

Table 14.1 includes human type insulins, prepared from enzyme-modified pork insulin (emp), or by pro-insulin recombinant biosynthesis (prb) or via yeast precursor DNA technology (pyr). These forms are used in much the same doses as other highly purified insulins, and are said to be less immunogenic.

ORAL HYPOGLYCAEMIC AGENTS[1]
Tolbutamide § (dose: 0.5–1.5 g daily)

Brand name: Rastinon §

Many attempts have been made to find orally active hypogly-

410 DRUGS AND PHARMACOLOGY FOR NURSES

caemic drugs, and thus avoid the need to inject insulin, but no real success was obtained until tolbutamide was discovered.

Tolbutamide is a sulphonylurea, and brings about a lowering of the blood glucose level by stimulating the release of endogenous insulin from the still-functioning beta-cells of the pancreas. It is not an orally-active insulin substitute, and is of no value in the absence of functioning beta-cells.

Tolbutamide is most effective in middle-aged and elderly patients, who are well stabilized on low doses of insulin, or who fail to respond solely to dietary restrictions. Therapy with tolbutamide or related drugs is not suitable for juvenile or unstable diabetics.

Transfer from insulin to tolbutamide should be made slowly over a few days, and the initial doses depend to some extent on the dose of insulin being given. With small insulin requirements (less than 20 units daily), the insulin may be withdrawn and the change-over commenced with an initial tolbutamide dose of 1 g twice a day, reduced steadily to a maintenance dose of 1 g daily or less.

Larger doses, or a reversion to insulin, may be necessary during illness and other periods of stress. Tolerance to tolbutamide may occur in a few patients after treatment for some months, necessitating a change of therapy.

Tolbutamide is well tolerated, and may be preferred in renal impairment, as it is largely metabolized in the liver.

Occasional **side-effects** are gastrointestinal disturbances, skin rash and weight gain, and it should be used with care in liver disease. Depression of bone marrow activity is uncommon, especially with low doses. Hypoglycaemia is indicative of overdose, requiring prompt adjustment.

Chlorpropamide § (dose: 250–500 mg daily)

Brand names: Diabinese §, Glymese §

Chlorpropamide is similar in action to tolbutamide, but with a more prolonged effect owing to a slower rate of excretion. It is less suitable for the elderly, or those with some renal impairment.

---

[1]These drugs are not hormones, but are considered here because of their therapeutic connection with insulin.

The maximum response may not occur for 4–7 days, and adjustment of dose is then necessary. Some patients with low insulin requirements can be transferred to chlorpropamide and stabilized on a single daily dose of 100–400 mg at breakfast and patients who fail or cease to respond to tolbutamide may also be controlled by chlorpropamide.

Side-effects are those common to the sulphonylureas generally. Occasionally, chlorpropamide may cause a prolonged hypoglycaemia in the elderly and for such patients a shorter-acting drug such as gliclazide is preferred. It is contraindicated in patients with renal failure. An occasional side-effect with chlorpropamide, but seldom with other sulphonylureas, is an intolerance of alcohol, characterized by a marked flushing of the face if alcohol is taken.

The hypoglycaemic action of chlorpropamide and related compounds may be increased by propranolol and other drugs, and decreased by the thiazide diuretics. Adjustment of dose may be required during such combined therapy.

Chlorpropamide is also used as an alternative to vasopressin in the treatment of diabetes insipidus (p. 365). It appears to act by potentiating the effect on the renal tubules of any still available endogenous vasopressin, and is given in daily doses of up to 350 mg daily, and up to 200 mg daily for children, but the dose must be adjusted to avoid any hypoglycaemic side-effects.

The range of sulphonylureas and other agents now available is indicated in Table 14.2.

Metformin § (dose: 1–2 g daily)

Brand name: Glucophage §

Metformin differs both chemically and pharmacologically from the sulphonylureas as it belongs to the biguanide group. It does not influence the islets of Langerhans to produce more insulin, but appears to act by reducing the absorption of glucose from the gut, and increasing its utilization by the tissues.

Maturity-onset diabetes may result from a disturbance of the sugar-regulating mechanism, and not a lack of insulin, and metformin may correct this disturbance. Like the sulphonylureas, the biguanides are active only when functioning pancreatic islet cells are present.

Table 14.2 Oral hypoglycaemic drugs (sulphonylureas and biguanides)

Approved name	Brand name	Daily dose range
chlorpropamide	Diabinese	100–500 mg
glibenclamide	Daonil, Euglucon, Libanil, Malix, Calabren	5–15 mg
gliclazide	Diamicron	40–320 mg
glipizide	Glibenese, Minodiab	2.5–30 mg
gliquidone	Glurenorm	45–180 mg
tolazamide	Tolanase	100 mg–1 g
tolbutamide	Rastinon,	500 mg–2 g
biguanide:		
metformin	Glucophage	1.5–3 g

Metformin is given in initial doses of 500 mg two or three times a day, gradually increasing over a period of 10 days according to response to a maximum dose of 3 g daily. Metformin is usually well tolerated, but it may cause some metabolic abnormalities, such as *lactic acidosis*, especially in patients with renal failure, for whom it should not be prescribed.

The main value of metformin is in the treatment of non-insulin-dependent diabetics who have failed to respond to sulphony-lureas and dieting, although it is also useful in overweight diabetics.

Side-effects are nausea, anorexia and diarrhoea. Lactic acidosis requires withdrawal of the drug.

Points about oral hypoglycaemic agents

(a) Effective only when some residual beta-cell activity is present.
(b) Insulin therapy may be required during illness, surgery and pregnancy.
(c) Elderly more at risk of hypoglycaemia, particularly with long-acting sulphonylureas.
(d) Alcohol may cause facial flushing if taken with chlorpropamide.

SUPPLEMENTARY HYPOGLYCAEMIC AGENTS

Acarbose (dose: 100–200 mg daily)

Brand name: Glucobay

Acarbose, obtained from cultures of actinomycetes, is an inhi-bitor of alpha-glucosidase. That enzyme is involved in the breakdown of dietary carbohydrates into monosaccharides such as glucose that can be readily absorbed. Acarbose binds with alpha-glucosidase, and so slows down the rate of carbohydrate break-down, which in turn reduces the immediate amount of glucose available for absorption. The use of acarbose leads to smoother daily blood glucose levels, and reduces the post-food peaks of hyperglycaemia that normally occur. Acarbose is indicated in the long-term treatment of non-insulin-dependent diabetes mellitus (NIDDM) in patients not otherwise adequately controlled, and is given initially in doses of 50 mg three times a day, just before or with food, and with water. The dose is increased after 6–8 weeks up to 300 mg daily according to need and response, as individual intestinal levels of glucosidase activity may vary widely. **Side-effects** are flatulence, abdominal discomfort and diarrhoea.

Clissold S P, Edwards C 1988 Acarbose. Drugs 35: 214–243

Guar gum (dose: 21 g daily)

Brand names: Guarem, Guarina

Guar gum has been used for many years as a thickening agent in food preparation, but if taken in large doses it retards the subsequent absorption of glucose. It is used in the treatment of diabetes mellitus, especially in diabetics poorly controlled by standard therapy, as it complements the hypoglycaemic action of insulin, the sulphonylureas and biguanides.

It may also have a supplementary action in promoting the lowering of plasma cholesterol levels, as such levels are often elevated in diabetes mellitus, and may be a factor in the development of atherosclerotic disease in diabetics. Guar gum is given as granules in doses of 7 g three times a day, and half a dose should be taken before a meal with at least 100 ml of fluid, with the other half sprinkled over the food. An adequate fluid intake with each dose is essential. Treatment is continued for 6 weeks initially, after which the dose is reduced to 7 g twice a day.

Side-effects are flatulence, which may be marked, abdominal discomfort and intestinal obstruction.

HYPERGLYCAEMIC AGENTS

Glucagon § (dose: 0.5–1 mg by injection)

An overdose of insulin in a diabetic patient causes a lowering of the blood-sugar level. If mild, this hypoglycaemia may be controlled by oral glucose, but if severe, or a state of insulin coma has occurred, prompt reversal of the hypoglycaemia is essential, and as an alternative to intravenous dextrose, glucagon may be given and is often a first-choice drug.

Glucagon is a hormone secreted by the *alpha* islet cells of the pancreas, and increases blood glucose concentrations by a rapid mobilization of liver glycogen and release of glucose. A dose of 0.5–1 mg by injection brings about a rapid rise in the blood-sugar level, which in hypoglycaemia should be supported by the administration of glucose to prevent a relapse. The dose of glucagon, which may be given by subcutaneous, intramuscular or intravenous injection, may be repeated if required after an interval of 20 minutes. It is ineffective in chronic hypoglycaemic states.

Diazoxide § (dose: 5 mg/kg daily)

Brand name: Eudemine §

Diazoxide is a synthetic drug that inhibits the release of insulin, and as a result, the blood-sugar level rises. It is of value in restoring a normal blood-sugar level in cases of hypoglycaemia associated with abnormally high insulin secretion due to islet-cell hyperplasia or pancreatic tumours, and also in the severe idiopathic hypoglycaemia of infancy. It is given orally in divided doses of 5 mg/kg daily, initially adjusted as soon as possible according to need and response.

Side-effects of diazoxide include nausea, common in the early stages of treatment, oedema, hypotension, which may be severe and require treatment, tachycardia and extrapyramidal symptoms. Blood examinations are necessary during prolonged treatment. Care is necessary in cardiac disease, renal impairment and pregnancy. Diazoxide is of no value in the treatment of acute hypoglycaemia.

The use of diazoxide in hypertensive crisis is referred to on page 212.

15

Antirheumatic and uricosuric agents

ANTIRHEUMATICS

Rheumatoid arthritis is a disease characterized by inflammation and destructive changes in the synovial lining of the joints generally, whereas osteoarthritis is mainly confined to the weight-bearing joints. The cause is unknown, but once inflammation is initiated, it may become self perpetuating. Inflammation is a defence reaction in which the immune system is involved, and is mediated by a variety of factors including histamine, serotonin, bradykinin and prostaglandin. Local vasodilatation causes an increase in capilliary pressure which results in inflammatory oedema and the accumulation of cell debris, and mobility is reduced by a reflex contraction of muscle around inflamed joints. The inflammatory process also causes pain by stimulating sensory nerve endings. In time, erosion of cartilage and bone occurs with permanent damage.

Although aspirin and related drugs have some useful anti-inflammatory as well as analgesic properties, in severe inflammatory conditions such as rheumatoid arthritis, reliance is largely placed on a group of drugs referred to as NSAIDs (non-steroidal anti-inflammatory drugs).

The corticosteroids (Ch. 13) are now less widely used except for acute conditions, and the powerful agents such as gold and penicillamine, which have more influence on the disease process, are used only when treatment with a NSAID is no longer effective.

The NSAIDs act by reducing the biosynthesis of prostaglandin by inhibiting cyclo-oxygenase (p. 421) and so interrupt the inflammatory response to mediators of inflammation such as bradykinin and histamine. They also appear to inhibit inflammatory cell migration, as well as preventing the release of other inflammatory factors, and their value in rheumatoid conditions is increased by their intrinsic analgesic potency. Their action is palliative, as they do not alter the underlying disease process.

Although all NSAIDs appear to have the same basic mechanism of action, individual members of the group vary in activity, and there is also a wide variation in individual response to therapy. Some differences in action may be due to variations in the degree of tissue binding, or the subsidiary mechanisms that may contribute to the overall anti-inflammatory response, and the best drug is the one that gives the individual patient optimum relief of symptoms with minimal side-effects.

The NSAIDs generally have a number of **side-effects**, which may be severe, including gastric irritation with nausea and vomiting which may lead to gastric erosion, and bleeding. Such reactions are linked with the inhibitory effects of NSAIDs on the synthesis of prostaglandins E and F, which normally inhibit gastric acid secretion and control mucosal blood flow. These gastric irritant side-effects can be reduced by administration of the drug with food or milk, and patients should be advised accordingly. More recently misoprostol (p. 327) has been used for the prophylaxis of NSAID-induced gastroduodenal ulceration. Other side-effects include headache, vertigo, tinnitus and dizziness that may interfere with driving. Care is also necessary in renal and hepatic impairment. Of particular importance is the risk of hypersensitivity reactions such as bronchospasm, angioneurotic oedema and rash. NSAIDs should be avoided in asthmatic patients, especially if it is known that the asthma is provoked by aspirin. Some NSAIDs may become highly protein bound, and the doses of oral anticoagulants and hyperglycaemic agents may require adjustment.

Many NSAIDs are derivatives of phenylpropionic acid. A few examples of representative compounds are discussed on pages 418 and 420, and Table 15.1 indicates the wide range available, but it should be noted that etodolac, although used in the treat-

Table 15.1   Non-steroidal anti-inflammatory drugs (NSAIDs)

Approved name	Brand name	Average daily dose
acemetacin	Emflex	120 mg
azapropazone	Rheumox	600 mg–1.2 g
diclofenac[a]	Voltarol	75–150 mg
diflunisal	Dolobid	500 mg–1 g
etodolac	Lodine	400–600 mg
fenbufen	Lederfen	600–900 mg
fenoprofen	Fenopron, Progesic	900 mg–2.4 g
flurbiprofen	Froben	150–300 mg
ibuprofen	Brufen, Apsifen, Tenbid, Lidifen, Motrin, Paxofen	600 mg–1.2 g
indomethacin[a]	Imbrilon, Indocid, Mobilan	50–200 mg
ketoprofen[a]	Alrheumat, Orudis, Oruvail	100–200 mg
mefenamic acid	Ponstan	1.5 g
nabumetone	Relifex	1 g
naproxen[a]	Naprosyn, Synflex	500 mg–1 g
piroxicam[a]	Feldene	20–40 mg
tenoxicam	Mobiflex	20 mg
sulindac	Clinoril	200–400 mg
tiaprofenic acid	Surgam	600 mg
tolmetin	Tolectin	600 mg–1.8 g

[a] Suppositories available for use at night to reduce morning stiffness.

ment of rheumatoid arthritis, has little analgesic activity. A recent development is the *local* use of certain NSAIDs for the symptomatic relief of rheumatoid and muscular pain and soft tissue inflammation. Representative products are Feldene Gel (piroxicam), Proflex Cream (ibuprofen), Traxam (felbinac) and Voltarol Emulgel (diclofenac). Small amounts should be rubbed into the affected areas three or four times a day, but occlusive dressings should not be used.

Points about NSAIDs

(a) Treatment should be initiated at a low dose level.
(b) Patients vary considerably in response, and a change of drug may be necessary to obtain the optimum response.
(c) Should not be given in active peptic ulcer or a history thereof or to the elderly unless other therapy is ineffective.
(d) *All* NSAIDs are contraindicated in patients hypersensitive to aspirin.
(e) Some NSAIDs can be obtained without prescription; deterioration in the condition of an asthmatic patient may be due to self-medication with a NSAID.
(f) Photosensitivity may occur with azapropazone (Rheumox); patients should be advised accordingly.

Aspirin (dose: 2–8 g daily)

The use of aspirin (acetylsalicylic acid) as a mild analgesic as well as its side-effects are referred to on page 101, but its associated anti-inflammatory action is of value in the treatment of the pain and inflammation of rheumatoid disease and musculoskeletal disorders generally. It is given in doses of 0.5–1 g up to 4-hourly, but in acute inflammatory conditions doses up to 8 g daily may be required to obtain an adequate response. Doses of 3 g daily or less have little anti-inflammatory activity.

Aspirin is also given for Still's disease (juvenile rheumatoid arthritis) in doses varying from 80–130 mg/kg daily, but otherwise it is now recommended that aspirin should not be given to children under 12 years of age, as there is a possible link between the use of aspirin and Reye's syndrome (acute encephalopathy with fatty degeneration of the viscera).

Benorylate, in which aspirin is combined with paracetamol, is also used in the treatment of the pain and inflammation of rheumatic disorders.

Salsalate, or salicylosalicylic acid (Disalcid) has analgesic and anti-inflammatory properties similar to those of aspirin, and is given in similar doses.

Naproxen § (dose: 500 mg–1 g daily)

Brand names: Naprosyn §, Nycopren §, Synflex §

Naproxen is one of the most widely used non-steroidal anti-inflammatory drugs (NSAIDs). It has analgesic as well as anti-inflammatory and anti-pyretic properties, and although rapidly absorbed, much of the drug becomes bound initially to plasma proteins, followed by relatively slow release. In rheumatoid conditions, naproxen is given as an initial dose of 250 mg twice a day, later increased to 500 mg twice daily. When morning stiffness causes difficulties the daily dose can be so divided that a larger dose is taken at night. Alternatively, suppositories of 500 mg can be used at night for a prolonged action and they are also useful when naproxen is not well tolerated orally.

Naproxen is also of value in the symptomatic treatment of acute gout, and is then given in doses of 750 mg initially, followed by 250 mg 8-hourly. It has also been used for the relief of the pain of dysmenorrhoea.

Side-effects of naproxen are those of the NSAIDs generally. As cross-sensitivity to aspirin and other NSAIDs may exist, naproxen should not be given to patients known to be sensitive to such drugs. Some reversible hair loss has occurred in children receiving naproxen.

Napratec § is a combination pack containing misoprostol tablets 200 micrograms together with naprosyn tablets 500 mg.

Fenbufen § (dose: 600–900 mg daily)

Brand name: Lederfen §

Fenbufen is an example of a pro-drug, as it is not effective until activated after absorption into active metabolites. It has the analgesic and anti-inflammatory properties of naproxen, and in rheumatoid disease and musculoskeletal disorders it is given in doses of 450 mg twice daily, or 300 mg and 600 mg morning and evening respectively.

It has the side-effects and hypersensitivity risks of the NSAIDs, although rash is more common, in which case the drug should be withdrawn immediately, as an allergic lung reaction may follow. Ibuprofen is a related drug now used more extensively as a mild analgesic (p. 103).

Indomethacin § (dose: 50–200 mg daily)

Brand names: Artracin §, Imbrilon §, Indocid §

Indomethacin is a derivative of indole-acetic acid, and is a potent anti-inflammatory agent with analgesic properties. It is used in the treatment of the inflammation and pain of rheumatoid arthritis and other musculoskeletal disorders, and is effective in doses of 25 mg two to four times a day with food, increased if necessary up to 200 mg daily. For a longer action in the control of night pain and morning stiffness, indomethacin may be used at night as a suppository of 100 mg. It is sometimes used in the treatment of acute gout in doses of 50 mg four times a day. Indomethacin has been used in the relief of the pain of dysmenorrhoea in doses of 25 mg three times a day.

Side-effects of indomethacin are those of related NSAIDs, including hypersensitivity reactions, which are a contraindication, as is peptic ulcer. Headache is common with initial treatment, but if it persists, the drug should be withdrawn. Ocular side-effects and corneal deposits have occasionally been reported.

Piroxicam § (dose: 20–40 mg daily)

Brand names: Feldene §, Larapam §

Piroxicam is an analgesic/anti-inflammatory agent with the advantage of a longer action that permits a single daily dose. In rheumatoid conditions it is given in doses of 20–30 mg daily, but in acute gout piroxicam is given in doses of 40 mg daily for 4–6 days. It is usually well tolerated, but extended treatment with doses of more than 30 mg daily may increase the incidence of gastrointestinal disturbances. Suppositories containing 20 mg of piroxicam are also available. In acute conditions it is sometimes given by deep intragluteal injection in doses of 20 mg. Feldene Melt is a tablet product designed to melt and dissolve in the mouth.

Phenylbutazone § (dose: 400–600 mg daily)

Brand name: Butacote §

Phenylbutazone has powerful anti-inflammatory and analgesic properties, but its value is limited by its **side-effects**. These include an acute pulmonary syndrome, fluid retention that can lead to cardiac failure, agranulocytosis and aplastic anaemia. The use of phenylbutazone is now restricted to the hospital treatment of ankylosing spondylitis. It is then given in doses of 100 mg two or three times a day, but prolonged treatment may be necessary.

PROSTAGLANDINS

As the prostaglandins are closely concerned with the onset and maintenance of the inflammatory processes, and many anti-inflammatory agents such as the NSAIDs act by inhibiting prostaglandin biosynthesis, it is convenient briefly to review here that interesting group of substances.

The prostaglandins are derivatives of arachidonic acid, a long-chain unsaturated fatty acid, linked with phospholipids, present in many body cells. Their release is mediated by the enzyme phosphatase A_2, and they are then metabolized by prostaglandin synthetase, also known as cyclo-oxygenase, to prostaglandin endoperoxides, which are later differentiated into a number of separate prostaglandins (Fig. 15.1).

As a group, the prostaglandins are concerned in the regulation of almost all biological functions, and have widely varying actions, as they are involved in the contraction and relaxation of smooth muscle in the blood vessels, bronchi and uterus, affect blood platelet aggregation and the inhibition of gastric secretion. Some important members of the group are designated as PGE, PGF, prostacyclin and thromboxane A_2 (TXA_2), and are sometimes referred to collectively as the prostanoids. PGE and PGF have been differentiated into certain sub-groups represented by PGE_1 and PGF_2. The latter have a powerful influence on the

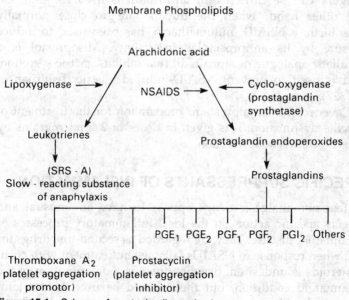

Figure 15.1 Scheme of prostaglandin synthesis.

inflammatory process, and cause a local vasodilatation, an increase in permeability, release of lyosomal enzymes, and the migration of other factors that play a part in the inflammatory response.

Leukotrienes are associated substances formed from arachidonic acid by lipoxygenase and also have inflammatory and allergic properties. The slow-reacting substance of anaphylaxis (SRS-A) is one of the leukotrienes.

Many anti-inflammatory drugs, including aspirin and the NSAIDs, prevent the synthesis of prostaglandins by inhibiting the action of cyclo-oxygenase, and so interrupt the development of the inflammatory process at an early stage. Other prostaglandins of interest include epoprostenol (prostacyclin) and thromboxane A_2 which are concerned with the maintenance of blood flow (p. 311). Prostaglandins with a selective action on the uterus are referred to on page 450.

Prostaglandins are also involved in the patency of the ductus arteriosus, which normally closes soon after birth with the changes in oxygen tension that occur. Babies born with congenital heart defects may still require a patent ductus for adequate oxygenation, and to maintain such patency until corrective surgery can be carried out, alprostadil is used (p. 452). On the other hand, when the ductus fails to close normally after birth, a NSAID, indomethacin, has been used to induce closure by its antiprostaglandin activity. Misoprostol is a synthetic analogue of alprostadil that inhibits gastric secretion, and is used to prevent NSAID-induced gastric disturbances (p. 327).

Caverject § is an alprostadil preparation for the treatment of erectile dysfunction. It is given in doses of 2.5 micrograms by direct intracavenous injection.

SPECIFIC SUPPRESSANTS OF INFLAMMATION

A few non-analgesic drugs appear to have an unusual and largely specific action on the local inflammatory processes of rheumatoid disease. They are regarded as second-line drugs for use when response to NSAIDs fails, when treatment with corticosteroids is undesired, or when there is a deterioration of the rheumatoid condition, but they should be used before joint damage has become irreversible. They are powerful drugs with which extended therapy is required, and their use requires care.

Points about gold, penicillamine and related drugs
(a) Used only in active inflammatory joint disease when NSAID treatment is ineffective.
(b) Treatment should be initiated before joint damage becomes irreversible.
(c) Response is slow and may take 4–6 months to appear with gold therapy, 6–12 weeks with penicillamine.
(d) If no benefit after 6 months with gold, 1 year with penicillamine, discontinue treatment.
(e) Development of a rash requires withdrawal of the drug.
(f) Relapse after gold treatment should be avoided, as response to a second course of gold therapy is usually poor or absent.
(g) Blood counts are necessary at regular intervals.
(h) Long treatment with chloroquine carries risk of retinal damage; regular eye tests necessary.

Penicillamine § (dose: 0.25–1 g daily)

Brand names: Distamine §, Pendramine §

Penicillamine, a chelating agent obtained by the acid degradation of penicillin, was introduced to increase the urinary excretion of copper in Wilson's disease, but it is also useful in some cases of severe active rheumatoid arthritis as an alternative to gold therapy. The adult dose is 250 mg daily before food, increasing at monthly intervals to a maintenance daily dose of 500 mg or more. Treatment may be required for 6–12 weeks before a response is obtained, and not all patients respond. Penicillamine is also used in juvenile chronic arthritis (Still's disease). It is also used in the control of chronic active hepatitis with initial doses of 125 mg three times a day, rising to maintenance doses of 1.25 g daily.

Penicillamine is potentially toxic, and regular blood and urine tests are essential. Blood dyscrasias and kidney damage require cessation of treatment, but therapy can be recommenced after a rest period if renal function and blood counts return to normal. Other **side-effects** include nausea, rash and proteinuria. Loss of taste may occur in the early weeks of treatment, but usually returns later. Hypersensitivity reactions or a late-occuring rash may require withdrawal of the drug.

Sodium aurothiomalate § (dose: 10–50 mg weekly by injection)

Brand name: Myocrisin §

This gold compound is used as an alternative to penicillamine for its anti-inflammatory action in active rheumatoid arthritis and Still's disease. It is most effective in severe conditions, when joint inflammation is progressive, but treatment must be commenced before irreversible joint damage has occurred. Sodium aurothiomalate is also useful in patients with severe rheumatoid arthritis requiring large doses of corticosteroids to control the symptoms, as it may permit a reduction in the dose of such steroids. Gold therapy is ineffective in other forms of arthritis, and is of no value when extensive deformities have developed.

Treatment with sodium aurothiomalate is commenced with a test dose of 10 mg to assess tolerance. It must be given by deep intramuscular injection, and the area should be massaged gently. If the drug is well tolerated, treatment is continued with increasing doses up to 50 mg weekly until remission of symptoms occurs or a total dose of 1 g has been injected. The response to treatment is slow, and may not occur until 500 mg have been given, but when it occurs, the interval between doses may be increased to 2–4 weeks.

A remission, once achieved, should continue to be treated with the effective dose for prolonged periods for 5 years or more. Maintenance of therapy is important, and if a relapse occurs, the dose should be increased at once to 50 mg weekly to regain control, after which the dose may be reduced to the previous maintenance level. The response to a second course of gold therapy after a complete relapse is seldom satisfactory.

Blood and urine tests should be carried out before each injection, as the **side-effects** of sodium aurothiomalate are sometimes severe and include skin reactions, oedema and renal disorders and pruritus. Blood disorders that may occur can require intensive supportive therapy if a fatal outcome is to be avoided. The drug should be withdrawn if a rash develops after prolonged treatment, and it is contraindicated in renal or hepatic disease, blood disorders, severe anaemia or dermatitis.

Auranofin § (dose: 6–9 mg daily)

Brand name: Ridaura §

Auranofin is a water-soluble gold compound with the actions, uses and side-effects of sodium aurothiomalate, and the advantage of being active orally. It is used in severe and progressive rheumatoid arthritis when other drugs are ineffective. It is given in doses of 3 mg after food twice daily initially, which, if well tolerated, may then be given as a single daily dose of 6 mg.

The response to treatment is slow, and if a 6 mg daily dose of auranofin is ineffective, 3 mg may be given three times a day, withdrawn after 3 months if the response remains unsatisfactory. Blood counts and tests for proteinuria should be performed throughout treatment, and auranofin should be withdrawn if thrombocytopenia occurs or is suspected.

The most common **side-effect** of auranofin is diarrhoea, which may be severe enough in some patients to require withdrawal of the drug. Other side-effects include rash, mouth ulcers, nausea, intestinal pain and pruritus. Blood and urine tests should be carried out monthly, as blood disorders sometimes develop suddenly.

Auranofin should be used with caution in patients with renal or hepatic disease, a history of bone marrow depression or rash. It does not interfere with the action of oral contraceptives.

It is of interest that the **Ridaura** product of auranofin is presented as a tablet of unusual shape that permits easy handling by arthritic patients, as the tablet tilts when placed on a flat surface.

Chloroquine § (dose: 150 mg daily)

Brand names: Avloclor §, Nivaquine §

Some antimalarials such as chloroquine may evoke a response in severe active rheumatoid arthritis similar to that induced by penicillamine, auranofin or sodium aurothiomalate. Chloroquine is given in doses of 150 mg daily after food, but prolonged treatment for up to 2 years may be necessary.

A potential danger with such long treatment is the risk of irreversible retinal damage, although the risk is slight when the dose does not exceed 4 mg/kg daily, or when the total cumulative dose does not exceed 100 g. As a precaution, an 8-week rest period from treatment every year has been recommended. In all cases, a full ocular examination is advisable before treatment, and twice-yearly thereafter.

Other **side-effects** include nausea, diarrhoea, pruritus, skin reactions, tinnitus, photosensitization, corneal opacities and blood disorders. Chloroquine should be used with caution in elderly patients, as it may be difficult to distinguish drug-induced retinopathy from age-related ocular changes.

Hydroxychloroquine (Plaquenil §) is a related drug with similar actions, uses and side-effects. Dose 200–400 mg daily, after food.

Sulphasalazine § (dose: 2–3 g daily)

Brand name: Salazopyrin §

Sulphasalazine, used chiefly in ulcerative colitis (p. 330) is sometimes effective in suppressing the inflammatory symptoms of rheumatoid arthritis. It is given in doses of 500 mg initially, increased up to 2–3 g daily over 4 weeks but haematological disturbances may occur, and full blood counts are necessary, particularly during the first 6 months of treatment. Liver function tests should also be carried out. Patients should be warned to report immediately if soreness of the throat, fever or malaise occurs, as blood disorders require prompt withdrawal of treatment.

For other side-effects see page 331.

IMMUNOSUPPRESSANTS

Several immunosuppressants represented by azathioprine, which is used to prevent rejection in transplant surgery (p. 560), have an action similar to that of gold and chloroquine in rheumatoid arthritis and other conditions thought to be auto-immune in character. They are sometimes useful as alternative therapy in patients not responding to other drugs.

Azathioprine (Imuran §) is given in doses of 1.5–2.5 mg/kg daily, but as the drug causes some bone marrow depression, blood counts should be carried out monthly. Nausea and diarrhoea may occur in the early stages of treatment, and may be severe enough to require withdrawal of the drug.

Chlorambucil (Leukeran §) is an alkylating agent (p. 279) with an action in rheumatoid arthritis similar to that of azothioprine, and is given in doses of 2.5–7.5 mg daily. Blood counts are necessary during treatment. Cyclophosphamide § (Endoxana §) (p. 279) has a similar action, and is given in doses of 1–5 mg/kg daily.

Methotrexate (Maxtrex §) is a cytotoxic agent (p. 284) with immunosuppressant properties. In severe active rheumatoid arthritis not responding to other therapy it is given in doses of 7.5 mg once weekly initially, rising according to need and response to a maximum dose of 30 mg weekly. Full blood counts and liver function tests are essential during methotrexate treatment. **Side-effects** include myelosuppression and mucositis, which can be reduced by folinic acid (p. 284). Methotrexate is contraindicated in marked renal impairment.

Cyclosporin (Sandimmun), the immunosuppressive agent referred to on page 560, is also used in the treatment of severe, active rheumatoid arthritis in adult patients resistant to other therapy. The initial dose is 2.5 mg/kg daily, and after 6 weeks the dose can be increased according to need and response, but should not exceed 4 mg/kg daily. Cyclosporin may be used with care together with a NSAID, but combined treatment increases the risks of renal and liver damage.

URICOSURIC DRUGS

Uricosuric drugs are used mainly in the treatment of gout, which is a painful metabolic disorder characterized by deposits of sodium urate crystals in the joints and tendons. Gout is caused by an excessive production of purines or a reduced renal clearance of uric acid, and an inflammatory response to the deposits of sodium urate causes the typical attack of acute gout, which usually arrives without warning. The long-continued deposit of the crystals results in the tophi of chronic gout as well as erosive damage to and deformity of the joints.

Some NSAIDs such as naproxen and indomethacin are used to relieve the inflammatory symptoms of acute gout, as is colchicine, but for chronic gout allopurinol is preferred. In all treatment with uricosuric agents, a high fluid intake is essential, and the urine made alkaline with sodium bicarbonate or potassium citrate to prevent the re-crystallisation of urates during excretion.

Points about gout treatment
(a) Acute attacks are treated with colchicine or NSAIDs, but not with aspirin.
(b) Colchicine is preferred in patients with heart failure as it does not cause fluid retention or affect anticoagulant therapy.
(c) Allopurinol, probenecid and sulphinpyrazone are used for chronic gout only.
(d) If given in acute gout they may prolong the attack.

Colchicine §

Colchicine is the alkaloid obtained from the autumn crocus, and is an old but specific drug for the treatment of acute gout. It is given in doses of 1 mg initially, followed by doses of 500 micrograms every 2–3 hours until relief is obtained, or until a total dose of 10 mg has been given. The response is usually dramatic, although sometimes adequate dosing is limited by the onset of vomiting and diarrhoea.

Colchicine is also used in doses of 500 micrograms two or three times a day to prevent the attacks of acute gout that may occur during the initial stages of treatment of chronic gout with allopurinol, or uricosuric drugs such as probenecid (but not aspirin or other salicylates). It should be used with care in the elderly, and in cases of renal impairment.

Allopurinol § (dose: 200–600 mg daily)

Brand names: Zyloric §, Caplenal §, Aluline §, Aloral §

Allopurinol has a unique action in the treatment of chronic gout. It inhibits xanthine oxidase, an enzyme linked with the formation of uric acid from purines, and so reduces the plasma concentration of that acid by a different mechanism from that of the uricosuric drugs. Allopurinol is widely used in the prolonged treatment of chronic gout, and may be of particular value in patients with impaired renal function not responding to uricosuric agents as it bypasses such impairment by its different mode of action.

Allopurinol is given in doses of 100 mg daily initially (after any attack of acute gout has subsided), and slowly increased over 3 weeks to a dose of 300 mg or more daily. The dose is later adjusted until the plasma uric acid level falls to 60 micrograms per ml, with maintenance doses of 200–300 mg daily. As allopurinol may precipitate an attack of acute gout during initial therapy, combined treatment with colchicine or a NSAID for at least 4 weeks is recommended. A high fluid intake and alkalization of the urine are necessary during allopurinol therapy. Allopurinol is also used to control the hyperuricaemia that may follow the use of some cytotoxic drugs, and should be commenced before such treatment is given.

Allopurinol is usually well tolerated, but intestinal disturbances may occur and alopecia has been reported. A rash with fever indicates withdrawal of treatment.

Probenecid § (dose: 1–2 g daily)

Brand name: Benemid §

Probenecid influences renal tubular activity, as it increases the rate of excretion of some substances such as uric acid and so is of value in the treatment of chronic gout. It is given in doses of 250 mg twice daily initially, increased as required up to a maximum of 2 g daily. Dosage should be adjusted later according to the plasma uric acid level.

Probenecid is generally well tolerated, but headache, flushing and dizziness may occasionally occur. It should be noted that in the initial stages of treatment, probenecid may precipitate attacks of acute gout as the stores of urate are mobilized and excreted. Such attacks may be controlled by colchicine or naproxen, but salicylates should not be used, as the uricosuric action of probenecid would then be reduced.

Sulphinpyrazone § (dose: 200–800 mg daily)

Brand name: Anturan §

Sulphinpyrazone promotes the renal excretion of urates by inhibiting tubular re-absorption. It brings about a lowering of uric acid level in the blood and the mobilization of urate tophi in the tissues that is of value in the treatment of chronic gout. Unlike the NSAIDs, it has no analgesic properties, and is of no value in acute gout.

Sulphinpyrazone is given for chronic gout in doses of

100–200 mg daily initially, with food, but as it may precipitate attacks of acute gout, colchicine or a NSAID such as naproxen may be given concurrently for a time to reduce the risks of such attacks. Subsequently, increasing doses of sulphinpyrazone up to 600 mg daily may be given, and adjusted later to a maintenance dose of 200 mg or more daily as required. In resistant gout, combined treatment with allopurinol is sometimes effective.

Sulphinpyrazone is usually well tolerated, but it may cause occasional gastrointestinal disturbances, and it should not be used in cases of peptic ulcer. It should be noted that sulphinpyrazone may influence the action of oral anticoagulants and sulphonylureas, and an adjustment of dose of those drugs may be necessary.

16

Allergy, antihistamines and associated drugs

ALLERGY

In allergic individuals certain tissues of the body become sensitive to various substances, collectively termed allergens. These substances are frequently but not necessarily protein in nature, and function as antigens that in turn lead to the formation of neutralizing antibodies or reagins. In allergic states these antibodies belong to the immunological Class E (IgE) (p. 557). Subsequent re-exposure to the offending allergen results in an antigen–antibody reaction, initiated when the antigen combines with and bridges adjacent IgE on cell walls. That bridging leads to an increased permeability of the mast cell wall, degradation of the granules and release of histamine and other spasmogens (Fig. 16.1). The released histamine binds with H_1-receptors on target organs and precipitates the allergic response. In order to control allergic states, the chain reaction of antigen–antibody–histamine release binding to the target organ must be broken at some point. If the allergen is a food, it can be removed from the diet, but often that relatively easy escape is not possible, and for the symptomatic relief of many allergic conditions, such as urticaria, hayfever, rhinorrhea, angioedema and anaphylaxis, reliance is largely placed on the group of drugs referred to as antihistamines. Acute and severe allergic attacks (anaphylaxis) are medical emergencies, and require immediate treatment with adrenaline (p. 233).

Occasionally the patient may be desensitized by a course of injections of weak solutions of the offending allergen. In some cases, as in hay fever, when due to a clear sensitivity to grass pollens, desensitization with a grass pollen vaccine may be successful. When a number of allergens are involved desensitization is more difficult, and the results are usually less satisfactory. (Pharmalgen is used for desensitization against bee and wasp stings.)

It is now recommended that desensitizing vaccines should only be used in seasonal allergic hay fever that has not responded to other treatment. Patients with asthma should not be so treated, as they are more susceptible to adverse reactions, the exception being patients hypersensitive to bee and wasp venoms, as reactions to such venoms may sometimes be life-threatening. Desensitization should only be carried out where facilities for full cardio-respiratory resuscitation are immediately available. Anaphylaxis may occur within 30 minutes of the injection of the vaccine, bronchospasm may develop within 1 hour, and patients should be monitored accordingly. Desensitizing vaccines should be avoided in pregnancy, and when beta-blockers are being taken.

 CSM. Current Problems in Pharmacovigilance 1993; 19:7

ANTIHISTAMINES

These drugs act by occupying the H_1-receptor sites, and by blocking the access of histamine to the target receptors, they inhibit the development of the allergic response. Their action is therefore palliative and not curative, and treatment must be continued throughout the period of exposure to the offending allergen. Nasal allergies and allergic rhinitis usually respond well to antihistamines, as do urticaria and other allergic skin reactions, drug allergies and insect bites, but they are of no value in asthma. The local use of antihistamines is no longer recommended, as paradoxically some may cause skin sensitization.

Side-effects. The main side-effects of most antihistamines are drowsiness, dizziness and lassitude, which may be increased by alcohol. Patients should be warned accordingly about car-driving and other machine-related activities. Anticholinergic effects are dryness of the mouth, blurred vision and gastrointestinal disturbances. Large doses may precipitate convulsions in epileptic patients. Older children usually tolerate antihistamines in suitable doses, but in young children they may have a central stimulant action, and cause hyperpyrexia and convulsions. There is no pharmacological antidote to the antihistamines, and overdose may require removal of any unabsorbed drug from the stomach, and the injection of a short-acting barbiturate or diazepam to control convulsions. Histamine itself is not an antidote, and its use may cause severe bronchospasm and circulatory collapse. Some of the newer antihistamines, such as astemizole and terfenadine, do not pass the blood–brain barrier so easily as the older drugs, and so have a reduced sedative action, but may be of less value in itching atopic eczema. On the other hand, in high doses they may cause ventricular arrhythmias, and the recommended doses should not be exceeded.

Points about hayfever treatment

(a) First-line treatment is with antihistamines.
(b) Drowsiness is a common side-effect of which patients should be warned.
(c) Recommended doses of astemizole and terfenadine should not be exceeded.
(d) Sympathomimetic nasal decongestants are useful; use intermittently to avoid rebound congestion.
(e) Intranasal corticosteroids used prophylactically; useful when pollen count likely to be high and when symptoms not fully controlled by other means.
(f) Sodium cromoglycate eye-drops for supplementary treatment of ocular symptoms.

Other actions

Some antihistamines are useful for sedative pre-medication before surgery; others have useful anti-emetic properties, and are used in nausea, vomiting and travel sickness (p. 332) as well as in Meniere's disease.

The following notes refer to some individual antihistamines, and Table 16.1 indicates the range available.

Diphenhydramine

Diphenhydramine was one of the first antihistamines, but its use

Table 16.1 Antihistamines

Approved name	Brand name	Oral daily dose range
acrivastine[a]	Semprex	24 mg
astemizole[a]	Hismanal, Pollon-Eze	10 mg
azatadine	Optimine	2–4 mg
brompheniramine	Dimotane	12–32 mg
cetrizine	Zirteck	10 mg
chlorpheniramine	Piriton	12–16 mg
clemastine	Tavegil	1–2 mg
cyproheptadine	Periactin	4–20 mg
loratadine	Clarityn	10 mg
mequitazine	Primalan	5–10 mg
oxatomide[a]	Tinset	60–120 mg
phenindamine[a]	Thephorin	100–200 mg
pheniramine	Daneral SA	75–150 mg
promethazine	Phenergan	20–75 mg
terfenadine[a]	Triludan	60–120 mg
trimeprazine	Vallergan	30–100 mg
triprolidine	Pro-Actidil	10–20 mg (long-acting)

[a]Antihistamines with reduced sedative effects.

has declined as drugs with a less marked sedative action have been introduced. It survives as Nytol, used for temporary sleep disorders, and as a constituent of some proprietary cough preparations represented by **Benylin**.

Acrivastine § (dose: 24 mg daily)

Brand name: Semprex §

Acrivastine is one of the antihistamines that does not pass the blood–brain barrier easily, and so has reduced sedative effects. It also has little anticholinergic or antimuscarinic potency, and is less likely to have **side-effects** such as dryness of the mouth, blurred vision or drowsiness. It is given in doses of 8 mg three times a day, but the onset of action is slow. It may have corresponding value when taken before an attack. Acrivastine is not recommended for children under 12 years of age.

Promethazine (dose: 25–75 mg daily)

Brand names: Phenergan; Sominex

Promethazine is one of the most effective and long-acting of the antihistamines. It is widely used in the treatment of hay fever, urticaria, and other allergic conditions in doses of 10–25 mg three times a day. It may also be given as a single dose of 25–50 mg at night, and such a dose may be given when a simple sedative effect is required as in mild insomnia. It is also given by intramuscular or slow intravenous injection in the supportive treatment of anaphylactic emergencies and severe allergies, but great care is necessary to give intravenous injections slowly, and to avoid extravasation, as severe chemical irritation may result.

Promethazine also potentiates the action of some analgesic drugs and it has been given by injection with chlorpromazine and pethidine for pre-anaesthetic medication. The central effects of promethazine are also useful in the auxiliary treatment of parkinsonism.

Astemizole (dose: 10 mg daily)

Brand name: Hismanal

Astemizole is an antihistamine with reduced sedative side-effects, as its penetration into the central nervous system is poor.

It is used for the symptomatic treatment of allergic conditions generally, and is given in daily doses of 10 mg before food. In severe conditions, it may be given initially in single doses of up to 30 mg daily for not more than 7 days, after which the maximum dose of 10 mg daily **must not** be exceeded, as high doses may have cardiotoxic side-effects. Combined treatment with macrolide antibiotics, antipsychotics, antidepressants and anti-arrhythmic drugs should also be avoided. See terfenadine, page 436.

Chlorpheniramine (dose: 12–16 mg daily)

Brand name: Piriton

Chlorpheniramine is a potent antihistamine, and effective in doses of 4 mg three or four times a day. A prolonged action tablet is also available. Chlorpheniramine is the preferred antihistamine for allergic emergencies, and is then given by intramuscular or slow intravenous injection in doses of 10–20 mg after an injection of adrenaline solution (1–1000) in a dose of 0.5–1 ml (see p. 233).

Chlorpheniramine is less likely to cause drowsiness, but care is necessary with intravenous injections, as the drug may cause transient hypotension, and the solution is potentially irritating.

Cyproheptadine (dose: 8–32 mg daily)

Brand name: Periactin

Some allergic and pruritic conditions are not always completely controlled by antihistamines as allergic reactions may be associated with the release of serotonin as well as histamine.

Serotonin resembles histamine in its wide distribution in the tissues, and is also linked in some way with certain allergic conditions, as serotonin antagonists can sometimes increase the response to antihistamines.

Cyproheptadine has both antihistamine and antiserotonin properties, is given in doses of 4 mg three or four times a day, and may be effective in allergic conditions not responding to conventional antihistamine treatment. It has also been used in 4 mg doses for the treatment of refractory migraine.

Side-effects of cyproheptadine are those of the antihistamines generally. It may increase the appetite and cause weight gain, and on that account it has been used as an appetite stimulant in underweight patients.

Phenindamine (dose: 100–150 mg daily)

Brand name: Thephorin

Phenindamine is one of the older antihistamines, but is exceptional in having a mild central stimulant action. It is given in doses of 25–50 mg up to three times a day.

Terfenadine (dose: 120 mg daily)

Brand name: Triludan

Terfenadine has the general properties of the antihistamines, and is used in the symptomatic treatment of allergic conditions, including hay fever and urticaria. It is given in doses of 60 mg twice a day, or as a single morning dose of 120 mg.

Like astemizole, terfenadine is less likely to cause sedation than older antihistamines, and in standard doses it is well tolerated, with few side-effects. In high doses, particularly when given with certain other drugs, it may prolong the QT interval with a consequent risk of inducing ventricular arrhythmias. Terfenadine is metabolized in the liver, and hepatic impairment, or use with drugs that inhibit hepatic metabolism, may lead to a rise in the plasma level of terfenadine (as with astemizole) and a similar risk potential. Combined therapy with macrolide antibiotics, anti-arrhythmics, antidepressants, antipsychotics, diuretics and oral antifungal drugs is therefore contraindicated.

Trimeprazine § (dose: 30–100 mg daily)

Brand name: Vallergan §

Trimeprazine is an antihistamine with sedative properties. It is used in the treatment of pruritus and related conditions in doses of 10 mg three times a day, up to a maximum of 100 mg daily. Trimeprazine is also used as a pre-operative sedative for children in doses of 2–4 mg/kg.

ANTI-ALLERGIC DRUGS WITH A PROPHYLACTIC ACTION

Sodium cromoglycate §[1] (dose: 20 mg four times a day)

Brand names: Intal §, Intal Compound §, Rynacrom §

Antihistamines are of little value in the treatment of allergic asthma and bronchitis, partly because spasmogens other than histamine may be involved, but in the prophylactic control of such conditions, sodium cromoglycate is widely used and frequently effective. Sodium cromoglycate has an unusual action, as it is not a bronchodilator, neither has it any anti-inflammatory properties, but it interferes in some way with the release of pulmonary spasmogens from the mast cells following an antigen–antibody reaction. It may also block the sensory nerves of the mucosa.

The spasmogens are contained in the mast cells as granules, and in sensitized patients these mast cells are coated with the immunoglobulin IgE. Contact with allergen or antigen results in an antigen–antibody reaction, which is followed by a degranulation of the mast cells, and release of the spasmogens. The reaction can be shown diagrammatically as in Figure 16.1.

After the reaction, the mast cells slowly regenerate. Sodium

---

[1]Sodium cromoglycate is not an antihistamine, but is included here because of its value as a prophylactic in hay fever.

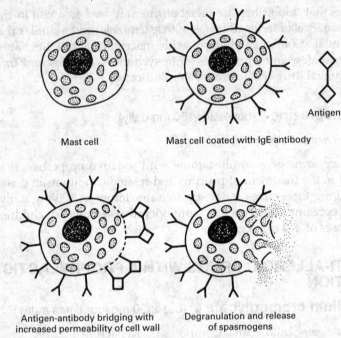

Mast cell

Mast cell coated with IgE antibody

Antigen

Antigen-antibody bridging with increased permeability of cell wall

Degranulation and release of spasmogens

Figure 16.1 Diagram of mast cell–antigen–antibody reaction.

cromoglycate strongly inhibits the release of the spasmogens after the antigen–antibody reaction by stabilizing the mast cell membrane, but is unable to antagonize any released spasmogen.

Sodium cromoglycate is used prophylactically in the control of allergic asthma, in the prevention of exercise-induced asthma and in the prophylaxis of allergic rhinitis. As it is not absorbed when given orally, it is administered by the inhalation of the powder from a 'spin-inhaler'. Each dose of 20 mg is contained in a gelatin capsule, which is pierced automatically to release the powder for inhalation as it is placed in the inhaler. As some patients may experience transient bronchospasm after inhalation of the powder, a compound capsule containing isoprenaline 100 micrograms is also available to offset any local irritation, but pretreatment with an inhalation of salbutamol is often preferred.

Sodium cromoglycate is given in doses of 20 mg by oral inhalation four times a day, and increased in severe conditions up to eight times a day. It may also be administered from a metered dose aerosol delivering 1 mg per puff in doses of 8–16 mg daily. For the prevention of exercise-induced asthma, sodium cromoglycate is given as a single dose half an hour before the anticipated exercise. A solution for use with a powered nebuliser is also available. All patients should be given full instruction in the proper use of sodium cromoglycate inhalation products if the optimum response is to be obtained, and regular use to maintain prophylaxis is essential.

Sodium cromoglycate is largely free from **side-effects**, but cough, irritation of the throat and transient bronchospasm may occur. Initially the treatment should be continued for 1 month, but the drug should then be withdrawn if the response is inadequate or absent.

Sodium cromoglycate is also given orally as **Nalcrom** § for the treatment of food allergies in doses of 200 mg four times a day, as it appears to have a stabilizing effect on the local inflammatory reaction in the gastrointestinal tract. The use of sodium cromoglycate as a nasal spray for the extended prophylaxis of seasonal rhinitis is referred to briefly on page 441. It is also used as Opticrom in allergic conjunctivitis (p. 525).

Ketotifen § (dose: 2–4 mg daily)

Brand name: Zaditen §

Ketotifen has an action similar to that of sodium cromoglycate in stabilizing mast cell membrane, although the mechanism of action appears to be different. It has the advantage of being active orally, and in the prophylactic treatment of asthma it is given in doses of 1 mg twice daily initially, increasing to 2 mg twice daily if necessary. The onset of action is slow, and some weeks may elapse before full protection is obtained, so any other anti-asthmatic therapy such as sodium cromoglycate, should be continued for 2–3 weeks. Ketotifen is of no value in acute asthma.

Side-effects. Ketotifen has antihistaminic properties, and may cause drowsiness, dry mouth and sedation, and potentiate the effects of alcohol, and patients should be warned accordingly about car driving.

Nedocromil § (dose: 8–16 mg daily)

Brand name: Tilade §

Nedocromil is used like sodium cromoglycate in the prophylactic treatment of asthma. It is considered that as reversible obstructive airway disease is associated with bronchial inflammation, the prevention and reduction of such inflammation could reduce the symptoms of the disease. Nedocromil has some of the required anti-inflammatory properties, as it inhibits the release of various mediators of inflammation in the bronchial tract, and as pulmonary function improves, the frequency of asthmatic attacks is reduced.

Nedocromil is given by oral aerosol inhalation in doses of 4 mg (two puffs), usually twice daily, but up to four times a day if necessary. A response should be obtained within 1 week, and extended therapy usually reduces the bronchial hyper-reactivity of reversible obstructive airway disease. It is of no value in the treatment of acute asthma, and at present it is not recommended for children under 12 years of age.

Side-effects are transient headache and nausea.

Seasonal rhinitis

Seasonal rhinitis, commonly known as hay fever, is an allergic reaction in sensitive subjects that follows exposure to plant pollens. It is frequently treated with antihistamines and mild nasal decongestants as sprays or drops, which often give rapid but transient symptomatic relief. Severe nasal congestion may be less easily relieved, and such treatment is of no value in prophylaxis. Those individuals who are known to be subject to hay fever

Table 16.2 Products used for seasonal rhinitis

Approved name	Brand name	Product
azelastine▼	Rhinolast▼	Spray 0.1%
beclomethasone	Beconase	Spray 50 micrograms
betamethasone	Betnesol	Drops 0.1%
	Vista-Methasone	Drops 0.1%
budesonide	Rhinocort	Spray 50 micrograms
flunisolide	Syntaris	Spray 25 micrograms
fluticasone	Flixonase	Spray 50 micrograms
ipratropium	Rinatec	Spray 20 micrograms
oxymetazoline	Afrazine	Spray 500 micrograms
sodium cromoglycate	Rynacrom	Spray 4%
xylometazoline	Otrivine	Spray and drops 0.1%

Dexa-Rhinospray is a mixed product containing dexamethazone, tramazoline and neomycin.

can be treated prophylactically with locally applied cortico-steroids or sodium cromoglycate, but the patient must be well motivated to obtain the best response. It is necessary to commence treatment at least 2–3 weeks before hay fever attacks are anticipated, as it may take time for protection to develop, and treatment must be continued regularly for some months, or even longer. Sufferers should remember to keep treatment supplies always readily available, and in severe cases, study pollen distribution maps before considering holidays abroad. The products in use are given in Table 16.2.

Brydon M J 1993 Management and treatment of seasonal rhinitis. Professional Nurse 8: 662–666

17

Respiratory stimulants, expectorants and mucolytics

RESPIRATORY STIMULANTS

Respiratory stimulants, by the nature of their action on the respiratory centre, have some central stimulant properties, and they have a limited place in therapeutics. They are used mainly by injection in ventilatory failure and postoperative respiratory distress, under close supervision, and with physiotherapeutic support. They are of no value in chronic respiratory disease.

The dose must be carefully adjusted to need and response as excessive doses may cause restlessness and even convulsions. Their activity depends on adequate oxygenation, and may be reduced in severe hypoxaemia. In the respiratory depression due to narcotic overdose, a specific antagonist such as naloxone should be used (p. 99).

Doxapram § (dose: 0.5–4 mg)

Brand name: Dopram §

Doxapram is a short-acting respiratory stimulant used mainly in postoperative respiratory depression. It is given by intravenous injection in doses of 0.5–1 mg/kg, repeated if neccessary after 1 hour. In acute respiratory failure it may be given by intravenous infusion in doses of 1.5–4 mg per minute according to need based on arterial blood gas measurements. It has a more selective action than naloxone (p. 99) as it does not antagonize the analgesic action of opioids; on the other hand it also has a stimulant action and may cause bronchospasm and tachycardia in some patients.

Care is necessary in cardiac disease and epilepsy. Doxapram is contraindicated in severe hypertension, status asthmaticus and thyrotoxicosis.

Ethamivan § (dose: 5–10 mg per kg)

Brand name: Clairvan §

Ethamivan is a respiratory stimulant with a mild pressor action. It has been used for respiratory depression in barbiturate poisoning, and other hypoventilatory states. Ethamivan is usually given by slow intravenous drip infusion as a 5% solution in doses of 100 mg, repeated as required according to response.

Nikethamide (dose: 0.5–2 g) has also been given intravenously as a respiratory stimulant, but the use of both drugs has declined as their value is limited and the margin between effective doses and those that may precipitate convulsive side-effects is too small.

EXPECTORANTS

Expectorants are drugs which increase the amount of sputum and tend to reduce the viscosity of bronchial secretion. An increase in the amount of sputum stimulates the cough centre by a reflex action, and thus helps to clear the bronchial tract by the act of coughing. A reduction in the viscosity of tenacious sputum is also a help in the treatment of the symptoms of respiratory disease.

Expectorants represent one of the older aspects of therapeutics. In recent years their effectiveness and value have been questioned, but expectorants are still widely prescribed.

Many proprietary cough remedies contain a variety of constituents, including an antihistamine, cough suppressants and bronchodilators. Some such products contain pseudoephedrine, and may cause *hallucinations* when given to young children. Any such reaction is an indication for withdrawal of the drug or a careful adjustment of dose.

Cough suppressants, represented by codeine and pholcodine, act centrally by a depressant effect on the cough centre, and are used mainly for the relief of useless cough, as **Codeine Linctus** (15 mg/5 ml) and **Pholcodine Linctus** (5 mg/5 ml). They have the disadvantage of causing constipation.

Ipecacuanha

Ipecacuanha is the root of a South American plant and the principal active constituent is the alkaloid emetine. In small doses it increases bronchial secretion and it is used in the treatment of cough where sputum is tough and scanty. Ipecacuanha is often used in association with alkalis such as ammonium bicarbonate, which are also said to liquefy bronchial secretions and Ammonia and Ipecacuanha Mixture is a familiar expectorant cough mixture containing these traditional drugs. Large doses of ipecacuanha have an emetic action (p. 575).

Potassium iodide (dose: 250–500 mg)

Potassium iodide is rapidly absorbed orally, and is partially excreted in the saliva and bronchial secretions and the amount and fluidity of the secretions are said to be increased. Potassium iodide has a traditional place with other expectorants in cough mixtures and in preparations for bronchitis and asthma, but is now used less frequently.

MUCOLYTICS

One of the symptoms of bronchitis is the increased production of thick sputum, and some of the older expectorants are not very effective in loosening and liquefying such sputum. This viscosity of sputum is associated with the formation of polysaccharide fibres, and some mucolytics are said to act by inhibiting the formation of these fibres, and thus tend to liquefy sputum by an indirect action. In practice, their value has been questioned, and it has been stated that some are little more effective than the time-honoured steam inhalations. The following products remain in use.

Acetylcysteine § (dose: 600 mg daily)

Brand name: Fabrol §

Acetylcysteine is a mucolytic agent that is said to act by splitting disulphide bonds in mucus glycoprotein, and it is used in the treatment of acute and chronic bronchitis and other conditions where mucolytic therapy is required, including cystic fibrosis.

It is given as granules in doses of 200 mg, to be taken with water three times a day. The duration of treatment varies according to need, and in chronic conditions it may be given for a period of months.

It may cause some gastrointestinal irritation, and other **side-effects** are urticaria and tinnitus. Acetylcysteine is also used by intravenous injection in the treatment of paracetamol poisoning (see p. 581).

Carbocisteine § (dose: 1.5 g daily)

Brand name: Mucodyne §

Carbocisteine reduces the viscosity of bronchial secretions, and so facilitates expectoration. It is said to produce a sputum with more normal characteristics, and is given in a variety of respiratory tract disorders requiring a reduction in sputum viscosity. Carbocisteine is given initially in doses of 750 mg three times a day, later reduced to doses of 500 mg three times a day. Children's doses are 20 mg/kg daily.

Gastrointestinal irritation and rash are **side-effects**.

Dornase alfa §▼ (dose: 2500 units daily by inhalation)

Brand name: Pulmozyme §▼

A recent development in the treatment of cystic fibrosis is the use of a recombinant form of human deoxyribonucease (rhDNase). The illness is associated with the formation of viscous purulent secretions in the airways, which reduce lung efficiency and exacerbate infection. Leukocytes accumulate in response to infection, and the viscous sputum contains large amounts of DNA released from degenerating leukocytes. Such extracellular DNA can be broken down with a reduction in sputum viscosity by dornase alfa, given by daily inhalation in doses of 2500 units by a suitable compressed air nebulizer. Continuous daily inhalation is necessary, as the improvement in pulmonary function brought about by the inhalation of dornase alfa subsides rapidly if treatment is withdrawn. As dornase alfa is an enzyme product, it should be refrigerator stored, and used as the supplied solution, and not mixed with any other drugs. **Side-effects** are few, but some pharyngitis and hoarseness of the voice have been reported.

Ranasinha C et al 1993. Efficacy and safety of short-term administration of aerolised recombinant human DNase I (rhDNase) in adults with stable stage cystic fibrosis. Lancet 342: 199–202

Methylcysteine (dose: 300–800 mg daily)

Brand name: Visclair

Methylcysteine has the actions and uses of carbocisteine, and is given in doses of 100–200 mg three or four times a day. For long-term prophylactic treatment during winter, alternate day administration is recommended.

Benzoin

Gum benzoin is a natural balsamic resin and is the main constituent of that time-honoured remedy known as Friar's Balsam, which is still widely used as an inhalation for the treatment of bronchitis (p. 24).

Drugs acting on the uterus and vagina

The oestrogenic and other hormones play an important part in the development and continuing function of the uterus, but there are also a few unrelated compounds that have a powerful action on the pregnant uterus. Of chief value are those that increase uterine contractions once labour has commenced, and those that inhibit premature labour. Of the former group, sometimes referred to as myometrial stimulants, ergot is one of the most effective drugs.

Ergot is a fungus that develops in the ear of rye and some other cereals, when instead of the normal grains, dark-coloured, long and tapering 'grains' are produced. These fungal bodies contain the alkaloids ergometrine and ergotamine. The former is widely used in the later stages of labour and in the control of post-partum haemorrhage; ergotamine is used in migraine (p. 106).

Flour made from infected rye can cause severe ergot poisoning, and epidemics due to such poisoning have often occurred in the past, and are not unknown today. This poisoning, once known as 'Saint Anthony's Fire' is characterized by extreme pain in the limbs, which is eventually followed by gangrene, and also by epileptiform convulsions.

Ergometrine maleate (dose: 0.5–1 mg orally; 0.2–1 mg by injection)

Ergometrine is the principal alkaloid of ergot, and is used mainly during the third stage of labour. Following oral doses of 0.5–1 mg, uterine contractions commence within a few minutes, and persist for about an hour. When there is a high risk of post-partum haemorrhage, or in emergency, ergometrine may be given intravenously in doses of 125–250 micrograms. Oral ergometrine is also of value in the control of minor post-partum haemorrhage in doses of 500 micrograms three times a day for up to 3 days.

Oxytocin, the pituitary hormone (p. 367), in doses of 5–10 units is an alternative to ergometrine, and the two drugs may be given together when a prompt and sustained action is required. **Syntometrine** § is a product formulated on that basis for intramuscular injection, and contains ergometrine 500 micrograms with 5 units of oxytocin.

PROSTAGLANDINS

Before the properties of the prostaglandins were discovered (p. 420), no drugs were known that could act on the uterus in the early stages of pregnancy, and cause expulsion of the contents, without highly dangerous toxic effects. This position changed dramatically with the introduction of prostaglandins with myometrial stimulating properties. Some are used for the induction of labour, others for post-partum haemorrhage, and others for drug-induced abortion.

Carboprost §

Brand name: Hemebate §

Carboprost has an action on the uterus similar to that of ergometrine and oxytocin, and is used in the control of post-partum haemorrhage not responding to those drugs. It is given by deep intramuscular injection in doses of 250 micrograms at intervals of 90 minutes, or less according to need, but a total dose of 12 mg should not be exceeded, i.e., 48 doses. Nausea, diarrhoea and flushing are among the many **side-effects** of carboprost.

Dinoprost §

Brand name: Prostin F2 alpha §

Dinoprost is a prostaglandin used for the induction of labour as well as for the therapeutic termination of pregnancy and abortion. It is given by intra-amniotic injection as well as intravenously, but intravenous injection is associated with an increased risk of **side-effects** such as shivering, pyrexia, dizziness and diarrhoea.

Dinoprostone §

Brand names: Prepidil §, Prostin E2 §

Dinoprostone is a prostaglandin used for the induction of labour as well as for the termination of pregnancy and for abortion. It is given orally in doses of 500 micrograms at hourly intervals up to a total of 1.5 mg, and as a vaginal gel containing 400 micrograms/ml, and as vaginal tablets containing 3 mg. For abortion it is given by intravenous infusion or slow extra-amniotic injection, under close hospital supervision.

Note. Prepidil cervical gel is used for cervical softening and dilation before induction; Prostin E2 vaginal gel is for the induction of labour. Prostin E2 vaginal tablets are used for the same purpose, but contain different doses of dinoprostone, and must not be regarded as equivalent products. Specialist literature should be consulted.

Gemeprost §

Brand name: Cervagem §

Gemeprost is a prostaglandin used to dilate the cervix uteri and facilitate operation in first trimester abortion, and is given as a 1 mg pessary 3 hours before surgery. For details of dose and risks, specialist literature should be consulted.

Mefipristone §▼

Brand name: Mefegyne §▼

Mefipristone is an antiprogestogen used in the termination of pregnancy (up to 63 days duration). It is given under close control as a single oral dose of 600 mg. If abortion is not complete after 36–48 hours, a pessary of genoprost (1 mg) should be used, but careful observation of the patient is necessary for 6 hours, as genoprost may cause hypotension. Both smoking and alcohol should be avoided by patients likely to need genoprost, and the drug is contraindicated in patients over 35 years who smoke.

Side-effects include nausea, diarrhoea, shivering and pyrexia. Severe uterine pain and bleeding may also occur.

 J Guillebaud 1990 Medical termination of pregnancy. British Medical Journal 301: 352–354

Alprostadil §

Brand name: Prostin VR §

Alprostadil or prostaglandin E_1 is used only to maintain the patency of the ductus arteriosus in neonates with ductus dependent heart defects, who are awaiting corrective surgery. It is given by intravenous infusion in doses of 50–100 nanograms/kg/minute, reduced according to need.

Alprostadil has many **side-effects**, and intensive care facilities must be available.

Indomethacin has the opposite action, and is used under specialist supervision when closure of the ductus arteriosus is required.

 Rennie J M Cooke R W I 1991 Prolonged low-dose indomethacin for ductus arteriosus of prematurity. Archives of Disease in Childhood 66: 55–58

PREMATURE LABOUR

To prevent premature labour a drug is required that has a powerful and selective relaxant action on the uterus, and is free from toxic side-effects. Suitable myometrial relaxants are few, but some of the required uterine muscle-relaxant properties are found among some sympathomimetic drugs with a selective action on the β_2-adrenoceptors (p. 241). They are indicated in the control of uncomplicated premature labour between the 24th and 33rd weeks, but the use of these drugs requires care, and the dose must be adjusted to need and response, and attention should be paid to the fetal as well as the maternal heart rate. Tachycardia is a common **side-effect**, and may increase to a serious extent if atropine has already been given during premedication. They are contraindicated in haemorrhagic conditions.

Ritodrine §

Brand name: Yutopar §

Ritodrine also has a relaxant action on uterine muscle, and is given by intravenous infusion as soon as possible after the onset of premature labour in doses of 50 micrograms/minute, increased as required up to 150–350 micrograms/minute. The optimum dose should be continued for 12–48 hours after the contractions have been brought under control, and the response maintained by intramuscular doses of 10 mg 4-hourly before transfer to oral therapy with doses of 10 mg as required, and continued as long as necessary. Intravenous doses of 50 micrograms/minute are also given in cases of fetal asphyxia due to uterine hypertonicity while preparing for delivery.

Side-effects are those of the sympathomimetic agents and include tachycardia, nausea, hypotension and flushing. Ritodrine is contraindicated in eclampsia, cardiac disorders and antepartum haemorrhage.

Salbutamol §

Brand name: Ventolin §

Salbutamol has the actions, uses, and side-effects of related drugs used in the control of uncomplicated premature labour. It is given by intravenous infusion in doses of 10 micrograms/minute initially, gradually increased to 45 micrograms/minute until contractions have ceased. Dosage can then be slowly reduced according to response, and intramuscular injections in doses of 100–250 micrograms may be given before oral therapy in doses of 4 mg 6–8 hourly.

Terbutaline §

Brand name: Bricanyl §

Terbutaline resembles salbutamol in its action and is given by intravenous infusion in doses of 5 micrograms/minute for

20 minutes, and gradually increased to 10 micrograms/minute until contractions have ceased. Later treatment is the subcutaneous injection of the drug in doses of 250 micrograms 6-hourly for 3 days, when oral therapy with 5 mg doses 8-hourly may be maintained up to the 37th week of pregnancy.

Side-effects of terbutaline are similar to those of other sympathomimetic agents used in the treatment of premature labour.

ENDOMETRIOSIS

Endometriosis is a painful condition that occurs mainly in women of the 25–35-year age group, and is due to the presence of endometrial tissue in extra-uterine sites. Treatment is with drugs that depress gonadotrophin production by the pituitary gland and so break the pituitary–ovarian link, which in turn inhibits ovarian steroid synthesis. Danazol is a synthetic steroid with some anti-oestrogenic properties; others such as buserelin depress gonadotrophin activity.

Buserelin § (dose: 900 micrograms daily)

Brand name: Suprecur §

Buserelin is a synthetic analogue of gonadotrophin that indirectly suppresses ovarian steroid production and is used as a nasal spray for the symptomatic relief of endometriosis. A dose of 150 micrograms is sprayed into each nostril three times a day, starting on the first day of the menstrual cycle. Prolonged treatment for up to 6 months may be required. A second course is inadvisable, as buserelin may bring about a reduction in bone density. From the nature of its action buserelin has many **side-effects** including menstrual and menopause-like symptoms, breast tenderness, nervousness and mood changes.

Danazol § (dose: 200–800 mg daily)

Brand name: Danol §

Danazol is a steroid with androgenic properties that has a suppressive action on gonadotrophin secretion. It is used mainly in endometriosis; other therapeutic applications are menorrhagia, gynaecomastia and hereditary angio-oedema. In endometriosis it is given in doses of 100–200 mg four times a day, starting on the first day of the cycle, and continued for some months. **Side-effects** are linked with its androgenic action, and include weight gain, oedema, acne and voice changes.

Gestrinone § (dose: 5 mg weekly)

Brand name: Dimetriose §

Gestrinone is an antiprogestogen that appears to have a multiple action in endometriosis. It is believed to reduce gonadotrophin activity and subsequent ovarian steroid production, to increase androgen levels and to have a direct effect on endometrial tissues. It is given in doses of 2.5 mg twice a week, starting on the first day of the cycle, with the second dose 3 days later. As with other drugs used in endometriosis, treatment for 6 months may be required. Care is necessary in patients with cardiac or renal disease as gestrinone may cause some fluid retention. Diabetic patients and those with hyperlipideamia require increased monitoring during gestrinone treatment. **Side-effects** are similar to those of danazol.

Goserelin §

Brand name: Zoladex §

Goserelin has the actions, uses and side-effects of buserelin, but differs in being given by subcutaneous injection into the anterior abdominal wall in doses of 3.6 mg every 28 days, starting on the 1st–5th day of the cycle. Like buserelin, treatment for up to 6 months may be required. It may cause local irritation at the injection site, and the use of a local anaesthetic may be necessary. Leuprorelin (Prostap SR) has a similar action and is given by subcutaneous or intramuscular injection in doses of 3.75 mg every 28 days. Goserelin is also used in the treatment of advanced premenopausal breast cancer (p. 295).

Nafarelin §

Brand name: Synarel §

Nafarelin, like buserelin, is given in endometriosis as a spray of

200 micrograms in one nostril each morning, and a similar dose in the other nostril in the evenings for a maximum period of 6 months. **Side-effects** are similar to those of buserelin.

VAGINAL THERAPY

Most of the drugs referred to in this section are those used locally for vaginal candidiasis or mixed infections. Those agents that are given orally and have a systemic action are dealt with in more detail in Chapter 5.

Clotrimazole

Brand name: Canestan

Clotrimazole is a synthetic antifungal agent used topically in various dermatomycoses, but it is also useful in candidal or mixed candidal–trichomonal vaginal infections. It is used as a vaginal tablet containing 100 mg of the drug, for insertion high in the vagina at night for at least 6 nights. A cream is available for more frequent use.

Metronidazole §

Brand names: Flagyl §, Femeron §

Metronidazole is used orally in the treatment of infections caused by the flagellate protozoan *Trichomonas vaginalis*. That organism causes a low-grade vaginitis, which may be treated with metronidazole in oral doses of 200–400 mg three times a day for 7–10 days, or 800 mg in the morning and 1200 mg at night for 2 nights.

For vaginitis of combined trichomonal and candidal origin, a mixed product of metronidazole and nystatin is available as **Flagyl Compak**. The use of metronidazole in systemic anaerobic infections is referred to on page 150.

Miconazole

Brand names: Gyno-Daktarin, Monistat

Miconazole is an antifungal agent that is mainly used systemically (p. 168), but it is also effective when used locally in the treatment of vulvo-vaginal candidiasis. It is used both as a pessary (100 mg) and as a vaginal cream (2%) and two pessaries or two applications of the cream should be used nightly for 7 nights, and subsequently repeated if necessary. Tampons impregnated with miconazole are also available.

Nystatin §

Brand name: Nystan §

Nystatin is an antifungal antibiotic used orally in intestinal candidiasis (p. 169) but it is also effective in vaginal candidiasis. It is used mainly as pessaries containing 100 000 units, two of which should be inserted high in the vagina nightly for 14 nights. Cream, gel and ointment are available for intravaginal or local use.

Econazole (Ecostatin; Pevaryl), **isoconazole** (Travogyn), **ketoconazole** (Nizoral) and **amphotericin** (Fungilin §) are other products used locally for vaginal infections. Clindamycin (Dalacin cream 2%) is used in bacterial vaginosis.

19

Anthelmintics, antimalarials and drugs used in tropical diseases

WORMS AND ANTHELMINTICS

The worms which have selected man as their unwilling host rarely cause severe disease but in some areas they can cause a great amount of chronic ill health. Infestation with parasitic worms is the most common disease in the world, and even when adequate medication is available, social conditions in some areas are such that re-infestation is almost impossible to prevent. Paradoxically, some irrigation schemes to increase soil fertility may bring about an extension of infestation by providing more favourable conditions for the development of some parasites.

Human parasitic helminths or worms can be classified as in Figure 19.1.

The life cycle of many of these parasites is very complex, and

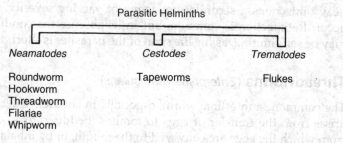

Figure 19.1 Classification of parasitic helminths.

an intermediate host may be involved before development from egg to mature worm in the human host can occur.

Roundworms (*Ascaris lumbricoides*)

The adult worms are some 10–15 cm long, and are usually found in the small intestine. The eggs are excreted in the faeces. Development occurs if the eggs are ingested by eating contaminated food, and larvae, about 0.25 mm long, penetrate the intestinal wall, pass into the liver, and make their way to the lungs. Later, the still immature worms reach the oesophagus and develop into adult worms in the small intestine. They may be present in numbers large enough to cause abdominal pain or even small bowel obstruction, and migration to liver ducts may occur.

Toxocariasis results from the invasion of the viscera by the larvae of *Toxocara canis* or *catis*, common roundworms of dogs and cats. It occurs mainly in young children, and is acquired by contact with infected dog or cat faeces. The larvae are widely spread through various tissues by the circulation, but do not complete their development in the human body. Toxocariasis is characterized by a persistent eosinophilia with heptomegalia and fever. Ocular lesions may also occur.

Hookworms (*Ancylostoma duodenale, Necator americanus*)

The eggs hatch in the soil, and the larvae gain access to the body by penetrating the skin, during which they may cause a local reaction. They enter the veins and lymphatics, reach the lungs, pass into the bronchi, and eventually migrate to the alimentary tract. There they attach themselves, and feed on the blood of the host. They cause abdominal pain and general debility, and in heavy infections a secondary anaemia of varying severity may occur. Re-infection is common, but in its absence the condition may be self-limiting, as the life span of the parasites is short.

Threadworms (*Enterobius vermicularis*)

The commonest intestinal worm, especially in children. Infection arises from the transfer of eggs to fomites (bedding, toys, etc.), from which the eggs are conveyed to the mouth, or by inhalation of airborne eggs. The adult females are 8–13 mm in length, and emerge from the anus, usually at night, to lay eggs on the adjacent skin. This causes an intense itching, with consequent scratching, and the infection is maintained by transference of the eggs to the mouth by the fingers. As the life span of adult worms is only 6 weeks, a high degree of social cleanliness to avoid re-infection is an essential part of any eradication treatment.

Whipworm (*Trichocephalus trichiuris*)

This worm is common in warm humid countries, and is often associated with hookworm. Infestation occurs from contaminated food and water. The symptoms are often mild but very heavy infestations may cause abdominal pain, diarrhoea and intestinal blood loss.

Filariae

Filariasis is due to invasion by *Wuchereria bancrofti*. The eggs develop into microfilariae, which are found in the peripheral blood, where they are picked up by mosquitoes. When the mosquito bites another host, these immature microfilariae are released into the blood. They migrate to the lymphatic vessels, where they develop into the adult parasites. Their presence causes inflammation and fibrosis of the lymphatics, leading to the progressive obstruction and subsequent blocking of the lymphatics, a condition that in its late stages is referred to as elephantiasis.

The microfilariae of *Onchocerca volvulus* are the cause of oncho-ceriasis or river blindness, a disease of West Africa spread by the bites of infected flies. The worms develop in the subcutaneous tissues and cause intense itching and disfiguring skin changes, but microfilariae in the eye set up an inflammatory focus that may cause sclerosing keratitis and blindness.

Tapeworms

The most common are the beef tapeworm (*Taenia saginata*), the pig tapeworm (*Taenia solium*), and the fish tapeworm (*Diphyllobothrium latum*). Infestation usually arises from eating undercooked meat or fish containing the larvae of the worm. The adult tapeworm, which develops in the intestines, is a segmented ribbon-like organism that may be several metres in length in the case of *T. saginata*, but the fish tapeworm and the pork tapeworm are much smaller, being only some 60 cm in length. The small head is firmly attached to the intestinal mucosa, and separation of the body from the head by an anthelmintic merely leads to regeneration of the worm.

Hydatid disease is due to the presence in the body of larval cysts of *Echinococcus granulosus*, a tapeworm found in dogs, with sheep as an intermediate host. The larvae do not develop into worms in the human host, but the cysts may increase considerably in size, and cause symptoms suggestive of liver abscess and multiple emboli.

Creeping eruption

Also known as cutaneous larva migrans, creeping eruption is caused by *Ancylostoma braziliense*, a hookworm of the dog and cat. The disease is spread by contact with larvae from infected dog faeces. When a larva penetrates the skin, it burrows in the epidermis, and its presence is shown by a winding, threadlike trail of inflammation with marked itching.

Schistosomes or blood flukes

Schistosomes are non-segmented flatworms, and the most important are the blood flukes, common in Egypt and some parts of Asia, and the cause of schistosomiasis or bilharziasis. The flukes of *Schistosoma haematobium* are usually found in the veins of the genito-urinary system, those of *Schistosoma mansoni* occur mainly in the veins of the large bowel, but *Schistosoma japonicum* is more likely to be found in the veins of the portal and alimentary systems. The spines of the eggs damage the walls of the veins which eventually ulcerate, and the eggs reach the bladder or intestines, and are excreted.

The larval forms can only undergo further development in the body of a suitable snail, so the disease is restricted to those areas in which such snails are found. A free-swimming form of the parasite is liberated from the snail, and that organism can penetrate the skin of the human host, enter the blood stream, mature in the intra-hepatic portal circulation, and then migrate to the venous system. Schistosomiasis may therefore be acquired by bathing in infected water. In some parts of the world schistosomiasis is a major public health problem.

ANTHELMINTICS

In recent years new and more specific compounds have been introduced, and the treatment of worm infestation is now much more effective and reliable, although the problem of mass treatment to eradicate the parasites remains to be solved.

Antimony sodium tartrate §

This old compound has a toxic action on the blood flukes causing schistosomiasis. It was once the drug of choice for *Schistosoma japonicum* but is now largely replaced by less toxic compounds.

Albendazole §▼ (dose: 800 mg daily)

Brand name: Eskazole §▼

Albendazole is chemically related to mebendazole and is one of the few drugs of value in hydatid disease (p. 462). It is given in doses of 400 mg twice a day for 28 days followed by a rest period before treatment is repeated for three cycles. It is also given in similar doses as an adjunct to the surgical removal of hydatid cysts. **Side-effects** include gastric-intestinal disturbances, headache, rash and occasional alopecia. Blood counts and liver function tests should be carried out during treatment.

Diethylcarbamazine citrate

Brand names: Banocide, Hetrazan

Diethylcarbamazine is one of the few compounds effective in the treatment of filariasis. It is active orally, and a standard dose is 6 mg/kg body weight daily in divided doses for 3 to 4 weeks. It induces rapid destruction of the microfilariae by the immune system of the body, but the death of the parasites often leads to a very severe allergic reaction, the Mazzotti reaction, with severe itching, rash, fever, pruritus and hypotension. It is now used less frequently.

Ivermectin §

Brand name: Mectizan §

Ivermectin is a derivative of a natural substance produced by an actinomycete, and has a selective action on the microfilariae of *Onchocerca volvulus*. It is now the preferred drug. Unlike diethylcarbamazine, it is well tolerated and is effective in onchocerciasis in a single dose of 150 micrograms/kg. It does not kill the adult worms or larvae, but appears to paralyse the nerve system of the microfilariae and prevent their development. Treatment should be repeated annually until the adult worms die out, which may take 20 years, but such dosage may eradicate one of the most serious of helminth diseases.

Levamisole

Brand name: Ketrax

Levamisole is highly effective against roundworm, and acts by paralysing the worm by a process of enzyme inhibition. It is considered by some to be the drug of choice, and although used abroad, paradoxically it is not marketed in the UK.

Levamisole is given as a single dose of 120–150 mg for adults, with doses for children based on 3 mg/kg. In hookworm, doses of 2.5–5 mg/kg daily for 2–3 days have been given. It is usually well tolerated, but care is necessary in severe hepatic and renal disease.

Mebendazole §

Brand name: Vermox §

Mebendazole is effective against threadworm, whipworm, roundworm and hookworm. For the treatment of threadworm infestation, a single dose of 100 mg is given, repeated after 2 or 3 weeks for all patients over the age of 2 years. For other worm infestations, doses of 100 mg twice a day for 2 or 3 days are necessary. Mebendazole is usually well tolerated but is not recommended for children under 2 years of age.

Mepacrine §

This antimalarial drug is effective in removing tapeworm and has been used when other forms of treatment are not available. Doses of 100–200 mg as an aqueous suspension have been given at 5-minute intervals up to a total dose of 1 g followed by a saline purge. Mepacrine is also used in the treatment of *Giardia lamblia* infections in doses of 100 mg 8-hourly for 5–8 days.

Metriphonate §

Brand name: Bilarcil §

Metriphonate differs chemically from other anthelmintics in being an organophosphorus cholinesterase inhibitor and having a selective action against *Schistosoma haematobium*. In such infections it is given in doses of 7.5 mg/kg at intervals of 2 weeks for three doses. In view of its chemical structure, it should be used with care in patients likely to come in contact with organophosphorus insecticides.

Niclosamide §

Brand name: Yomesan §

Niclosamide is a widely-used and effective drug against tapeworms, and has a rapid killing action on the parasites. The adult dose is 1 g, taken in the morning after a light breakfast, followed by a similar dose after 1 hour (tablets should be chewed or crushed and taken with fluid). Alternatively, a single dose of 2 g may be given. A brisk purge should be given 2 hours later. Children of 2–6 years of age may be given half doses. The killed worms disintegrate, and there is no immediate proof of cure.

Niclosamide is well tolerated, and **side-effects** are not common.

Oxamniquine §

Brand names: Mansil §, Vansil §

Oxamniquine is the drug of choice for the treatment of *Schistosoma mansoni* infections, but it is of no value against other forms. It causes the flukes to migrate from the mesenteric veins to the liver, where they are killed. A standard dose is 15–30 mg/kg daily for up to 3 days which is well tolerated. It has also been given by intramuscular injection as a single dose of 7.5 mg/kg, but such injections are painful, and may cause a febrile reaction.

Piperazine

Piperazine is very effective for the expulsion of both roundworm and threadworm. For roundworm treatment in adults a single dose of 4 g is given; children's doses are relatively large, and a dose of 120 mg/kg may be given up to a maximum of 4 g.

The drug paralyses the worms, and they are removed by the peristaltic movements of the intestines and excreted in the faeces. As the worms are not killed, a purge may be necessary to ensure their expulsion before the effects of the drug wear off after about 5 hours.

In threadworm infestation a course of treatment for 1 week is given. Adults and children over 12 may be given doses of 2 g daily in divided doses; children 4–6 years half doses, and infants 9–24 months quarter doses. A second course may be given if required after an interval of a week. Threadworm infection is easily spread, and it is necessary to treat all members of a family at the same time to ensure eradication. Piperazine is well tolerated, but some nausea and giddiness may be experienced by a few patients on full doses. Pripsen is a mixed product containing piperazine 4 g together with a senna extract, and provides the anthelmintic and purge in a single dose.

Praziquantel §

Brand name: Biltricide §

Praziquantel is one of the most effective of schistosomicides available, as it is active against all human schistosomes and has few side-effects. Praziquantel is given in single oral doses of 40 mg/kg, but against *Schistosoma japonicum* doses of 20 mg/kg three times a day for 1 day may be necessary. It may prove the drug of choice for mass treatment. It is also effective in tapeworm infestations in single doses of 10–20 mg/kg.

Pyrantel §

Brand name: Combantrin §

Pyrantel is an anthelmintic with a range of activity that includes roundworm, threadworm and hookworm. It is given to adults and children over 6 months of age in single doses of 10 mg/kg, but in heavy infections a second dose may be given 2 weeks later.

Pyrantel acts by paralysing the worms, which are then expelled by peristalsis. It is well tolerated, and side-effects are few and transient.

Thiabendazole

Brand name: Mintezol

Thiabendazole is a wide range anthelmintic, effective against *Strongyloides*, roundworm, threadworms, whipworms, guinea worm and 'creeping eruption'. It is sometimes useful against refractory hookworm. It is given in doses of 25 mg/kg in the evening, followed by a similar dose next morning after breakfast, continued up to a maximum daily dose of 3 g for 2 or 3 days. In mixed threadworm infestation, a second course after 1 or 2 weeks may be required.

Side-effects are nausea, diarrhoea, dizziness and drowsiness. Hypersensitivity reactions with fever and rash may also occur.

ANTIMALARIALS AND OTHER DRUGS USED IN TROPICAL DISEASES

Those who live in temperate climates often find it difficult to realize that malaria is one of the greatest killing diseases in the world, and is responsible for more than a million deaths annually. Malaria was once rarely seen outside tropical and subtropical countries, but it is now met with elsewhere in increasing frequency as a direct consequence of high-speed travel from infected areas, and treatment is becoming increasingly difficult with the development of drug-resistance.

Plasmodial life-cycle

Malaria is a febrile disease, due to the presence in the blood of one or more species of the protozoan organism *Plasmodium*. These organisms are transferred to the unfortunate human victim by the bites of infected female mosquitoes of the genus *Anopheles*. The forms of the parasite present in the salivary glands of the mosquito, and injected into the host, are termed sporozoites. These organisms migrate to the liver and other tissues where they undergo further development. The liver or tissue stage of development is known as the exoerythrocyte stage.

After a few days the organisms leave the tissues and enter into the red cells of the blood. Here they increase in number by division to form merozoites, and when division is complete and the cell nutrient is exhausted, the cells burst, and the merozoites are set free to infect other red cells and so repeat the process. When the number of infected red cells approaches about 250 million or more, this bursting of the red cells and release of the merozoites result in the rise in temperature, rigor and sweating which characterize a malarial attack.

While this development in the erythrocytes is taking place some of the merozoites develop into the sexual forms (gametocytes). These gametocytes circulate in the blood, and if drawn up by an anopheline mosquito in the act of biting, develop in the stomach of the insect, and finally form more sporozoites. These in turn migrate to the salivary glands of the mosquito, ready to be passed on to another victim.

Three main varieties of the parasite are commonly associated with malaria, and they are differentiated mainly by the time taken for development and release of the merozoites in sufficient numbers to cause a malarial attack. The varieties are:

Plasmodium vivax, which takes about 48 hours to develop, and causes benign tertian malaria.

Plasmodium falciparum, which also develops in about 48 hours and causes malignant tertian malaria.

Plasmodium malariae, which takes about 72 hours to develop and causes quartan malaria.

The first two are the most common. Malignant tertian malaria is so called because in addition to the chill and fever of the so-called 'benign' form, the attacks may take a fulminating and rapidly fatal course. This complication is associated with diarrhoea, anaemia, dehydration, and cerebral disturbances, the latter being due to the obstruction of the small blood vessels by merozoite-containing blood cells.

Figure 19.2 indicates the general outline of the life cycle of the malarial parasites, and the points of attack of various drugs.

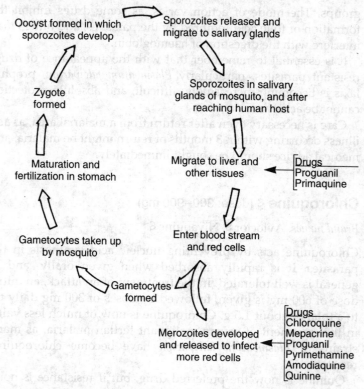

Figure 19.2 Life cycle of malarial parasites.

Treatment

So far, no vaccine against the malarial parasites has been developed, (although DNA recombinant technology suggests that the problem may not be insoluble) and no drug has yet been found that will kill the sporozoites as injected by the mosquito.

Treatment and prophylaxis are therefore directed against the organisms at a later stage of development. Drugs which act upon the parasites in the red blood cells are known as schizontocides, and those that attack the organisms in the tissues are referred to as tissue schizontocides.

The following drugs are of therapeutic importance, and are divided into two groups—those used mainly in the treatment of an acute attack of malaria, and those used both to suppress attacks and for prophylaxis. Some drugs have properties common to both groups. The mode of action varies, as some drugs inhibit the formation of folic acid required by the parasites, and others may interfere with the digestion of haemoglobin.

It is essential to remember that with the appearance of drug-resistant parasites, particularly *Plasmodium falciparum*, prophylaxis is becoming increasingly difficult, and absolute protection cannot be achieved.

Care is necessary even after return from a malarial area, as any illness occurring within 3 months of return might be malaria, and medical advice should be sought immediately.

Chloroquine § (dose: 300–900 mg)

Brand names: Avloclor §, Nivaquine §

Chloroquine acts by preventing nucleic acid synthesis in the parasites. It is rapidly absorbed when given orally, and in general is well tolerated. In the treatment of an attack, an initial dose of 600 mg is given, followed by doses of 300 mg daily up to a total of about 1.5 g. Chloroquine is now of much less value in the treatment of severe malignant tertian malaria, as many strains of *Plasmodium falciparum* have become chloroquine-resistant.

Quinine is now the preferred drug, but if resistance is not a problem, chloroquine may be given by intravenous infusion in doses of 10 mg/kg repeated after 8 hours, followed by three doses of 5 mg/kg. Intramuscular injections are also effective.

The suppressive treatment of malaria varies from continent to continent, and is linked with drug resistance, and up-to-date advice should always be sought. Where chloroquine is the drug of choice, it is given in weekly doses of 300 mg.

Side-effects. Chloroquine is usually well tolerated, apart from occasional gastrointestinal disturbance and pruritus, but full and extended treatment may cause corneal opacity and changes in pigmentation.

Halofantrine §▼ (dose: 1.5 g)

Brand name: Halfan §▼

Halofantrine resembles mefloquine in its pattern of activity, and is used in chloroquine-resistant falciparum and vivax malaria. It is given as three doses of 500 mg at 6-hourly intervals on an empty stomach, repeated after an interval of 1 week. **Side-effects** are nausea, abdominal pain and diarrhoea, but with halofantrine there is a risk of cardiac toxicity as it prolongs the QT intervals and may cause arrhythmias in sensitive patients. It should not be taken with food, which increases the absorption rate, or with any other potentially cardiotoxic drug.

Mefloquine § (dose: 250 mg weekly)

Brand name: Lariam §

Mefloquine is a rapidly-acting quinoline derivative effective in all forms of malaria, but in practice it is used for the prophylaxis of drug-resistant malaria due to *Plasmodium falciparum* and chloro-quine-resistant vivax malaria. For short-term prophylaxis extending over 3 months, mefloquine is given in doses of 250 mg weekly, starting 1–2 weeks before possible exposure to infection, and continuing for 4 weeks after leaving the area. **Side-effects** include gastrointestinal disturbances, and the drug should be withdrawn if any neuropsychiatric changes occur. It is contraindicated in pregnancy and patients with a history of psychiatric disturbances.

Mefloquine should not be given in association with quinine, and care is necessary in renal or hepatic impairment.

Primaquine § (dose: 15–60 mg daily)

Primaquine differs from most other antimalarials in acting upon the sporozoites in the liver and tissues, and on the gametocytes. It has little action on the erythrocytic forms of the parasites, and so is of no value alone in the treatment of acute malaria, but given after a course of chloroquine, which kills off the erythrocytic stages, primaquine will eradicate the remaining malarial parasites, particularly *Plasmodium vivax*.

It is thus of value in the definitive treatment (radical cure) of benign tertian malaria in those people returning from infected areas, who are unlikely to be exposed to the risk of further infection. The dose for such patients is 15 mg of primaquine daily for 2 weeks, after a standard course of chloroquine.

Quinine § (dose: 60–600 mg)

Quinine is an alkaloid obtained from cinchona bark, and is of historical interest as the first effective drug for the treatment of malaria. It suppresses the development of the malarial parasites in the blood, but has no action against those in the tissues.

For some time it was virtually replaced by the synthetic antimalarials such as chloroquine, but the situation has changed markedly with the emergence of chloroquine-resistant strains of *Plasmodium falciparum*. In severe resistant malignant tertian malaria, quinine dihydrochloride, given by intermittent intravenous infusion is now the drug of choice.

The standard dose is 10 mg/kg and three doses should be given at 8-hourly intervals up to a total dose of 1.8 g, but in less severe infection, quinine can be given orally in doses of 600 mg three times a day for 7 days. Following a course of treatment with quinine, it has been recommended that treatment should be concluded with a single dose of pyrimethamine 50–75 mg with sulfadoxine 1.5 g (equivalent to 3 tablets of Fansidar).

Suppressive treatment

In areas where malaria is common, re-infection may occur so easily after treatment that the prolonged use of a drug that will prevent development of the disease is essential. Chloroquine, already described and used mainly in the treatment of malarial attacks, is also used as a suppressive agent in weekly doses of 300 mg, but other useful prophylactic drugs are proguanil and pyrimethamine. Treatment should be commenced a week before possible exposure.

Proguanil § (dose: 100–300 mg daily)

Brand name: Paludrine §

Proguanil inhibits the development of the malarial parasites at several points, but in practice this action is too slow to be of value in the treatment of malaria attacks. Conversely, this slow action is of great advantage in suppressive treatment, and a daily dose of 200 mg will confer immunity on susceptible patients in some areas where malaria is common. In others, combined treatment with chloroquine 300 mg weekly may be necessary. Regular dosing is essential, as both *Plasmoduim falciparum* and *Plasmoduim vivax* may acquire a resistance to the drug if inadequate doses are given.

Pyrimethamine §

Brand name: Daraprim §

Pyrimethamine acts by interfering with the uptake of folic acid by the malarial organisms. Dapsone and sulphadoxine have a similar action but at a different stage of folic acid metabolism, and in practice pyrimethamine is always given in combination. Fansidar contains pyrimethamine 25 mg with 500 mg of sulphadoxine; Maloprim contains pyrimethamine 12.5 mg together with dapsone 100 mg. Fansidar is used in the single-dose treatment (three tablets) of falciparum malaria, but it is not recommended for prophylaxis as severe reactions have followed prolonged use. Maloprim has been used prophylactically in some areas, but it is contraindicated in early pregnancy, and if used in the second and third trimesters, folate supplements should be given and specialist advice should be obtained.

AMOEBIC DYSENTERY

Amoebic dysentery, also known as amoebiasis, is due to the presence in the intestinal tract of the protozoal organism *Entamoeba histolytica*. It exists both as the motile vegetative form and as cysts, and the disease is acquired by the ingestion of food or fluids contaminated with the cysts, or spread by symptomless human carriers of the disease. The cysts escape digestion in the stomach, but develop in the intestines and release active amoebae. These penetrate the mucosa of the lower intestines and set up an ulceration and chronic diarrhoea. In severe conditions large areas of the bowel become ulcerated, with consequent bleeding and sloughing of tissues. Occasionally some organisms penetrate the damaged intestinal mucosa, reach the portal vein, and are carried to the liver, and may cause amoebic abscesses.

In some patients the disease runs a mild course, with apparent recovery. Some of these patients still harbour the cysts, and may transmit the disease to others, and are referred to as 'carriers'.

Emetine §

Emetine is the principal alkaloid of ipecacuanha, and was once the standard drug for amoebiasis. It was given by subcutaneous or intramuscular injection in doses of 60 mg daily for 4–5 days, but severe **side-effects** required bed-rest during treatment and it has now been superseded by metronidazole and diloxanide.

Diloxanide furoate § (dose: 1.5 g daily)

Brand name: Furamide §

Diloxanide furoate has a specific action against *Entamoeba histolytica*, and is effective in the treatment of intestinal amoebiasis. It is the preferred drug in the control of chronic infections in which the cystic forms of the organism are passed in the faeces.

The standard adult dose of diloxanide is 500 mg three times a day for 10 days in chronic infections, and it is also used after acute infections have been controlled to clear any remaining cysts from the intestines. Diloxanide is of no value alone in the treatment of hepatic amoebiasis.

Side-effects are mild, but some flatulence, nausea and pruritus may occur.

Metronidazole § (dose: 1.2–2.4 g daily)

Brand name: Flagyl §

Metronidazole is the standard drug in the treatment of invasive amoebiasis, as it is effective at all sites of infection. In acute intestinal amoebiasis it is given in doses of 800 mg three times a day for 5 days, but in chronic conditions, and in amoebic liver abscess, doses of 400 mg three times a day are preferred. For symptomless carriers of the disease, doses of 400–800 mg three times a day for 5–10 days are given.

Metronidazole is much less effective in chronic intestinal forms of the disease, when diloxanide is the preferred drug. Entamizole is a mixed product containing metronidazole 200 mg and diloxanide 25 mg. Tinidazole (Fasigyn) (p. 151) has a similar action to that of metronidazole.

LEISHMANIASIS

This disease, of which the visceral form is known as kala-azar, occurs in Africa, China, India and some Mediterranean countries. It is due to protozoal organisms such as *Leishmania donovani*, which are transmitted by sand flies. The disease is characterized by an irregular but recurrent fever, enlarged liver and spleen, anaemia and other constitutional disturbances. A cutaneous form of the disease (oriental sore) also occurs, but may disappear without specific treatment.

Sodium stibogluconate § (dose: 20 mg/kg daily by injection)

Brand name: Pentostam §

Sodium stibogluconate (sodium antimony gluconate), is the standard drug for the treatment of visceral and cutaneous leishmaniasis. It is given in doses of 20 mg/kg daily up to a maximum of 850 mg daily by intramuscular or intravenous injection. A further course may be given after a rest period. A 10-day dosage course is used in cutaneous leishmaniasis.

Anorexia, vomiting and diarrhoea are **side-effects**; cough and substernal pain may also occur, especially if the intravenous injection is given too quickly.

The form of kala-azar that occurs in the Sudan is resistant to antimony compounds, but may respond to **pentamidine isethionate** (p. 477).

LEPROSY

This disease, although uncommon in the UK, may be seen more frequently than in the past as a consequence of easy air-travel from infected areas. It is caused by the bacterium *Mycobacterium leprae*, which resembles in some ways the tubercle bacillus, and two main forms of the disease are distinguished, tuberculoid leprosy and lepromatous leprosy. The infection is usually acquired by contact, and contrary to popular belief, the infectivity is normally low, although susceptibility may vary.

Tuberculoid leprosy is characterized by a marked cellular reaction to the bacterial invasion, with consequent skin lesions. Few bacteria are found in these lesions, which suggests that the skin reaction is an attempt to limit the disease, and chemotherapy, commenced at an early stage, can control the infection, and prevent subsequent neural damage. When such damage occurs, it is followed by the wasting of muscle and the deformities characteristic of untreated leprosy.

In lepromatous leprosy, the tissue reaction may be slight or absent, and bacterial invasion of the mucous membranes may continue unchecked. On that account, lepromatous leprosy is more contagious than the tuberculoid type. As with tuberculosis, prolonged multi-drug treatment is required, usually with dapsone, clofazimine and rifampicin. It should be noted that anaemia is frequent in leprosy, and the best response to treatment may not occur until the anaemia has been relieved.

Dapsone §

Dapsone is a sulphone derivative with bacteriostatic properties, and is considered to act by preventing the uptake of metabolites essential for the development of the leprosy bacillus. It is given in doses of 100 mg daily, with rifampicin 600 mg monthly, together with clofazimine 50 mg daily. Treatment with dapsone and other drugs must be prolonged up to 2 years or more.

Side-effects are allergic dermatitis, anorexia and anaemia. Neuropathy is a late complication of prolonged dapsone therapy.

Clofazimine §

Brand name: Lamprene §

Clofazimine is given in doses varying from 50 mg daily to 100 mg three times a week, but long-term treatment in association with other drugs is necessary. For lepra reactions doses of 300 mg daily for 3 months may be required. As it has some anti-inflammatory properties, it may give relief from the pain in swollen nerves that may occur in tuberculoid leprosy. Following absorption, the drug is deposited in the subcutaneous fat, and slowly released.

It may cause a red pigmentation of the skin, and the lesions may acquire a bluish-black colour that may persist for some months after the course of treatment has ended.

TRYPANOSOMIASIS

This disease, also known as African sleeping sickness, is due to the presence in the blood of a flagellate parasite, either *Trypanosoma gambiense*, or *Trypanosoma rhodesiense*. These parasites are transmitted from infected animals by the bite of the tsetse fly. The disease is characterized by a prolonged intermittent febrile condition, followed by a slow progressive mental and physical deterioration, ending in coma and death. The range of effective drugs is very limited, and early treatment is necessary.

Pentamidine isethionate § (dose: 4 mg/kg daily by injection)

Brand name: Pentacarinat §

This organic chemical is effective in the early stages of trypanosomiasis, but as it cannot cross the blood–brain barrier it is of much less value once the central nervous system has been invaded by the parasites. It is given by deep intramuscular or intravenous injection in doses of 4 mg/kg daily or on alternate days, up to a total of ten injections. The course is repeated after a rest period of some weeks. For prophylaxis, a dose of 300 mg may be given every 6 months.

Pentamidine is also used in the treatment of *Pneumocystis carinii* pneumonia, sometimes referred to as pneumocystosis. The organism is a common cause of pneumonia in immunocompromised patients and in AIDS, and for treatment, the standard dose of pentamidine should be given daily for 14 days. Pentamidine has also been used in the treatment of leishmaniasis.

Pentamidine has many and serious **side-effects**, including hypotension, hypoglycaemia, blood disorders and arrhythmias. The blood pressure should be monitored during administration of pentamidine, and regularly during treatment.

Suramin § (dose: 1 g weekly)

Suramin, once known as Antrypol, resembles pentamidine in

its general properties and is most effective in the early stages of trypanosomiasis. After an initial test dose of 200 mg, doses of 20 mg/kg (up to 1 g) by slow intravenous injection are given at weekly intervals for 5 weeks. In the later stages of the disease it may be used in association with tryparsamide.

Suramin may cause vomiting and paraesthesia but a serious **side-effect** is albuminuria, and urine tests should be carried out during treatment. It is contraindicated in renal disease.

Melarsoprol § (dose: 3.6 mg/kg intravenously)

Melarsoprol is an arsenical trypanocide that is effective in all stages of trypanosomiasis, but it is used mainly in the later stages of the disease in which the parasites have invaded the CSF. It is given by intravenous injection in doses of 3.6 mg/kg up to a maximum of 200 mg daily for 3 days, and repeated after a rest period of 7–10 days.

Side-effects are common, and may be severe, and include hypersensitivity reactions. Another severe reaction, which has proved fatal, is a reactive encephalopathy, characterized by tremor, convulsions and coma, which is thought to be a Herxheimer reaction caused by antigens released from dead trypanosomes.

20

The vitamins

Experiments during the early part of the present century showed that artificial diets containing adequate amounts of protein, fats, carbohydrates, minerals and water could not maintain growth and health. Some other factors present in normal diets were necessary, and these factors are now well known as vitamins.

They differ very widely in chemical constitution, and although in some cases their exact function is still obscure, they appear to be closely concerned with the action of enzymes in the body cell. When first discovered their chemical nature was unknown, and they were identified by letters. Many have now been synthesized, and are referred to by their chemical names as well as by the older letters. Reference will be made mainly to vitamins A, B, C, D, E and K.

VITAMIN DEFICIENCY

A good mixed diet provides adequate amounts of vitamins so vitamin supplements are normally unnecessary, and are of no value as 'tonics'. Restricted diets, or defective absorption or utilization of food result in vitamin deficiencies which lead to a number of recognizable conditions (Table 20.1) and require the administration of the appropriate vitamins.

Deficiencies may occur in alcoholics, food faddists, and in the elderly on poor diets, and also when natural demands for vitamins are increased, as in fevers, pregnancy and metabolic disorders such as diabetes. A deficiency of vitamin B_{12} invariably develops after total gastrectomy and may also occur in

Table 20.1   Vitamins

Vitamin	Some deficiency symptoms	Some effects of overdose
Vitamin A[a] (retinol)	Night blindness, drying of mucous membranes, uncommon in the UK	Rash, pruritus, liver disease
Vitamin B_1 (thiamine) (aneurine)	Beri-beri, polyneuritis, uncommon in the UK	
Vitamin B_2 (riboflavine)	Cracking of corners of the mouth, uncommon in the UK	
Vitamin B_3 (nicotinamide)	Pellagra, a syndrome of dermatitis, diarrhoea and delirium, uncommon in UK	Peptic ulcer, hypotension, pruritus Hepatotoxicity
Vitamin B_6 (pyridoxine)	Polyneuritis, uncommon in the UK	Peripheral neuropathy
Vitamin B_{12} (cyanocobalamin)	Pernicious anaemia	
Vitamin C (ascorbic acid)	Scurvy, easy bruising	Oxalate stones in susceptible individuals
Vitamin D[a] (calciferol) (cholecalciferol)	Rickets, osteomalacia, common in steatorrhoea	Hypercalcaemia, renal calcinosis, hypertension
Vitamin E[a] (tocopherol)	Unknown	Potentiation of oral anticoagulants
Vitamin K_1[a] (phytomenadione)	Prolonged bleeding, easy bruising	Haemolytic anaemia

[a]Fat-soluble vitamins.

vegans (pure vegetarians). Drugs which have a bactericidal action on the organisms normally present in the intestines, such as some oral antibiotics, may also indirectly cause a vitamin deficiency.

In such circumstances relatively small doses of vitamins are adequate to rectify the deficiency, but in certain unrelated conditions some vitamins are given in large doses, and should then be regarded as therapeutic agents, and not as dietary supplements and in overdose may have toxic side-effects (Table 20.1).

Vitamins present in food can be divided into two classes, the fat-soluble and the water-soluble vitamins. The fat-soluble vitamins include vitamins A, D, E and K; the water-soluble vitamins are represented by vitamins B and C.

As many vitamins are now made synthetically, and water-soluble derivatives are often available, this distinction between fat-soluble and water-soluble vitamins has become less important.

> ### Points about vitamins
>
> (a) Used in specific deficiency states, most of which are uncommon in the UK.
> (b) Usually unnecessary if a good mixed diet is taken.
> (c) Of no value as 'tonics'.
> (d) Excessive doses of vitamins A and D have toxic effects.
> (e) Treatment of pernicious anaemia with vitamin B$_{12}$ is for life.

VITAMIN A

Vitamin A (retinol) (prophylactic dose: 4000 units; therapeutic dose: 50 000 units daily)

Brand name: Ro-A-Vit

Vitamin A may be present in various foods as such, or as the closely related compound carotene, from which the vitamin can be formed in the body. Dietary sources of the vitamin include milk, butter, carrots and green vegetables, and vitamin A deficiency is uncommon. Fish liver oils contain large amounts together with vitamin D.

Vitamin A is concerned with the growth and maintenance of the epithelial tissues, as well as with normal vision, as it plays an essential part in the formation of the visual purple. A deficiency may lead to night blindness and if prolonged, to a keratinized condition of the cornea (xerophthalmia) which cannot be relieved by subsequent treatment with vitamin A.

The chief value of vitamin A is in deficiency states such as coeliac disease and sprue, or where absorption has been reduced by the excessive use of liquid paraffin as a laxative. It may be given as capsules of halibut liver oil, containing 4000 units, as cod liver oil or as the synthetic vitamin. In severe deficiency states vitamin A can be given by deep intramuscular injection in doses of 150 000–300 000 units monthly. Overdose causes toxic effects such as rough skin, enlargement of the liver and serum calcium disturbance. Care is necessary to avoid overdose with vitamin A supplements in pregnancy as high levels of the vitamin may cause birth defects.

VITAMIN B GROUP

This group or complex includes several water-soluble vitamins that usually occur together in various foods, and are concerned with the metabolism of proteins, fats and carbohydrates. The term 'vitamin B' was originally applied to what was thought to be a single substance, distinguished later as vitamins B_1, B_2, B_6, B_{12}, etc. Since then more specific names have been introduced. Deficiency rarely occurs singly, and administration of all the main vitamins of the group is usually advisable.

Thiamine (dose: prophylactic, 2–10 mg daily; therapeutic: 25–100 mg daily, orally or by intramuscular injection)

Brand name: Benerva
Brand names of some B-complex products: Becosym, Benerva Compound, Pabrinex, Parentrovite

Thiamine, also known as vitamin B_1 and aneurine, is essential for the utilization of carbohydrates and the nutrition of nerve cells. It is present in egg, liver, yeast and wheat germ, but is now made synthetically. Severe deficiency, which is uncommon in the UK, results in beri-beri, a condition characterized by peripheral neuritis, cardiac enlargement, oedema and mental disturbances. Nausea and vomiting occur during the early stages of thiamine deficiency, and thus lead to further losses of the vitamin. In such conditions, thiamine is given in doses that may vary from 25–300 mg daily according to the severity of the deficiency, and doses of 200–300 mg may also be given daily by intramuscular injection.

Thiamine is also given in the treatment of the various manifestations of polyneuritis, in gastrointestinal disorders, and during the administration of wide-range antibiotics. In alcoholism and severe deficiency states, large doses of thiamine are usually given by intramuscular or slow intravenous injection in association with other vitamins of the B group, and with vitamin C in products such as **Pabrinex** and **Parentrovite**. Severe allergic reactions may occur during or soon after thiamine injections, and anaphylactic therapy must be immediately available.

Riboflavine (prophylactic dose: 1–4 mg daily; therapeutic dose: 5–10 mg daily)

A deficiency of riboflavine (vitamin B_2) results in a syndrome, characterized by cracking of the lips and of the skin at the corners of the mouth (angular stomatitis), photophobia and other visual disturbances. Treatment with a mixed vitamin B preparation is usually required.

Nicotinic acid (prophylactic dose: 15–30 mg daily; therapeutic dose: 50–250 mg daily)

Nicotinic acid is present in liver, yeast, and unpolished rice but it is now made synthetically. Lack of nicotinic acid, often associated with a maize-rich diet, results in the deficiency disease known as pellagra, characterized by diarrhoea, dermatitis and dementia. These symptoms, as well as the mental confusion, respond rapidly to nicotinic acid and associated vitamins.

Nicotinic acid also has vasodilatory properties, and has been used in Meniere's disease, peripheral vascular disorders and chilblains (p. 217) and as a blood-lipid lowering agent (p. 224).

Nicotinamide is closely related to nicotinic acid, and is used in pellagra and other deficiency states when the vasodilator action of the acid is not desired or proves an embarrassment. **Ronicol** (p. 217), although related to nicotinic acid, has no vitamin properties.

Pyridoxine (vitamin B₆)(dose: 50–150 mg daily)

Brand name: Benadon

Pyridoxine is concerned with the metabolism of proteins, amino acids and fats, and is present in a wide variety of foods. Deficiency results in peripheral neuritis, which although uncommon, may arise during treatment with isoniazid as well as in sideroblastic anaemia. Pyridoxine has been used empirically in the nausea of pregnancy, in irradiation sickness and alcoholism, and in premenstrual syndrome, but not with marked success. Pyridoxine may reduce the response to levodopa in Parkinson's disease.

Cyanocobalamin (vitamin B₁₂) § (dose: 1 mg by injection)

Brand name: Cytamen §

Cyanocobalamin is the anti-anaemia factor, and its use in pernicious anaemia is discussed on page 497. It has virtually been replaced by hydroxocobalamin.

VITAMIN C

Ascorbic acid (therapeutic dose: 200–600 mg daily; prophylactic dose: 25–75 mg daily)

Brand name: Redoxon

Ascorbic acid is the water-soluble vitamin present in oranges and other citrus fruits, blackcurrants and green vegetables. It is essential for the development of collagen, cartilage and bone, and is concerned in haemoglobin formation and tissue repair.

Deficiency of ascorbic acid, if severe, results in the once dreaded disease of scurvy, characterized by subcutaneous haemorrhage, due to capillary fragility. Scurvy was once common on sailing ships with restricted supplies of fresh fruit and vegetables, but it is now rarely seen.

Mild deficiency states may occur during pregnancy and in patients on restricted diets, and chronic marginal deficiency of vitamin C, especially in the elderly, may be more common than is normally suspected. Infantile scurvy may sometimes occur in bottle-fed infants. Vitamin C requirements are increased during infections and following trauma, and the drug has been given to promote wound healing. Very large doses have been used in the treatment of the common cold, but the response is not impressive.

VITAMIN D

Calciferol (vitamin D_2) [therapeutic dose: 5000–50 000 units (125 micrograms–1.25 mg) daily; prophylactic dose: not more than 800 units (20 micrograms) daily]

The term vitamin D includes several related substances, of which calciferol, also known as ergocalciferol (vitamin D_2), is the most important. Vitamin D is found mainly in dairy products, and it is also formed as cholecalciferol, vitamin D_3, in the body by the action of sunlight on the skin. Although fish liver oils are a rich source, calciferol is now prepared synthetically. It is an essential factor in the absorption of calcium and phosphorus from the gastrointestinal tract, and thus in the formation of bone.

In children, a deficiency of calciferol results in rickets, a disease characterized by weak bones, bowed legs and deformities of the chest. In confirmed rickets in children, the standard treatment is a daily dose of 1000–1500 units of calciferol, but occasionally a single dose of 300 000 units is given by intramuscular injection. Calciferol is also used in certain other conditions associated with calcium deficiency as in coeliac disease, and in the low blood calcium due to parathyroid deficiency.

In general, the vitamins are well tolerated even in very large doses, but calciferol is the main exception, as **toxic effects** may follow the prolonged administration of high doses. Thirst, drowsiness and gastrointestinal disturbances, which may be severe, are among the symptoms of overdosage, and continued administration may result in the release of calcium from bone and its storage in the tissues, kidneys and arterial vessels, causing renal damage and hypertension.

The following products are available:

Strong calciferol tablets 250 micrograms/10 000 units.

High strength calciferol tablets 1.25 mg/50 000 units.

Calciferol injection 7.5 mg/300 000 units.

Whenever *strong* calciferol tablets are prescribed, confirmation should be sought that the 1.25 mg product is in fact required, as errors have occurred.

Calcium with vitamin D tablets: calciferol 10 micrograms/400 units, calcium lactate 300 mg, calcium phosphate 150 mg.

Calcichew: calciferol 5 micrograms/200 units, calcium carbonate 1.26 g.

Chocovite: calciferol 1.25 micrograms (50 000 units) calcium gluconate 500 mg.

Alfacalcidol § (dose: 0.25–5 micrograms daily)

Brand names: Alfa D §, One-Alpha §

The action of calciferol is mediated by its conversion in the kidneys and liver to the much more potent hydroxylated metabolite calcitriol. In renal impairment that conversion may be incomplete, and the response to calciferol less satisfactory. It is the cause in part of vitamin D resistance. Alfacalcidol is a calciferol derivative which bypasses the renal stage of vitamin D metabolism, and is converted in the liver to the final and most active metablite calcitriol (dihydroxyvitamin D_3). Alfacalcidol is indicated in a variety of conditions associated with disturbances in the biosynthesis of calcitriol, including renal osteodystrophy, osteomalacia, vitamin D resistance and hypoparathyroidism. The response to alfacalcidol is prompt and more controllable than that of slower-acting forms of vitamin D. It is given initially in doses of 0.5 microgram daily (half doses for the elderly), subsequently adjusted according to response as shown by changes in the plasma calcium levels, with maintenance doses of 1–3 micrograms daily. In severe conditions, similar doses may be given by intravenous injection. Absorption may be impaired by aluminium-based antacids, and the risks of hypercalcaemia are increased in patients taking thiazide diuretics or any calcium-containing products. The main side-effect is hypercalcaemia, which requires withdrawal of treatment, after which the normal plasma calcium level returns in about a week, when treatment can be resumed with half doses.

Calcitriol § (dose: 0.5–1 microgram daily)

Brand name: Rocaltrol §

Calcitriol (dihydroxyvitamin D_3) is the metabolite derived from calciferol formed in the liver, and is characterized by its high potency. Like alfacalcidol, it is used to correct abnormalities of calcium and phosphate metabolism, mainly when such abnormalities are associated with chronic renal failure as in renal osteodystrophy. Calcitriol reduces the associated hypocalcaemia, and relieves the symptoms of bone disease. The initial dose is 250 nanograms daily or on alternate days, slowly increased as required by increments of 250 nanograms at intervals of 3–4 weeks. As with alfacalcidol, dosage requires careful and continued control.

Dihydrotachysterol § (dose: 200 micrograms–2 mg)

Brand name: AT10 §

Dihydrotachysterol is related to calciferol, but it has an action resembling that of the parathyroid hormone. It increases the absorption of calcium, and is used together with calcium gluconate in the hypocalcaemia due to parathyroid deficiency. It is given initially in doses of 200 micrograms daily, but maintenance doses vary from 200 micrograms to 1 mg or more adjusted to the serum calcium levels. Excessive doses lead to decalcification of bone, hypercalcaemia and renal damage.

VITAMIN E

Tocopherol (dose: 10–200 mg daily)

Brand name: Ephynal

Tocopherol, also known as vitamin E, is present in wheat germ, soya-bean, lettuce and other green leaves, but the synthetic drug is referred to as alpha tocopherol acetate.

The vitamin has some general action on the metabolism of fats, carbohydrates and proteins but a deficiency is not followed by any clear symptoms. Tocopherol has been used empirically in muscular dystrophy, angina, Dupuytren's contracture, vascular disease and in certain anaemias in children, and for malabsorption in cystic fibrosis. In general, the response to tocopherol treatment is variable and often disappointing.

Mixed vitamin products

Many mixed vitamin products are available, often containing mineral supplements. These mixtures are mainly of value in the treatment of deficiencies due to restricted diets but have no 'tonic' properties. A few are useful during the prenatal period, but their value in other conditions where full diets are available is problematical.

Some polyvitamin preparations are represented by Abidec, Concavit, Orovite and Tonivitan.

Foreceval and Ketovite are multivitamin products with mineral supplements. They are used mainly in association with restricted diets.

VITAMIN K

Vitamin K is essential for the formation of prothrombin in the liver, as well as the production of accessory factors essential for the functioning of the blood-clotting system (p. 303).

Lack of vitamin K leads to hypoprothrombinaemia, or deficiency of prothrombin, resulting in delayed clotting of the blood and, if severe, to spontaneous haemorrhage.

The natural vitamin which is present in green vegetables and eggs, and is formed in the intestines by bacteria, is fat-soluble, and bile is essential for its absorption. A deficiency may therefore arise, even during an adequate dietary intake, in such conditions as obstructive jaundice or coeliac disease.

Deficiency may also occur during treatment with anticoagulants, which reduce vitamin K metabolism, and with antibacterial drugs which interfere with vitamin K synthesis by intestinal bacteria. Salicylates and clofibrate may also decrease the availability of vitamin K. Synthetic water-soluble compounds with a similar but more controllable action are now used instead of the natural vitamin.

Menadiol (dose: 10–40 mg daily)

Brand name: Synkavit

Menadiol sodium diphosphate is a water-soluble analogue of vitamin K, and is suitable for the treatment of most forms of hypoprothrombinaemia. It is also used for the prophylaxis of haemorrhagic conditions associated with obstructive jaundice, or following the prolonged administration of salicylates or other drugs that may extend the bleeding time. Menadiol is given orally in doses of 10–40 mg daily according to need. Care is necessary in G6PD deficiency (p. 501) as there is some risk of haemolysis.

Phytomenadione (dose: 5–20 mg orally, or by intramuscular or slow intravenous injection)

Brand name: Konakion

Phytomenadione is a natural form of vitamin K, and is also referred to as vitamin K_1. It is an essential co-factor in the hepatic synthesis of prothrombin and other clotting factors, and its physiological function is the maintenance of the normal level of prothrombin in the blood. Therapeutically it is used to counteract the haemorrhage that may occur during oral anticoagulant therapy with synthetic drugs. (It is not an antidote to heparin.) In such cases, phytomenadione acts more rapidly than the water-soluble synthetic drugs such as menadiol, and the action is more prolonged.

In severe haemorrhage, an initial dose of 10–20 mg may be given by slow intravenous injection. The prothrombin level should be determined 3 hours later, and subsequent doses adjusted according to need. For less severe conditions, phytomenadione may be given orally in doses of 10 mg, or by intramuscular injection. (Tablets should be chewed or allowed to dissolve in the mouth.)

In the prophylactic treatment of haemorrhagic disorders of the newborn, the drug may be given to the mother by intramuscular injection in doses of 1–5 mg before delivery. It may also be given to the baby as a single dose of 0.5–1 mg, especially if intracranial or other haemorrhage is anticipated.

Opinion is still divided on the safety and route of administration of vitamin K_1, and local practice should be followed.

21

Anti-anaemic and haematopoietic agents

Anaemia can be broadly defined as an insufficiency of mature red cells in the blood. The most frequent and important cause is impaired blood formation, but excessive blood loss or destruction of red cells may also lead to anaemia. The blood cells or erythrocytes begin in the bone marrow as large cells, termed megaloblasts, which gradually diminish in size as they mature, and are then referred to as normoblasts.

At a later stage these normoblasts acquire haemoglobin (the red iron-containing protein of the blood cells), and then enter the circulation as fully developed and mature erythrocytes. Haemoglobin is concerned with the transport of oxygen from the lungs to all the body tissues, and iron is an essential element of its constitution.

Anaemia can therefore arise simply from a deficiency of iron, and in such iron-deficiency anaemias an adequate number of normoblasts may develop, but they lack the oxygen-carrying capacity of the mature red cells. Other and more serious forms of anaemia are due to a true deficiency of fully developed and mature erythrocytes owing to impaired cell formation by the bone marrow.

IRON-DEFICIENCY ANAEMIA

In health the loss of iron from the body is less than 2 mg daily, as almost all the iron released by the breakdown of red blood cells is re-absorbed, and the daily loss of iron is rarely more than 2 mg, which is normally replaced by dietary iron. Iron requirements are increased during pregnancy and childhood but iron-deficiency anaemia is usually due to excessive blood loss in conditions such as profuse menstruation and haemorrhage due to peptic ulcer. On the other hand, iron overload may occur after repeated blood transfusions. Most dietary iron is in the non-absorbable ferric state, and is excreted in the faeces after combination with dietary substances such as phosphate as insoluble iron salts. A small amount of ferric iron is converted to the ferrous state by the acid nature of the gastric contents, and it should be noted that antacids may reduce the formation of ferrous iron. The ferrous iron is absorbed by the mucosal cells of the small intestine where it combines with a protein (apoferritin) to form ferritin, in which the iron is stored within a protein shell. When the body stores of iron are adequate, there is little free apoferritin available for the further take-up of iron, a state sometimes referred to as mucosal block. When the iron stores are low, transferritin functions as a transport protein for the take-up of iron by the bone marrow for subsequent conversion to haemoglobin and other factors such as myoglobin and iron-containing enzymes. Ferritin also functions as a re-cycling agent, as it is concerned with the re-use of iron released by the breakdown of red blood cells.

The treatment of iron deficiency is basically replacement therapy, and the following products are in use.

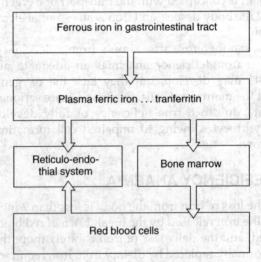

Figure 21.1 Diagram of iron transport and utilization.

Ferrous sulphate (prophylactic dose: 200 mg daily; therapeutic dose: 600–900 mg daily)

Ferrous sulphate is one of the most widely used therapeutic forms of iron, as it is soluble, effective and inexpensive. It is usually given as tablets containing 200 mg, equivalent to 60 mg of elemental iron. The drug is astringent and may cause occasional gastric disturbance, which can be reduced by taking the tablets after food. Ferrous sulphate may also be given in solution as Ferrous Sulphate Mixture (Paediatric), which is a very suitable product for the administration of iron to small children. Iron salts should not be given with the tetracycline group of antibiotics, as the absorption of both drugs may be mutually reduced.

Many alternatives have been introduced with the aim of reducing the side-effects associated with ferrous sulphate, although some better tolerated products merely contain smaller doses of iron. A few, such as Feospan, Ferrograd and Slow-Fe contain ferrous sulphate in a slow-release form.

Tablets of ferrous sulphate are usually coated to prevent oxidation, and have been taken by children in mistake for sweets. Such an overdose may cause severe gastrointestinal damage, leading to haematemisis, shock and cardiovascular collapse. Many deaths have occurred in small children from this cause. Immediate treatment includes emetics, gastric lavage and treatment with desferrioxamine (Desferal).

Desferrioxamine is a chelating agent that binds iron as a water-soluble non-toxic complex which is excreted in the urine. In iron poisoning it should be given as a dose of 2 g as soon as possible by intramuscular injection, followed by doses of up to 15 mg per kg body weight hourly by intravenous drip infusion up to a total dose of 80 mg/kg in 24 hours, to eliminate any absorbed iron. The further absorption of any iron remaining in the stomach may be prevented by giving an oral dose of 5 g of desferrioxamine dissolved in 50–100 ml of water.

Iron overload may also occur after repeated blood transfusions, and desferrioxamine has been given in doses up to 2 g with each transfusion. It is also given by subcutaneous infusion in doses of 20–40 mg/kg daily for 5–7 days. The effects in iron overload can be increased by the oral use of ascorbic acid (vitamin C) in doses of 200 mg daily between meals. Desferrioxamine is also useful in the treatment of aluminium overload in patients on maintenance haemodialysis.

Ferrous gluconate (prophylactic dose, 600 mg daily; therapeutic dose, 1.2–1.8 g daily)

Ferrous gluconate has the same action as ferrous sulphate, but is less irritant and is often acceptable when ferrous sulphate is not tolerated. Weight for weight it contains less iron than the sulphate, so that larger doses are required (300 mg is equivalent to 35 mg of iron).

Ferrous gluconate is present in a number of proprietary iron preparations, many of which contain vitamins. Such vitamin supplements, with the exception of vitamin C, do not increase the absorption of the associated iron compound and are of little therapeutic value.

Other iron salts

Ferrous fumarate and ferrous succinate are other iron salts with reduced side-effects, and are present in a number of proprietary anti-anaemic preparations. They are useful for patients who cannot tolerate other forms of iron, but have few other advantages.

Sodium iron-edetate (Sytron) is a liquid preparation in which the iron is combined as an organic complex. It breaks down in the body and releases the iron in an absorbable form. It is useful when gastric intolerance to other oral iron preparations is severe.

Some iron deficiency is common in pregnancy, and if associated with a folic acid deficiency, it may manifest itself in late pregnancy as a folate-deficiency-megaloblastic anaemia. Several preparations of iron and folic acid are now available for prophylactic use throughout pregnancy, and are often used routinely. Representative products include Fefol, Pregaday and Meterfolic. The use of these products in older patients is not advised, as in undiagnosed pernicious anaemia, neurological symptoms could be precipitated.

Iron by injection

In very severe iron deficiency, or when oral iron is not tolerated, or when the patient fails to cooperate with oral treatment, it may be necessary to give iron by injection. Solutions of ordinary iron salts are too toxic, but injectable products are available in which the iron is bound up in a complex with various carbohydrates. Preparations of this type are tolerated fairly well, and are of value in the treatment of severe iron deficiency. As such iron injections bypass the mechanism that normally controls the degree of iron absorption, the total dose must be based on the actual iron deficiency as shown by laboratory tests, otherwise an overdose may be given. The rate of response is comparable with that to oral therapy.

Iron-sorbitol injection §

Brand name: Jectofer §

This product is a complex of iron, sorbitol and citric acid,

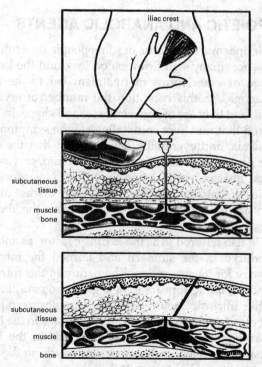

Figure 21.2   Injection of iron. (Reproduced by kind permission of Fisons Pharmaceuticals, Loughborough.)

stabilized with dextrin (1 ml = 50 mg iron). It is given under haematological control in doses equivalent to 1.5 mg of iron per kg daily by deep intramuscular injection. (It is not suitable for intravenous use and care must be taken to avoid unintentional injection into a vein.) The total dose given is based upon the degree of haemoglobin deficiency.

Deep intramuscular injection is necessary to reduce the risk of subcutaneous staining, and should be made only into the muscle mass of the upper and outer quadrant of the buttock, employing a Z-track injection technique. That involves a lateral displacement of the skin before the needle is inserted (Fig. 21.2) and, after injection of the drug, pausing for a few seconds before withdrawing the needle. That will allow the muscle mass to accommodate the volume of the injection, and so minimize the risk of leakage up the injection track. To further minimize the risk, the patient should be warned not to rub the injection site.

HAEMATOPOIETIC AND ANABOLIC AGENTS

A megaloblastic anaemia may occur in some people on a full diet even in the absence of any significant blood loss, and the lack of response to iron or other forms of treatment led to the term 'pernicious anaemia'. In this condition the number of erythrocytes is reduced, and they are of abnormal size and shape. In 1926 it was discovered that raw liver could alleviate the symptoms of pernicious anaemia, and eventually it was found that the anti-anaemic factor present in liver was cyanocobalamin, or vitamin B_{12}. Pernicious anaemia can be relieved by injections of cyanocobalamin, so that basically it is a deficiency disease due to an inability to absorb vitamin B_{12} obtained from the diet or formed by intestinal bacteria.

The vitamin is also referred to as the extrinsic factor, as another substance, produced in the stomach and termed the intrinsic factor, is necessary for its absorption. The nature of this intrinsic factor is not known, but it appears to be a glycoprotein. Vitamin B_{12} binds to the intrinsic factor, and the complex is rapidly absorbed and bound to plasma protein before storage in the liver, and released as required for red cell production in the bone marrow. It is partly excreted in the urine, and partly in the bile. The process is summarized in Figure 21.3.

A deficiency of cyanocobalamin not only causes a megaloblastic

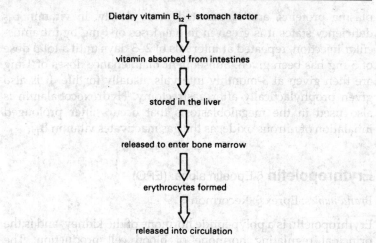

Dietary vitamin B_{12} + stomach factor

⬇

vitamin absorbed from intestines

⬇

stored in the liver

⬇

released to enter bone marrow

⬇

erythrocytes formed

⬇

released into circulation

Figure 21.3 Outline of vitamin B_{12} absorption and action.

anaemia, but may also bring about a degeneration of the spinal cord (combined subacute degeneration). Such neurological damage also responds slowly but not always completely to vitamin B_{12}.

In the UK cyanocobalamin has been replaced by hydroxocobalamin, but in the USA it remains the preferred drug, on the basis that antibodies to the hydroxocobalamin–protein complex could develop.

Cyanocobalamin § (dose: 250 micrograms–1 mg by injection)

Brand names: Cytamen §, Cytacon §

Cyanocobalamin, originally extracted from liver, is obtained as a by-product of the growth of various micro-organisms. It has been given in doses of 1 mg monthly by intramuscular injection. It is of no value orally.

Hydroxocobalamin (dose: 1 mg by injection)

Brand names: Neo-Cytamen §, Cobalin-H §

Hydroxocobalamin has the actions and uses of cyanocobalamin but it has a longer action, as it binds more firmly with specific plasma proteins, and is excreted more slowly. In vitamin B_{12} deficiency states it is given in initial doses of 1 mg by intramuscular injection, repeated at intervals of 2–3 days until a total dose of 5 mg has been given. Subsequent maintenance doses of 1 mg are then given at 3-monthly intervals, usually for life. It is also given prophylactically after gastrectomy. Hydroxocobalamin is also used in the megaloblastosis that occurs after prolonged inhalation of nitrous oxide, as the gas inactivates vitamin B_{12}.

Erythropoietin § Epoetin alpha: (EPO)

Brand names: Eprex §, Recormon §

Erythropoietin is a polypeptide hormone of the kidney, and is the principal regulating hormone of blood cell production. The kidneys are sensitive to the amount of oxygen in the circulation, and a reduction in the kidney-tissue oxygen supply stimulates the release of erythropoietin, followed by a rapid production of oxygen-carrying red cells by the bone marrow (erythropoiesis). The consequent improved transport of oxygen to the tissues by the red cells is also detected by the kidneys, and as a result the release of erythropoietin is inhibited. The feed-back mechanism is shown diagrammatically in Figure 21.4.

Natural erythropoietin is not readily available, but large amounts can now be obtained by recombinant DNA technology,

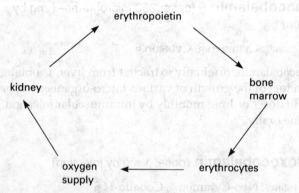

Figure 21.4 An oxygen deficiency stimulates the release of erythropoietin and the formation of more oxygen-carrying erythrocytes. As the lack of oxygen is relieved, the rate of erythropoietin production and release falls.

and the hormone is being used to control the anaemia associated with chronic renal failure in patients maintained by haemodialysis. Such patients become severely anaemic because they cannot produce erythropoietin naturally, and because of the blood loss associated with haemodialysis. Two forms of recombinant human erythropoietin are available, and although they are similar and clinically interchangeable, the dose differs according to the product used. Epoetin alfa (Eprex) is given by subcutaneous or intravenous injection in doses of 50 units/kg three times a week, slowly increased by 25 units/kg as required. Epoetin Beta (Recormon) is given similarly but in initial doses of 20 units/kg. Close haematological control is necessary during erythropoietin therapy, and specialist literature should be consulted for dosage details. Supplementary iron may be required by some patients, but provided adequate iron is available, the haemalogical response may be rapid.

Side-effects include headache, a dose-dependent increase in blood pressure and influenza-like symptoms. A sudden migraine-like pain may be a warning of an incipient hypertensive crisis. Seizures have occurred in patients with poor renal function.

 Winearls C G et al 1986 Effects of human erythropoietin derived from recombinant DNA on the anaemia of patients maintained by chronic haemodialysis. Lancet ii: 1175–1178

Erythropoietin may have other therapeutic applications, as some neonates lack both the hormone and red cells, and must be ventilated. Exogenous erythropoietin could supply the deficiency, and the anaemia associated with rheumatoid arthritis and cancer may also respond to erythropoietin.

Filgrastim §▼ (dose: 500 000 units by injection)

Brand name: Neupogen §▼

Neutropenia is an abnormal reduction in the number of circulating neutrophils, one of the forms of leucocytes concerned with phagocytosis and the removal of invading bacteria. In neutropenia, which is often caused by depression of bone-marrow activity by cytoxic drugs, the risks of infection are correspondingly increased. The production of neutrophils in the bone marrow is regulated by a factor referred to as the granulocyte colony-stimulating factor (G-CSF) and filgrastim is a recombinant form of human G-CSF that stimulates neutrophil production. In drug-induced neutropenia filgastrim is given in doses of 500 000 units/kg daily by subcutaneous injection or intravenous infusion beginning not less than 24 hours after the end of chemotherapy. The injections should be continued until the normal neutrophil count has been restored, which may take up to 2 weeks. **Side-effects** are muscle pain and dysuria. Molgramostim (Leucomax) is a recombinant form of human granulocyte macrophage-colony stimulating factor (GM-CSF) with similar properties and uses.

Lenograstim §▼

Brand name: Granocyte §▼

Lenograstim is a recombinant form of the granulocyte colony stimulating factor (G-GSF) with the actions and uses of filgrastim. In the treatment of drug-associated neutropenia in malignancy it is given in daily doses of 150 micrograms/m^2 of body area by subcutaneous injection, commenced the day after the end of the course of chemotherapy. Treatment should be continued until the neutrophil count has reached a satisfactory level for up to a maximum of 28 days. A similar course is given by slow intravenous injection after bone marrow transplantation. Full blood counts are necessary during lenograstim treatment.

Folic acid § (dose: 5–15 mg daily)

Folic acid is a member of the vitamin B complex, and is one of the many factors concerned in blood formation, particularly the maturation of red blood cells. Deficiency of folic acid may lead to a megaloblastic anaemia, and the administration of folic acid is of value in dietary deficiency anaemias, and in some disturbances of fat metabolism such as tropical sprue. Folic acid is also used prophylactically during pregnancy, and is given in doses of 200–500 micrograms daily, usually with iron (p. 494). When given to prevent neural defect, doses of 5 milligrams daily should be taken and continued until the twelfth week of pregnancy. Folic acid was used at one time in the treatment of pernicious anaemia, as it can restore the blood picture to normal, but such use may precipitate degeneration of the spinal cord, and the use of folic acid alone in pernicious anaemia has been abandoned.

Oxymetholone § (dose: 2–3 mg/kg daily)

Brand name: Anapolon §

Anabolic steroids such as oxymetholone have been used in high doses for the treatment of aplastic and haemolytic anaemias, but the mode of action is not clear, and the response is variable. Treatment for 3–6 months is necessary, and with such long therapy, virilizing side-effects are likely to occur.

Nandrolone § (Deca-Durabolin §) has similar properties, and is given by deep intramuscular injection in doses of 50–100 mg weekly.

GLUCOSE 6-PHOSPHATE DEHYDROGENASE DEFICIENCY

One form of haemolytic anaemia, found in some African and Asian populations, and also known to occur in the Mediterranean area, is due to a deficiency of the enzyme glucose 6-phosphate dehydrogenase (G6PD). That enzyme plays a key role in red blood cell (RBC) activity and integrity, and a deficiency of G6PD, which occurs mainly but not exclusively in males, leads to an increased sensitivity of the RBCs to the oxidative breakdown by certain drugs, resulting in an haemolytic anaemia. The degree of susceptibility is subject to individual variation, and may be dose-related to some extent, but care is necessary in treating any patient known to be G6PD deficient with sulphonamides, nalidixic acid and other quinolones, dapsone, nitrofurantoin, primaquine, pamaquin and methylene blue. Some patients may also be susceptible to aspirin, chloroquine, menadione, quinine and quinidine.

22

Fluid therapy and clinical nutrition

The metabolic processes of the body can only function normally when adequate supplies of tissue fluids of suitable consitution are available. In health the composition of the plasma and cell fluids is controlled by the kidneys within very narrow limits, and this control is capable of dealing with very variable physiological demands.

Some 70% of the body weight consists of water and dissolved electrolytes. Electrolytes are metallic salts which dissociate in solution to form ions, which may be positively or negatively charged. The principal electrolytes of the body are sodium, potassium, calcium and magnesium, present as chlorides, bicarbonates, sulphates and phosphates. In solution the metals form positively charged ions or cations, and the non-metallic radicals form negatively charged anions.

BODY WATER

Of the body water, some 50–60% exists within the cells, and is termed intracellular fluid; the balance, which is present in the blood, lymph and tissue spaces, is the extracellular fluid. The electrolyte composition of these fluids varies, as the intracellular fluid contains most of the potassium and phosphate, whereas the extracellular fluid contains the bulk of the sodium and bicarbonate. Normally, there is a dynamic balance between the concentration of the ions in these fluids, but this balance can be seriously disturbed by any severe loss of water and electrolytes. Loss of mineral salts is more serious than loss of water, which can be replaced easily. Thus prolonged vomiting causes a loss of chloride, potassium and sodium as well as water, as does excessive diuretic treatment. Diarrhoea results in a loss of water and bicarbonates, and severe burns also cause marked dehydration and loss of plasma and electrolytes.

Electrolyte balance and intravenous infusion fluids

In an attempt to maintain the electrolyte balance of the body in such conditions, marked changes in the relative proportions of the intracellular and extracellular water may occur. Water may leave the subcutaneous tissues and a large amount of dilute urine may be excreted in order to maintain the concentration of remaining electrolytes. In severe conditions such as diabetic coma this excretion of electrolytes, especially potassium, may lead to respiratory and circulatory collapse, and rapid restoration of the fluid and electrolyte balance is an essential therapeutic measure. Several standard fluid and electrolyte replacement solutions for intravenous infusion are in use (Table 22.1).

In this field, nurses can play an important part by monitoring the rate and volume of all intravenous fluids.

Hyaluronidase

Brand name: Hyalase

Sodium Chloride Injection and other electrolyte solutions are normally given by intravenous infusion. In young children and in older patients where intravenous infusion presents difficulties, subcutaneous infusion is a practical alternative when hyaluronidase is used to facilitate absorption by 'hypodermoclysis'.

Hyaluronidase is a mucolytic enzyme obtained from animal testes, and it has the power of causing a temporary decrease in the viscosity of the mucoprotein 'group substance' or 'cement' of the tissue spaces. This reduction in viscosity increases the speed of diffusion into the tissues of fluids injected subcutaneously and facilitates absorption.

The standard dose of hyaluronidase is 1500 units, and the enzyme may be given subcutaneously directly into the injection site, or added to 500–1000 ml of the injection solution. Absorption of the injection solution takes place at the rate of about 100 ml per

Table 22.1 Intravenous infusion fluids

Solution	Electrolyte content (mmol per litre)					Energy content per litre (k/cal)	Notes on use
	Na$^+$	K$^+$	Ca^{2+}	Cl	Bicarbonate or lactate		
Glucose 5%						200	Fluid and energy replacement
Glucose 2.5% with sodium chloride 0.45%	75			75		100	Fluid, energy and electrolyte replacement
Glucose 5% with sodium chloride 0.9%	150			150		200	Fluid and multiple electrolyte replacement
Hartmann's solution	131	5	2	111	29		
Mannitol 10%, 15%, 20%							Osmotic diuretic, contraindicated in congestive heart failure and pulmonary oedema

Table 22.1 (cont'd)

Solution		Electrolyte content (mmol per litre)					Energy content per litre (kcal)	Notes on use
		Na$^+$	K$^+$	Ca^{2+}	Cl	Bicarbonate or lactate		
Potassium chloride (in 5% glucose)	0.2%		30		30		200	For correction of potassium deficiency after severe diarrhoea, and vomiting, and diuretics
	0.3%		40		40		200	
Potassium chloride (in glucose 4% with sodium chloride 0.9%)	0.2%	150	30		180		160	Wherever possible these solutions should be used in preference to adding strong potassium chloride solution to other infusions
			30					
Potassium chloride (in 0.9% saline)	0.2%	150	30		150			Fluid and electrolyte replacement
	0.3%	150	40		150			
Ringer's Solution		147	4	2	155			
Sodium bicarbonate	1.4%	167				167		Treatment of metabolic acidosis. The stronger solutions are used in severe acidosis following cardiac arrest
	4.2%	500				500		
	8.4%	1000				1000		
Sodium chloride	0.45%	77			77			Fluid and electrolyte replacement. The stronger solutions are used to correct acute sodium loss while the weaker ones are used for maintenance therapy in secondary dehydration
	0.9%	150			150			
	1.8%	308			308			
	2.7%	460			460			
	5%	855			855			
Sorbitol 30%							1200	An alternative energy source

hour. Hyaluronidase is also used occasionally to facilitate the local diffusion and absorption of local anaesthetic and other injection solutions.

INTRAVENOUS INFUSION FLUIDS

The simple glucose and glucose/saline solutions are used mainly for fluid replacement and when there is some loss of sodium, but others are used to correct potassium and multiple electrolyte disturbances. The type and volume of the intravenous infusion used will depend on the individual patient's need and response, as overdose can occur with such solutions as with other drugs.

Additions are sometimes made to infusion solutions, as by that means a more steady plasma level of the added drug or drugs can be made, but such additions carry risks. Ideally, all solutions containing additive drugs should be prepared in the hospital pharmacy. When that is not possible, and nurses are expected to prepare such additive products, they should be aware of the risks, and employ a strict aseptic technique to avoid bacterial contamination.

No drug should be added to an infusion fluid unless it is known that all the constituents are compatible, and that no loss of potency of the added drug will occur. Intravenous infusion additive solutions are usually prepared with standard glucose or saline infusion fluids, and only one container should be prepared at a time, and used as soon as possible. Drugs should not be added to infusion solutions of sodium bicarbonate, amino acids, mannitol or blood products, and only specially prepared additive products should be added to intravenous fat emulsions.

Some infusion solutions must be protected from the light to reduce the risk of inactivation, and any change in colour or development of cloudiness in an infusion fluid is an indication to stop the infusion. The absence of any change in appearance is not an assurance that no loss of potency has occurred. Care must be taken to ensure thorough mixing of the additive before the infusion is commenced. An additional label should be placed on the container, indicating what additive and how much, the date of preparation, by whom it was prepared, and the name of the patient. In some cases, as with certain irritant drugs, the additive is not added to the bulk of the infusion fluid, but is injected into the tubing of a fast-running intravenous infusion, thus ensuring rapid dilution and a reduced risk of local irritation.

With drugs that are unstable in dilute solution, such as some antibiotics, intermittent infusion can be used, in which the drug is dissolved in about 100 ml of infusion solution, and injected over about 30 minutes. Table 22.2 gives some guidance on suitable infusion fluids for additives, in which G refers to glucose solution 5%, S to sodium chloride 0.9%, and W to Water for Injections, but Hartmann's solution and Ringer's solution, and sometimes dextran solution may also be suitable. CI indicates continuous intravenous infusion, VDT to injection via the infusion tubing, and I to intermittent infusion. When Water for Injection is used, the volume should be restricted to about 100 ml to avoid giving an hypotonic solution.

PLASMA AND BLOOD VOLUME EXPANDERS

In conditions of acute blood loss and low plasma volume, as after haematemesis, trauma and burns, there is a marked fall in the colloidal osmotic pressure of the blood. Intravenous fluids can bring about a temporary improvement, but their effect is soon lost unless plasma replacement treatment is also given. Plasma can be given as such, or as Plasma Protein Solution (4–5%), of which the principal protein is albumin, or as Human Albumin Solution, derived from plasma or placentae, containing 4–5% of protein, of which at least 95% is albumin. Albuminair and Buminate are concentrated products (20%).

Plasma and blood volume expanders such as dextran may be given without reference to the patient's blood group, but the latter are not suitable for maintenance use as plasma substitutes when the plasma loss is serious and continuing, as in severe burns.

Dextran

Brand names: Gentran §, Macrodex §

Dextran is a polysaccharide, formed in sugar solutions by a non-pathogenic coccus, *Leuconostoc mesenteroides*. Polysaccharides may be regarded as aggregations of sugar molecules linked together to form large units, and the physical properties of products such as dextran depend on the size and molecular weight of these large aggregate units.

Table 22.2 Drug additives to infusion systems

Drug	Infusion fluid	Method of use
acebutolol	S	I
aclarubicin	G or S	CI
actinomycin D	G or S	VDT
acyclovir	G or S	I
alfentanil	G or S	CI, I
alprostadil	G or S	CI
amikacin	G or S	I
aminophylline	G or S	CI
amiodarone	G	CI, I
amoxycillin	G or S	I
amphotericin	G	CI (protect from light)
ampicillin	G or S	I
amsacrine	G	I
ancrod	S	CI
aprotinin	G or S	CI or VDT
atenolol	G or S	CI
atracurium	G or S	I
azathioprine	G or S	VDT
azlocillin	G or S	I
betamethasone	G or S	CI or VDT
bleomycin	S	I
bromhexine	G or S	CI
bumetanide	G or S	I
calcium gluconate	G or S	CI (not with sodium bicarbonate)
carbenicillin	G	I
carboplatin	G or S	CI
carmustine	G or S	I
cefotaxime	G or S	I
cefoxitin	G or S	I, VDT
cefsulodin	G or S	I, VDT
ceftazidime	G or S	I, VDT
ceftizoxime	G or S	CI, VDT
cefuroxime	G or S	I, VDT
cephaloridine	G or S	I, VDT
cephalothin	G or S	I, VDT
cephamandole	G or S	I, VDT
cephazolin	G or S	I, VDT
cephradine	G or S	CI, I
chloramphenicol	G or S	I, VDT
cimetidine	G or S	CI, I
cisplatin	S	CI
clindamycin	G or S	CI, I

Key. S = sodium choloride 0.9%; G = glucose solution 5%; I = intermittent infusion; VDT = injection via infusion tubing; CI = continuous intravenous infusion; W = water for injections.

Table 22.2 *(cont'd)*

Drug	Infusion fluid	Method of use
clomipramine	G or S	I
clonazepam	G or S	I
cloxacillin	G or S	I, VDT
colistin	G or S	CI, I
co-trimoxazole	G or S	CI
cyclophosphamide	W	I, VDT
cyclosporin	G or S	CI
cytarabine	G or S	CI, I, VDT
dacarbazine	G or S	I
desferrioxamine	G or S	CI, I
dexamethasone	G or S	CI, I, VDT
diazepam	G or S	CI
digoxin	G or S	CI
dinoprost	G or S	CI
disopyramide	G or S	CI, I
dobutamine	G or S	CI (not with sodium bicarbonate)
dopamine	G or S	CI
doxorubicin	G or S	VDT
epirubicin	S	VDT
epoprostenol	S	I
erythromycin	G or S	CI, I
ethacrynic acid	G or S	VDT
etoposide	S	I
flecainide	G or S	CI, I
flucloxacillin	G or S	I, VDT
fluorouracil	G	CI, VDT
folinic acid	G or S	CI
frusemide	S	CI
fusidic acid	G or S	CI
gentamicin	G or S	I, VDT
glyceryl trinitrate	G or S	CI
heparin	G or S	CI
hydralazine	S	CI
hydrocortisone	G or S	CI, I, VDT
ifosfamide	G or S	CI, I, VDT
iron-dextran	G or S	I
isoprenaline	G or S	CI (well diluted)
isosorbide dinitrate	G or S	I
isoxsuprine	G or S	CI
kanamycin	G or S	I
labetalol	G or S	I
latamoxef	G or S	I, VDT
lignocaine	G or S	CI (well diluted)
mecillinam	G or S	I
melphalan	S	CI, VDT
mesna	G or S	CI, VDT
metaraminol	G or S	CI, VDT
methicillin	G or S	I, VDT
methocarbamol	G or S	I
methohexitone	G or S	I

Table 22.2 *(cont'd)*

Drug	Infusion fluid	Method of use
methotrexate	G or S	CI, VDT (well diluted)
methyldopa	G	I
methylprednisolone	G or S	CI, I, VDT
metoclopramide	G or S	I
metronidazole	G or S	I
mexiletine	G or S	CI
mezlocillin	G or S	CI
miconazole	G or S	CI, I
mithramycin	G	I (well diluted)
mustine	G or S	VDT
naloxone	G or S	CI
netilmicin	G or S	I, VDT
noradrenaline	G or S	CI (well diluted)
orciprenaline	G	I
oxpentifylline	G or S	CI
oxytocin	G or S	CI (well diluted)
phenoxybenzamine	S	I
phentolamine	G or S	I
phenylephrine	G or S	I
piperacillin	G or S	I
plicamycin	G	I (well diluted)
polymyxin B	G	CI
potassium chloride	G or S	CI (well diluted)
prednisolone	G or S	CI, VDT
propofol	G or S	VDT
quinine dihydrochloride	S	CI
ranitidine	G or S	I
rifampicin	G or S	VDT
ritodrine	G or S	CI (well diluted)
salbutamol	G or S	CI
sodium nitroprusside	G	CI (well diluted; protect from light)
streptokinase	S	CI
sulphadiazine	S	CI
suxamethonium	G or S	CI
terbutaline	G or S	CI
tetracosactrin	G or S	CI
tetracycline	G or S	CI
thiopentone	S	CI, VDT
thymoxamine	G	CI
ticarcillin	G	I
tinidazole	G or S	I
tobramycin	G or S	I
tocainide	G or S	I
treosulfan	W	VDT
trimethoprim	G or S	VDT
urea	G	CI
urokinase	S	CI
vancomycin	G or S	I
vasopressin	G	I
vecuronium	G or S	I

Table 22.2 *(cont'd)*

Drug	Infusion fluid	Method of use
verapamil	G or S	CI
vidarabine	G or S	CI (well diluted)
vinblastine	S	VDT
vincristine	S	VDT
vindesine	G or S	VDT
zidovudine	G	VDT

Solutions of certain fractions of dextran have some of the physical properties of plasma and are given by slow intravenous injection as temporary plasma substitutes in conditions of severe blood loss. Any blood cross-matching should be carried out *before* commencing the dextran infusion. These fractions are referred to as dextran 70, dextran 40 and the standard solutions contain 6% of the dextran in normal saline or 5% glucose solution.

Dextran solutions are valuable in haemorrhage, traumatic shock, and burns in doses of 500–1000 ml with a total dose in shock of 2000 ml, and up to 3000 ml in severe burns. Care should be taken to avoid overloading the circulation in renal damage or heart failure, and any patient receiving a dextran solution of the first time should be watched in case any signs of anaphylactic reactions occur.

Low molecular weight dextrans

Brand names: Gentran 40 §, Rheomacrodex §

Although the low molecular weight dextrans are eliminated from the circulation more rapidly than the standard dextran solutions, products such as dextran 40 are of value in improving blood flow in cases of intravascular aggregation or 'sludging' of blood cells. The dose range is from 500 ml initially to 1000–2000 ml daily by slow intravenous infusion.

The use of these solutions increases peripheral circulation, improves blood supply to crushed or damaged tissues, and may be of value in other conditions associated with local ischaemia where a decrease in blood viscosity and an improved blood flow is required.

Other blood volume expanders

A modified gelatin preparation, referred to as polygeline

(Haemaccel §) is also used as a plasma substitute in hypovolaemic shock and crush injuries, and occasionally for extracorporeal organ perfusion. It also promotes an osmotic diuresis, and so maintains kidney function. **Gelofusine** is a similar modified gelatin product. Modified starch preparations such as Elohes, Hespan and Pentaspan are also used as blood volume expanders for short-term use. With all these products, the possibility of allergic reactions should be borne in mind.

ENTERAL AND INTRAVENOUS NUTRITION

The stress of severe trauma or infection leads to an increase in body metabolism or catabolism. Energy needs may be increased very considerably in severe conditions, and if the need is not recognized and treated at an early stage, the body starts to draw on tissue stores to provide the necessary energy. The initial use of fat reserves causes few problems, but later the lean muscle protein is broken down and negative nitrogen balance may soon develop. Another important consideration is that the lean body mass contains 98% of the potassium reserves of the body, and any loss of such tissue will cause a loss of potassium.

The aim of treatment is to provide new energy sources such as amino acids and carbohydrates, so that replacement proteins can be built up to maintain the function of essential organs of the body.

Enteral feeding, sometimes referred to as tube-feeding consists of giving low-residue foods by naso-feeding tubes, and is a development of 'space-diets'. The system avoids many of the problems of intravenous feeding, although if necessary they can be given together, so the two systems are complementary. Diarrhoea and electrolyte disturbances are the most common side-effects of enteral feeding, but can be reduced with diluted feeds, or feeds given at a controlled rate by a feeding pump. Representative products are **Albumaid**, **Elemental**, **Clinifeed and Ensure**. It should be remembered that any non-sterile feeds are potential breeding grounds for bacteria, and it is now recommended that both bag and giving set for enteral feeds should be changed after 4–6 hours.

Oral rehydration

The loss of fluid and electrolytes by diarrhoea is a major health problem in some parts of the world. In theory, treatment is simple, but in undeveloped countries may be extremely difficult to apply. The absorption of supplementary electrolytes given orally is increased by the addition of glucose, and several standard formulations of Oral Rehydration Salts (ORS), containing sodium chloride, potassium chloride, sodium citrate and glucose have been devised. Proprietary products of basically similar compositions are represented by **Dextrolyte**, **Diorolyte**, **Electrolade** and **Rehidrat**.

After reconstitution of oral rehydration products with water, any unused solution, if not used within an hour of preparation, should be discarded, unless stored in a refrigerator for use or rejection within 24 hours.

Amino acids

In conditions of severe protein deficiency due to defective absorption, or after abdominal operation, it is sometimes necessary to bypass the digestive system, and to supply nitrogen and calories by the intravenous route. This can be achieved by the administration of solutions of selected amino acids essential for protein synthesis. Glucose may be added to such products as an additional source of calories, and so permit more amino acids to be used for protein synthesis. Some details of certain products are given on page 515 (Table 22.3).

Intravenous fat emulsion

Brand name: Intralipid §

Carbohydrate in the form of glucose is often given intravenously to provide calories, but in severe burns and other conditions a very high caloric intake is required. Fats provide a rich source of calories, and an emulsion of soya bean oil suitable for intravenous drip infusion is frequently used. Nothing should be added to or mixed with intravenous fat emulsion, with the exception of Vitilipid N, a specially formulated vitamin additive product for use with Intralipid.

Central venous feeding

This method of giving nutritional support, also known as Total

Table 22.3 Parenteral nutrients. This table lists some products commonly used in hospitals. More than one solution may be required to give a satisfactory balance of fluid, energy, nitrogen and electrolytes. Vitamin supplements are also needed. Most of the following nutrient solutions of amino acids are expensive, and their value in routine postoperative therapy has been questioned

Solution	Calorie source	Energy (kj/litre)	Nitrogen (g/litre)	Na+	K+	Mg²⁺	Ca²⁻	Acetate	Cl⁻	Other constituents
Aminoplasmal L 10	Amino acids		16.0	48	25	2.5		59	62	Phosphate
Aminoplex 14	Amino acids		13.4	35	30	2.5			79	Phosphate
Glucoplex 1000	Glucose	4200		50	30				67	Zinc
Intralipid 10%	Soya bean oil, egg lecithin and glycerol	4600								phosphate Phosphate
Synthamin 9			9.1	70	60	5		100	70	Phosphate
Vamin 9 Glucose	Glucose	1700	9.4	50	20	1.5	2.5		50	Phosphate

Parenteral Nutrition, or TPN, is a highly complicated one that is only used when conventional methods are inadequate. The solution used contains glucose and fat to provide energy, amino acids which are necessary to optimize protein production, together with electrolytes, vitamins and trace elements. It is given by a surgical technique which requires placement of a catheter in the superior vena cava, with adequate precautions against infection and consequent septicaemia.

The advantage of the method is that much stronger solutions of glucose and essential amino acids can be used, so a patient's total nutritional needs may be given in 2–3.5 litres of solution over 24 hours. If the TPN system is to be used for more than 7 days, the solution must provide all the calories, electrolytes and trace elements necessary for nutrition. If large amounts of glucose are administered it may be necessary to give insulin as well to prevent or control hyperglycaemia. Such insulin injections can be given by a syringe pump device, which permits simple adjustment of dose as indicated by blood-glucose measurements.

In most centres the so-called 'big bag' method is used. The required nutrient fluid is prepared daily in the hospital pharmacy and supplied as a sterile solution in a 3-litre container, together with the giving sets and connectors to the central venous catheter. Only one giving set change is made daily, thus minimizing the risks of contamination. The flow-rate must be carefully controlled, and it is standard practice to use an administration pump or electronic flow controller. Such equipment has sensors and alarms to warn both nurse and patient of problems such as air in the line or varying flow-rates.

Total parenteral nutrition is very much a team effort, as biochemical monitoring is necessary throughout; a high standard of pharmaceutical processing is required, as well as full nursing care. The method however, in spite of the problems, is a practical one, and TPN has been continued in some patients for weeks with regular checking of the serum levels of urea, sodium, potassium and glucose, as well as levels of magnesium and phosphate. With properly formulated solutions, the nutritional requirement can be spread easily and evenly over 24 hours. Utilization of the constituents of the solution appears to be consistent, and leads to an increase in the lean tissue mass. The technique is of wider application, as in addition to its use in severe trauma, it is of considerable value in conditions where complete bowel rest may be required, as for example, in Crohn's disease and severe ulcerative colitis.

A few patients may require TPN permanently and some are now being taught to carry out the necessary procedures at home. It is often possible to give the required level of nutrients over less than 24 hours, thus enabling the patient to lead a more nearly normal life by day, and self-administer the TPN solutions overnight.

Although outside the scope of this book it should be noted that special solutions are available for continuous ambulatory peritoneal dialysis (CAPD). These solutions provide an alternative to haemodialysis for patients with end-stage renal failure. CAPD enables patients to live and be treated at home, and have extended the availability of dialysis to diabetic and elderly patients previously excluded for various reasons, such as infection risks, from haemodialysis.

Most fluids for CAPD contain glucose, which is rapidly absorbed and so reduces the dialysis time, and with extended use may cause metabolic complications including obesity. Icodial is a recently introduced fluid for CAPD based on icodextrin, a glucose polymer obtained from maize starch, and has a longer action than conventional CAPD solutions that permit its overnight use.

23

Drugs used in ophthalmology

The drugs used in ophthalmic work fall into two main groups: (a) those applied locally, and (b) those used systemically. It should be noted that with some drugs used as eye-drops, systemic effects may sometimes occur from absorption of the drug into the circulation. Some eye-drops may damage soft contact lenses, and as a rule no contact lenses of any type should be worn during ophthalmic treatment.

Points about ophthalmic drugs

(a) Atropine may cause acute glaucoma in some elderly patients.
(b) Corticosteroids may cause 'steroid glaucoma' within a few weeks.
(c) Beta-blockers may precipitate asthma in sensitive patients.
(d) Some mydriatics may cause contact dermatitis.
(e) Every care should be taken to avoid contamination of eye-drops.

MYDRIATICS AND CYCLOPLEGICS

Mydriatics are drugs that dilate the pupil and cycloplegics are those that paralyse the accommodation. Some drugs have both effects.

Dilatation of the pupil is necessary for retinoscopy and to immobilize the iris and ciliary muscle, and eye-drops of atropine sulphate are widely employed for this purpose. **Atropine** is the most powerful and persistent of the mydriatics used therapeutically, as the effects may extend over several days. There is always the risk with some older patients that atropine may precipitate an attack of acute closed-angle glaucoma, and the synthetic compound **cyclopentolate** (Mydrilate) is often preferred.

Homatropine is related to atropine, but has a more rapid and less prolonged action, as the mydriatic effect fades after about 24 hours. **Hyoscine** also produces a more rapid mydriatic

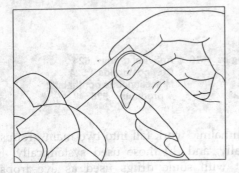

Holding the paper handle, remove the NODS unit taking care not to touch the medicated flag.

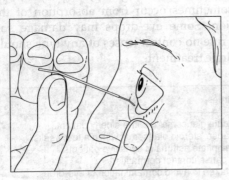

Place the medicated flag in the lower conjunctival sac and release the lower eyelid. Continue holding the paper handle for 2-3 seconds allowing the membrane to dissolve and flag to detach.

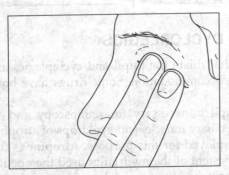

Closing the eye for a few seconds aids the dissolution of the medicated flag. NODS is well tolerated and any sensation of a foreign body will be transient.

Figure 23.1 Use of NODS. (Reproduced by permission of Chauvin Pharmaceuticals.)

response than atropine, with a correspondingly brief duration. Occasionally some patients have, or develop, a sensitivity to atropine and associated alkaloids, and in such cases a synthetic drug such as **lachesine** may be used.

Occasionally a drug is required, particularly in examination of the fundus, that has the mydriatic but not the cycloplegic effects of atropine, and so will dilate the pupil without paralysing the accommodation. **Phenylephrine** is often used in this way, in strengths ranging from 1 to 10%.

When a drug with a rapid action is preferred, **cyclopentolate** (Mydrilate, 0.5–1%), or **Tropicamide** (Mydriacyl 0.5–1%) may be used.

A highly interesting new method of using tropicamide is represented by the sterile single-dose NODS (*n*ovel *o*phthalmic *d*elivery *s*ystem) device. Each individual unit contains 125 micrograms of tropicamide in a water-soluble polyvinyl alcohol flag attached by a membrane to a paper handle. In use, the flag is touched on the surface of the lower conjunctival sac after drawing down the eyelid. On contact, the flag becomes detached from the membrane and dissolves with the release of the drug. It is claimed that the system permits greater ocular penetration and response, and that one unit will produce mydriasis and cycloplegia similar to that obtained by one drop of tropicamide 1% solution.

MIOTICS

Miotics are drugs that cause the pupil to contract, and they are widely employed in the treatment of simple glaucoma, which is an insidious disease of the elderly, characterized by an increased intraocular pressure. Such pressure, if high and sustained, causes damage at the junction of the optic nerve and retina, leading to blindness if untreated (Fig. 23.2). The contraction of the pupil facilitates drainage of the anterior chamber into Schlemm's canal, and so relieves the intraocular pressure, which is basically due to a reduction in the normal outflow of the aqueous humour as the inflow largely remains constant.

Physostigmine (eserine) as a 0.5% solution, was once widely used as a miotic as the effects are rapid and sustained for about 12 hours, but is now less popular. **Pilocarpine nitrate** (1%) has a similar but less prolonged action. **Ecothiopate iodide** (0.25–0.3%)

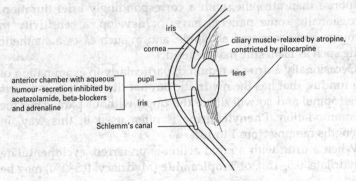

Figure 23.2 Diagram of eye with points of action of drugs in glaucoma.

(Phospholine iodide) has a more powerful and prolonged action, as one drop daily in the eye may be sufficient to produce an adequate lowering of intraocular pressure. As cataract formation is a side-effect, it is now available only on a named-patient basis.

Another method of using pilocarpine is represented by the long-acting device **Ocusert Pilo**, which has a central reservoir of pilocarpine contained in a slow-release form. In use, the device is placed in the conjunctival sac, and replaced with a new unit a week later. Care in positioning the unit is essential.

The beta-blockers are also used locally in the treatment of simple chronic glaucoma. They act by reducing the rate of formation of the aqueous humour, and are used as eye-drops twice a day. They include betaxolol 0.5% (Betoptic §), carteolol 1% (Teoptic §), metipranolol 0.1% and timolol 0.25% (Timoptol §) and Glaucol § 0.25% and 0.5%. Levobunolol 0.5% (Betagan §) has a longer action, and once-a-day use is often adequate to maintain a decrease in the intraocular pressure. Some systemic absorption may occur when beta-blockers are used as eye-drops, and the Committee on Safety of Medicines has advised that such drugs, even those said to be cardioselective, should not be used for patients with asthma or a history of obstructive airway disease unless no other treatment is available. If so used, the risk of drug-induced bronchospasm should be borne in mind.

Adrenaline also reduces intraocular tension, both by decreasing the production of aqueous humour and promoting its outflow, but standard solutions are too irritating for local use. Less irritant products containing adrenaline 1% are Eppy § and Simplene §.

Dipivefrine (Propine 0.1% §) is a pro-drug which passes readily into the chamber, and is converted to adrenaline. It is useful in some cases of intolerance to adrenaline solutions. Adrenaline eye-drops are contraindicated in closed-angle glaucoma as they have a mydriatic action.

Guanethidine, used in hypertension, also has applications in the treatment of glaucoma. As eye-drops (5%) it reduces intraocular pressure both by increasing the outflow of the aqueous humour and decreasing its formation. Ganda § is a mixed product containing guanethidine 1% and adrenaline 0.2%. The prolonged use of guanethidine may cause conjunctival fibrosis, and eye examinations should be made every 6 months.

A reduction in intraocular pressure can be obtained by the oral administration of a few drugs. Acetazolamide (Diamox §) reduces the amount of bicarbonate in the aqueous humour by inhibiting the enzyme carbonic anhydrase. It is given in doses of 250 mg two to four times a day. Acetazolamide is also given by intravenous injection in doses of 250–500 mg in the pre-operative treatment of closed-angle glaucoma. Dichlorphenamide (Daranide §) has similar actions and uses in oral doses of 100 mg twice daily.

Side-effects of both drugs, particularly in the elderly, include paraesthesia, hypokalaemia and drowsiness. Some drugs used as eye-drops are available as single-use pre-sterilized products referred to as Minims.

ANAESTHETICS

Cocaine once held a premier place as a local anaesthetic in ophthalmology, as it is very effective, and has the advantages of causing dilatation of the pupil and blanching of the conjunctiva. It is usually employed as a 2% solution, often in association with homatropine. The marked anaesthetic and vasoconstriction action of cocaine is not always necessary, and **oxybuprocaine** (Benoxinate 0.4%), **lignocaine** 2–4% and **amethocaine** 1% are often preferred. **Proxymetacaine** (Ophthaine 0.5%) is useful in children as it causes less initial stinging. In all cases, due protection should be given to the anaesthetized eye to avoid any trauma.

ANTIBACTERIAL DRUGS

Some antibiotics, particularly those seldom used systemically, are of value in ophthalmic infections. Chloramphenicol is used as eye-drops (0.5%) and ointment (1%), and other antibiotics with a wide range of activity include neomycin drops 0.5% and framycetin 0.5% (Soframycin). Gentamicin 0.3% (Cidomycin, Garamycin, Genticin) and tobramycin 0.3% (Tobralex) are effective against *Pseudomonas aeruginosa*. Propamidine 0.1% (Brolene) and fusidic acid 1% (Fusithalmic) are used in staphylococcal conjunctivitis. Tetracycline is also used locally as eye-drops and ointment 1%, and is effective in the prolonged mass treatment of trachoma. Ofloxacin 0.3% (Exocin) and ciprofloxacin 0.3% (Ciloxan) are used in external ocular infections such as conjunctivitis.

ANTIVIRAL DRUGS

Idoxuridine §

Brand name: Idoxene §

The virus of herpes may attack the eye, at first causing a superficial punctate keratitis, characterized by minute white plaques on the cornea. In severe cases the erosions coalesce to form a dendritic ulcer, and the specific treatment is the use of the antiviral drug idoxuridine.

Thymidine appears to be an essential metabolite for the virus, and idoxuridine, sometimes referred to as IDU, resembles thymidine in chemical structure, and by replacing thymidine in the metabolic process, can prevent development of the virus. The drug is effective only by local application, and hourly use as eye-drops (0.1% solution) or 0.5% ointment for application to the eye every 4 hours is essential to achieve the necessary high local concentration.

Acyclovir (Zovirax) is a pro-drug that is activated after penetration into herpes-virus infected cells (p. 159). It is used as a 3% ointment in the treatment of herpes simplex infections, and should be continued for at least 3 days after complete healing has occurred.

CORTICOSTEROIDS

Corticosteroids are used in ophthalmological practice in the treatment of a number of non-infective inflammatory conditions such as keratitis, uveitis and spring catarrh. For local use **hydrocortisone** as drops or ointment (1%) or **prednisolone** (Predsol 0.5%) or **dexamethasone** (Maxidex) 0.1% or **fluorometholone** (FML) 0.1% and betamethasone (Betnesol 0.1%) are satisfactory, but frequent use of the drops is necessary.

The local use of steroids requires care and they should not be used in herpetic or dendritic ulcers or undiagnosed 'red eye' as such inflammation may be linked with the herpes simplex virus. It should be noted that in some patients, a rise in intra-ocular pressure and the development of a 'steroid glaucoma' with irreversible damage may follow the prolonged use of corticosteroid eye-drops.

Sodium cromoglycate also has an anti-inflammatory action in allergic conjunctivitis when used as eye-drops (Opticrom).

Lodoxamide (Alomide) is a mast-cell stabilizer of the cromoglycate type. It has some anti-inflammatory properties, and is of value in allergic conjunctivitis as eye-drops 0.1% to be used four times a day.

MISCELLANEOUS OPHTHLAMIC PRODUCTS

Acetylcholine (Miochol 1% §) is used in cataract surgery when rapid miosis is required; chymotrypsin (Zonlulysin 300 units §) is used during intracapsular cataract extraction, diclofenac (Voltarol Ophta 0.1% §) and flurbiprofen (Ocufen 0.03% §) are useful when the inhibition of intra-operative miosis is required during cataract surgery. **Apraclonidine** (Iopidine 1% ▼§) is used to prevent the postoperative rise of intraocular pressure that may occur after laser ophthalmic surgery. It is given as one drop of the solution 1 hour before laser treatment and one drop immediately postoperatively.

Reduced tear production resulting in chronic soreness of the eyes may occur, often in rheumatoid arthritis, and products for tear deficiency include eye-drops of acetylcysteine 5%, hydroxycellulose 0.44%, hypromellose 0.5% and polyvinyl alcohol 1.4%.

Lime burns

Lime (calcium oxide) has caustic properties, and as it is used in the building trade, lime burns of the eye are not uncommon. Immediate irrigation is essential, but if lime particles are still present, they can be dissolved by trisodium edetate solution 0.4%. **Trisodium edetate** (Limclair) is a chelating agent, and dissolves metallic salts and removes them from the tissues as a soluble complex. In lime burns, the eye is first anaesthetized and the solution of trisodium edetate is then dropped on the denuded surface. Opacities due to calcium deposits soon dissolve.

Corneal staining

It is occasionally necessary to determine the nature and extent of damage to the corneal epithelium, and this can be done by staining with **fluorescein** solution (2%). Fluorescein is a yellow dye, and any areas of the cornea that have become denuded of epithelium by abrasions or ulcers, even if quite invisible to the naked eye, take up the dye, and are stained green. The undamaged epithelium remains unstained. **Bengal rose** solution (1%) may also be used as the dye stains damaged and devitalized cells a red colour.

Fluorescein has been given by intravenous injection as a 5% solution to facilitate examination of the retinal vessels. Such use is not without risk, as sudden collapse has occurred after intravenous fluorescein, and resuscitation facilities should be available.

Eye-drops and sterility

Infections of the eye are always potentially serious, particularly when due to *Pseudomonas aeruginosa*. As a precautionary measure, eye-drops are supplied as sterile solutions, but the possibility of subsequent contamination during use remains an ever-present risk. It has been recommended that eye-drop bottles should not be supplied complete with dropper, and that a separate sterile disposable dropper should be used for each application of the drops, particularly when the eye has been damaged.

As an extension of this safety measure, pre-filled single-use eye-droppers are available exemplified by the Opulet and Minims products. The range of drugs available in these special droppers is still limited, but the Ocusert and NODS devices indicate other advances in the presentation of ophthalmic drugs.

Ocular reactions to drugs

It should be noted that certain drugs can cause adverse ocular reactions. **Neomycin** and **framycetin** may cause a drug-induced conjunctivitis, as may atropine. Eye ointments generally tend to cause more irritation than eye-drops, and the prolonged use of ointments in conditions such as chronic blepharitis, should be avoided. **Chlorpromazine** and some related drugs may bring about a slate-blue discolouration of the eye lids, and the conjunctiva may develop a golden-brown pigmentation. Associated deposits of melanin in the cornea may cause blurred vision. **Chloroquine** in full doses has been known to result in corneal opacity and pigmentation, but such reactions are usually reversible when treatment is stopped. Retinopathy, on the other hand, although uncommon, is progressive and correspondingly serious.

Occasionally, deposits of a dark pigment (adrenochrome) may occur following the use of **adrenaline** drops in glaucoma. The use of local corticosteroids in dendritic ulcers may permit the spread of such ulcers. These steroids can increase intraocular pressure, particularly in patients with chronic open angle glaucoma. They may also cause lens opacity. Opacities may also follow the prolonged use of long-acting anticholinesterase drugs such as **phospholine iodide**. Visual disturbances have followed the use of **nalidixic acid**.

24

Drugs used in some skin disorders

The skin is that extensive organ that protects the body from its environment, but it is very far from being an inert barrier. It plays an important part in controlling the fluid balance of the body, and as it is subjected to internal and external stress, and is also influenced by many emotional factors, it is not surprising that the cause of some skin conditions is difficult to diagnose. The increasing sophistication of the environment, from clothing to cosmetics, may on occasion cause a baffling dermatitis, which clears readily when the offending substance is traced (which may be a very difficult process), so that further contact can be avoided.

Other conditions may be more easy to diagnose but no less difficult to treat, and therapy may be complicated by the fact that the base in which an active drug is incorporated may also play an important part in treatment, so before considering drugs, a brief survey of some dermatological formulations may be useful.

Dermatological product forms

Ointments are a common form of skin medication, and two main types may be distinguished, the greasy ointments containing soft paraffin, which tend to retain skin moisture and are useful in dry lesions, and the non-greasy ointments that contain emulsifying waxes as in Emulsifying Ointment, often used as vehicles for locally-acting drugs.

Pastes are stiff ointments containing a high proportion of zinc oxide and starch in a soft paraffin base. They are used as protective applications, mainly to limited areas, such as those occurring in psoriasis and chronic eczema, but they may also be used more extensively on inflamed and excoriated areas. Pastes should be applied thickly and liberally, and additional applications should be made without attempting to remove paste previously applied.

Creams are soft, water-containing products prepared either from an emulsifying wax, as Aqueous Cream, or from a lanolin or wool alcohol base, as Oily Cream. They are of value in cooling, softening and humidifying the skin, but it is worth noting that on occasion, lanolin-containing products can themselves cause a skin reaction.

Lotions are aqueous solutions or suspensions of locally-acting drugs, often used as wet dressings.

ANTIBIOTICS

Antibiotics are occasionally useful in skin infections where the causative organism is susceptible, but ideally, an antibiotic used topically should be one that is not used systemically, in order to reduce the risk of antibiotic resistance. Such resistance would restrict systemic therapy should it be required later.

Neomycin and the closely related **framycetin** (Soframycin) is too toxic for systemic use, but it has a wide range of activity and is present in some products for topical use in superficial bacterial infections such as impetigo, sycosis barbae and burns. It may cause sensitization, so prolonged local application should be avoided.

Gentamicin is also present in some creams and ointments, and with the above warning in mind, may be useful in local infections due to *Pseudomonas* and related organisms. **Fusidic acid** (Fucidin) is of value in staphylococcal skin infections, and **chlortetracycline** is sometimes used locally in the treatment of impetigo.

Mupirocin is an antibiotic unrelated to any others in current use, and is effective against a wide range of pathogens associated with skin infections. It is used as **Bactroban** §, an ointment containing 2% of mupirocin in a water-miscible base. It should not be used continuously for more than 10 days. Bactroban Nasal is used for the elimination of the nasal carriage of staphylococci.

Antiseptics

Very many antiseptic preparations are available for local use, intended for the prevention of sepsis and the treatment of wounds and burns. Time-honoured preparations such as Eusol, a solution of sodium hypochlorite, are still in use, and **iodine** has recovered part of its former popularity by presentation as **povidone-iodine** (Betadine), a slow-release form of iodine free from the disadvantages of older preparations.

Cetrimide is a mild antiseptic with some detergent properties but **chlorhexidine** is more effective and is used in the Hibitane–Savlon series of products for pre-operative preparation and prevention of sepsis generally. **Chloroxylenol** (Dettol) represents an older type of phenolic antiseptic with a more limited range of antibacterial activity.

Antifungal agents

Many antifungal preparations are available for the local treatment of fungal infections of the skin and nails such as candidiasis and some forms of ringworm (tinia). They vary from time-honoured drugs such as benzoic and salicylic acid (present in Whitfield's Ointment) to antibiotics represented by natamycin and nystatin, organic compounds such as the imidazoles, and metallic salts such as zinc undecenoate. They may be used as ointments, creams, lotions, sprays, paints or dusting powders. They are too numerous to refer to individually, but Table 24.1 indicates the range available. The use of griseofulvin and terbinafine orally in the treatment of ringworm of the skin and nails is referred to in Chapter 5, together with other antifungal agents that are taken orally for either systemic or superficial fungal infections.

CORTICOSTEROIDS

Corticosteroids are widely used in many inflamed skin conditions because of their powerful suppressive action on the inflammatory processes, but if used as the sole treatment, the condition may return when therapy is discontinued. They have no antibacterial properties, and should be used primarily for symptomatic relief, whilst the underlying cause of the inflammation is being treated by other means, i.e. by a systemic antibiotic if the cause is bacterial in origin. In addition, there is the risk that a locally applied corticosteroid may be absorbed in sufficient amounts to have undesirable systemic effects by distur-

Table 24.1 Antifungal preparations

Approved name (of main constituent)	Brand name
amorolfine▼	Loceryl
amphotericin	Fungilin
clotrimazole	Canestan, Masnoderm
econazole	Ecostatin, Pevaryl
ketoconazole	Nizoral
metronidazole	Metrogel
miconazole	Daktarin, Dermonistat
natamycin	Pimafucin
nystatin	Nystan
sulconazole	Exelderm
terbinafine	Lamisil
tioconazole	Trosyl
tolnaftate	Timoped
zinc undecenoate	Mycota, Tineafax

bance of the adrenal–pituitary balance, a risk that is increased if an occlusive dressing is used.

Local treatment with a corticosteroid should be with a weak drug in the lowest effective concentration, especially when treatment is likely to be prolonged. In severe conditions however, it may be necessary to initiate treatment with a potent product, but a change to a weaker preparation should be made as soon as possible.

Table 24.2 gives a general indication of the relative potency of some available products, but it does not include mixed products containing antibiotics. It should be noted that in preparations for local use, a derivative of the systemically active form of the corticosteroid may be used, as some derivatives have a more powerful local action. Hydrocortisone for example, is considered to have a 'low' local activity whereas hydrocortisone butyrate (**Locoid**) is regarded as 'potent'.

In order to keep Table 24.2 simple, only the name of the basic drug is given. The local activity may sometimes be increased by auxiliary substances such as urea. Urea is considered to increase skin penetration, and hydrocortisone with urea is placed in the 'medium' potency group. Topical corticosteroids are mainly used in severe eczema, psoriasis, resistant dermatoses and neurodermatoses, and are also of value in other inflammatory skin conditions. They are also useful in the control of allergic contact dermatitis, which may be due to one of several environmental factors, of which nickel, chromium and rubber additives are

Table 24.2   Corticosteroids for local use

Approved name	Strength	Brand name	Potency
hydrocortisone	1%	Efcortelan (and many others)	Low
alclometasone	0.05%	Modrasone	
methylprednisolone	0.25%	Neo-Medrone	
clobetasone[a]	0.05%	Eumovate	Medium
fluocortolone	0.1%	Ultradil	
flurandrenolone	0.0125%	Haelan	
hydrocortisone	1% + urea	Alphaderm; Calmurid HC	
beclomethasone[a]	0.025%	Propaderm	Potent
betamethasone[a]	0.1%	Betnovate	
budesonide	0.025%	Preferid	
desonide	0.05%	Tridesilon	
desoxymethasone	0.25%	Stiedex	
diflucortolone[a]	0.1%	Nerisone	
fluclorolone	0.025%	Topilar	
fluocinolone[a]	0.025%	Synalar	
fluocinonide[a]	0.05%	Metosyn	
fluticasone▼	0.05%	Cutivate▼	
hydrocortisone[a]	0.1%	Locoid	
triamcinolone[a]	0.1%	Adcortyl; Ledercort	
clobetasol[a]	0.05%	Dermovate	
diflucortolone[a]	0.3%	Nerisone Forte	
halcinonide	0.1%	Halciderm	

[a]Indicates those preparations containing a derivative with increased local activity.

common examples. As they act by controlling local inflammation, any local infection that may be present remains unchecked, and may spread unless suitably treated.

Side-effects include acne, thinning of the skin, mild depigmentation and increased hair growth.

ACNE

Acne is characterized by increased activity of the sebaceous glands and their blocking with sebum plugs and the presence of *Propionibacterium acnes*. Initial treatment is usually with peeling agents that remove superficial ketarinized cells and preparations of sulphur and salicylic acid and resorcin represent the traditional approach to the problem. **Benzoyl peroxide** is an antibacterial agent used in a wide range of proprietary products often as a 10% cream or lotion, but the response to treatment is slow. Azelaic acid § (Skinoren §▼) has a bacteriostatic action on

Propionibacterium acnes and *Staphylococcus epidermidis,* which are often present in sebum plugs. It is used as a 20% cream in mild to moderate acne applied to the skin once or twice a day, but prolonged action up to a maximum of 6 months may be required. A prolonged course of **tetracycline** therapy is often given in refractory acne. A different type of product is Dianette, which contains **cyproterone** and **ethinyloestradiol**. It is essentially an anti-androgen product, intended for use in females with severe acne refractory to prolonged treatment with tetracycline or other antibiotic.

A different approach is the use of **tretinoin** (Retin-A). Tretinoin is a derivative of vitamin A, and appears to promote the formation of a less cohesive epidermal layer as well as reducing the production of sebum. When applied to the affected skin as a cream, gel or lotion (0.025–0.05%) it produces an erythematous reaction similar to sunburn, with eventual peeling. Response to treatment is slow, and initially there may be an exacerbation of the localized mild inflammation.

Isotretinoin § (Roaccutane §) is a related but much more powerful drug used orally in doses of 500 micrograms/kg daily with food for 4 weeks, later adjusted according to response. Treatment should be continued for not more than 13 weeks, and repeated courses of isotretinoin therapy are not recommended. It is 'last-resort' treatment, and should be used only when all other drugs have failed to relieve the condition, and even then only under careful control. An exacerbation of symptoms may occur after a few weeks, but tends to subside as the treatment is continued.

Side-effects are numerous and often dose-related, and include dry lips, nose bleeding, visual disturbances and transient hair loss. It may cause liver disturbances, and both liver function and plasma lipid levels should be checked monthly. Isotretinoin is contraindicated in pregnancy and in renal and hepatic impairment. In less severe acne, isotretinoin can be used as a 0.05% gel (Isotrex), applied sparingly once or twice a day for 6–8 weeks. The gel should not be used near the eyes, mouth, mucous membranes or damaged or sunburnt skin, and exposure to ultraviolet light should be avoided.

Brasivol contains particles of aluminium oxide in a detergent base. It is an abrasive agent designed to remove the superficial keratin layer mechanically. **Zineryt** is an erythromycin–zinc acetate complex for the local treatment of acne vulgaris.

Points about acne treatment

Aims of treatment are to prevent scarring, reduce duration and limit psychological stress. Response to treatment is often slow, and co-operation of the patient with the treatment is necessary.

Mild acne
Benzoyl peroxide preparations (2.5–5%), apply once daily
Azaleic acid cream (20%) ⎫
Clindamycin lotion (1%) ⎪
Erythromycin solution (2%) ⎬ apply once or twice daily
Tetracycline solution (2%) ⎪
Tretinoin cream (0.025%) ⎭

Moderate acne
Local preparations as above
Oral treatment with
   doxycycline 50 mg once a day
   erythromycin 250 mg ⎫
   tetracycline 250 mg ⎬ three times a day

Severe acne
Hign-dose antibiotics
   cyproterone 2 mg with ethinyloestradiol 35 micrograms
   isotretinoin 500 micrograms/kg–1 mg/kg daily

Metronidazole is used as a 0.075% gel in acute acne rosacae, a chronic form of acne in adults that is characterized by telangiectasia, particularly of the nose.

PRURITUS

No specific treatment for this distressing itching condition has yet been found. The impulses that pass along nerve fibres to be experienced as itching pass along the same nerves as those that transmit pain sensation, yet analgesics are of little value, and morphine may even cause pruritus, possibly by releasing histamine. Once pruritus occurs, the itching may lead to scratching with temporary relief that may eventually make the condition worse.

Soothing lotions such as Calamine Lotion have some little value, and **crotamiton** (Eurax) is claimed to have some specific effect. The itch appears to be associated in some way with histamine release, as the antihistamines have some value in urticarial conditions, but the local applications of antihistamine creams is not recommended as they may themselves cause skin sensitization.

Trimeprazine (Vallergan) taken orally in doses up to 100 mg daily often gives relief in pruritic conditions, and its sedative effect may also be of value. **Cholestyramine** is sometimes of value in the severe pruritus associated with jaundice. In children, peri-anal itching at night may be due to threadworm.

PSORIASIS

Psoriasis is a chronic inflammatory skin disease which may affect 1–2% or more of the population. The condition is basically due to an excessive formation of epidermal cells. The normal turnover rate of such cells is about 28 days, but in psoriasis new cells may be formed every few days. Psoriasis is characterized by a rough thickening of the skin, and the most common form is plaque psoriasis with well defined patches, often on the elbows and knees. In guttate psoriasis, which occurs mainly in children, numerous very small patches appear over a wide area. The cause is unknown, and treatment is suppressive, not curative, and remissions and relapses may occur unexpectedly. Psoriasis may also be triggered off by certain drugs such as NSAIDs, chloroquine and lithium. For the treatment of mild psoriasis emollient preparations may be useful, and topical anti-inflammatory corticosteroids are of value in the short-term control of small lesions, but in more severe psoriasis, dithranol is often the first treatment. In the hospital control of severe, refractory or extensive psoriasis, methotrexate and cyclosporin have been used, but new treatments include acetretin, a vitamin A derivative, and the vitamin D analogue calcipotriol. Traditionally some coal tar products have been used, but the response is often poor and disappointing, and patient compliance with tar treatment is often inadequate.

Acitretin §▼ (dose: 25–50 mg daily)

Brand name: Neotigason §▼

Acitretin is a derivative of vitamin A with a marked action on keratinizing epithelial cells. It is used in severe and extensive psoriasis resistant to other treatment, but it is a powerful drug for use only under expert supervision. It is teratogenic even in therapeutic doses, and that action must be considered carefully before acitretin is given to a female patient of child-bearing age, and such patients should avoid pregnancy for at least 2 years after such therapy. Acitretin is given in oral doses of 25 mg daily, subsequently adjusted according to response up to 50 mg daily. The drug has many **side-effects**, and specialist literature should be consulted for details.

Lassus A et al 1987 Treatment of severe psoriasis with etretin (acitretin). British Journal of Dermatology 117: 333–341

Calcipotriol §

Brand name: Dovonex §

Calcipotriol is a vitamin D derivative and represents a different approach to the treatment of psoriasis. Human keratinocytes have vitamin D receptors, and some vitamin D derivatives are known to decrease the proliferation of such cells. Calcipotriol has a similar action with the advantage of having reduced hypercalcaemic effects, and it is now widely used for topical application as a cream or ointment containing 0.005% of the drug. It is used mainly in mild to moderate plaque psoriasis, including extensive lesions, and the cream or ointment should be applied to the affected areas twice daily up to a maximum weekly use of 100 g, but for no longer than 6 weeks. Calcipotriol has few **side-effects**, although some local irritation may occur and any elevation of the serum calcium level, which is uncommon with standard therapy, subsides rapidly when treatment is discontinued.

Hutchison P, Berth-Jones J 1991 Calcipotriol: a better treatment for psoriasis? Prescriber 5: 21–22

Cyclosporin § (dose: 2.5–5 mg/kg daily)

Brand name: Sandimmun §

Cyclosporin is an immunosuppressant (p. 560) and on the basis that psoriasis is due to some immunological abnormality, it is used orally in the short-term treatment of severe psoriasis resistant to conventional therapy. Cyclosporin is given initially in doses of 1.25 mg/kg twice daily, increased if the response is good to a maximum dose of 5 mg/kg daily. The treatment period should not exceed 8 weeks. The mode of action of cyclosporin is not clear, but it may inhibit the excessive production of epithelial cells by suppressing T lymphocyte activity in the epidermis. Cyclosporin should be used under expert supervision, as it has many side-effects, and for details specialist literature should be consulted.

Dithranol

Dithranol is a synthetic drug used solely for the treatment of psoriasis as it has some peripheral cytotoxic action. It has some local irritant properties, and may cause a burning sensation when applied to the skin. As some patients are exceptionally sensitive to dithranol, a preliminary test for sensitivity should be carried out on a small area of the skin with a low-strength preparation (0.1%) to assess tolerance. Dithranol is often used as a Dithranol Paste (dithranol 0.1% in Zinc and Salicylic acid Paste), and the strength of dithranol is slowly increased up to 1% according to response.

In the past, the paste was applied to the psoriatic lesion daily, but more reliance is now placed on short-term contact, in which a 0.5% preparation is applied to the lesion for 15 minutes. The dithranol preparation is then washed off in an emollient bath. The application is repeated daily, but the exposure time is increased by 15 minutes each day, up to a maximum exposure time, if tolerated, of 1 hour daily. The concentration of dithranol in the application is then increased to 1%, but the exposure time is reduced to 15 minutes, and gradually increased as before. If irritation or burning occurs, treatment should be suspended for 48 hours, and recommenced with a lower strength preparation. In some cases, a dithranol strength of up to 5% may be tolerated. Dithranol paste is sometimes used after a slight erythema has been produced by previous exposure to ultraviolet radiation (Ingram's method).

Care must be taken to apply dithranol preparations to the psoriatic lesions only, as normal skin is highly susceptible to irritation by the drug, and concentrations as low as 0.05% can cause erythema, especially on fair skin. Patients should be warned to wash the hands thoroughly after using a dithranol preparation, to avoid any eye contact, and advised that dithranol can stain clothing and other fabrics. Some proprietary preparations of dithranol, represented by Anthranol, may cause less staining than the standard dithranol paste. Exolan contains dithranol triacetate, and has similar properties and uses.

Cade oil

Cade oil is obtained by the destructive distillation of the branches of juniper. It is a time-honoured treatment for psoriasis and survives as a constituent of some proprietary remedies.

Coal tar

Crude coal tar has long been used in the treatment of psoriasis, especially for patients unable to tolerate dithranol. It is used as Zinc and Coal Tar Paste, or as ointments containing 10–20% of coal tar, but such preparations may be cosmetically unacceptable to some patients. Some proprietary products, containing coal tar extracts are less objectionable, but may be less effective. An alcoholic solution of coal tar is present in some shampoo products for the treatment of psoriasis of the scalp. Coal Tar has some sensitizing properties, so small amounts of a low-strength product should be used initially to assess the response. Official preparations include Calamine and Coal Tar Ointment and Coal Tar and Salicylic Acid Ointment.

Methotrexate § (dose: 10–25 mg weekly)

Brand name: Matrex §

Methotrexate is a cytotoxic agent (p. 284) that is occasionally used in severe psoriasis not responding to other treatment. It is given orally in doses of 10–25 mg once weekly according to response, but it has many and severe side-effects, and should be used only under specialist supervision. Blood counts are essential during methotrexate treatment, as suppression of haemopoiesis may occur without warning even after low doses. Liver function tests must also be carried out. Pulmonary toxicity may occur in rheumatoid arthritis, and methotrexate toxicity generally may be increased by aspirin or any other NSAID.

Methoxsalen

Methoxsalen is a photosensitizer that markedly increases skin reactions to long-wave ultraviolet light, leading to bonding of the drug with DNA, and to the inhibition of cell division. It has been given in a dose of 10–30 mg in PUVL (psoralen–ultraviolet light) in vitiligo and very resistant psoriasis under expert supervision. The skin and eyes must be protected from sunlight during methoxsalen treatment.

SOME OTHER DERMATOLOGICAL PRODUCTS

Aluminium acetate

Weak solutions of aluminium acetate have mild astringent and anti-inflammatory properties, and are used in dermatitis and suppurating wounds. Strong solutions (10–20%) are used in hyperhydrosis as antiperspirants but such strong solutions can be irritant.

Benzoyl peroxide

Benzoyl peroxide is an antiseptic and keratolytic agent, often used with sulphur and other substances in the treatment of acne.

Calamine

Calamine is a pink form of zinc carbonate, and has long been employed in association with zinc oxide as Calamine Lotion. It has a mildly astringent action on the skin, and is widely employed for the temporary relief of various forms of dermatitis. The lotion is also useful in the relief of sunburn.

Dimethicone

Dimethicone is a water repellent silicone product, and is used in a wide range of barrier cream preparations as a protective against skin irritants, for the prevention of bed sores and napkin rash, and colostomy discharge. **Siopel** represents one of the proprietary products containing dimethicone now available.

Formaldehyde and glutaraldehyde

These related compounds are used mainly as sterilizing agents, but they also have applications in the treatment of warts. **Formaldehyde** is used for plantar warts as a 3% solution or as a gel presentation (Veracur). **Glutaraldehyde** is applied as a 10% solution (Glutarol) or a gel form as Verucasep. These preparations are not suitable for the treatment of facial warts.

Gamolenic acid

Brand names: Epogam §, Efamast §

Gamolenic acid, which is present in evening primrose oil, is a prostaglandin precursor. It is used in the treatment of atophic eczema in doses of 160–240 mg twice a day; half doses are given for children. It is also given in doses of 120–160 mg twice daily for the treatment of mastalgia associated with disturbances of fatty acid metabolism. Its lack of anti-oestrogenic properties is of value in the treatment of young women.

Ichthammol

Ichthammol is a thick black liquid with mild tar-like properties. It has a traditional reputation as a mild antiseptic and skin stimulant, and is present in many products for the treatment of mild chronic eczematous conditions.

Minoxidil

Minoxidil has been found to have some stimulant effect on hair growth, and is used for the treatment of male pattern baldness (*alopecia androgenetica*). It is supplied as 2% solution (Regaine) of which 1 ml should be applied to the affected areas of the scalp twice daily. A spray applicator is also available. Extended treatment is usually necessary, but treatment should be discontinued if there is no response after 1 year. Local itching is an occasional side-effect. Potential systemic effects are possible from the nature of the drug (p. 213).

Podophyllum

An irritant plant resin with some antimitotic properties. When dissolved in Compound Benzoin Tincture, it is used as a paint

(15%) for the treatment of ano-genital and plantar warts. It is strongly irritant to normal skin and mucous membranes and should be washed off after 6 hours. Podophyllotoxin, the active principle, is available as a less irritant 0.5% solution (Condyline, Warticon) for the treatment of penile warts.

Resorcin

Also known as resorcinol, resorcin has exfoliative and keratolytic properties, and is a constituent of many preparations used as mild peeling agents in the treatment of acne.

Salicylic acid

Salicylic acid has a long established reputation as a mild keratolytic agent for softening and removing the horny layers of the skin. As Salicylic Acid Lotion or Ointment (2%) it is also used in various eczematous and psoriatic conditions, and is present in many preparations used for acne. Strong ointments and plasters are used to facilitate the reduction in size or removal of corns.

Selenium sulphide

Brand name: Selsun

This compound is used almost exclusively for the treatment of dandruff and seborrhoeic dermatitis of the scalp. It is available as a 2.5% suspension, and 5–10 ml are used as a shampoo, with a time of application of about 5 minutes. After thorough rinsing of the hair, further applications can be made at weekly or twice-weekly intervals according to the response.

Sulphur

Sulphur, like resorcin, has mild antiseptic and peeling properties. The two drugs are often employed together for the treatment of acne as Compound Sulphur Lotion.

Titanium dioxide

Titanium dioxide is similar in many respects to zinc oxide, and is used for the treatment of various exudative skin conditions and in pruritus, often as Titanium Dioxide Paste.

Zinc oxide

Zinc oxide is a heavy, white powder, widely used in dermatology as zinc cream, ointment and paste, and also as calamine lotion. It has a soothing and protective action in eczema and many other excoriated skin conditions.

Zinc sulphate

Zinc sulphate solution (1%) is sometimes used as an astringent application for indolent ulcers, and to assist granulation and wound healing. It is of interest that zinc sulphate has been given orally in doses of 220 mg for the same purpose, apparently with some success.

SKIN PARASITICIDES

Scabies is caused by the mite *Sarcoptes scabiei*. The female parasites burrow in the skin and the characteristic itch is thought to be due to hypersensitivity to the mites. The infection is easily transmitted by hand to hand contact, and an entire household may be infected very rapidly. The head is rarely infected, but the itch may persist long after the parasites have been eliminated. Pediculosis is caused by the head louse *Pediculus humanus capitis*, the body louse *Pediculus humanus corporis*, or the crab louse *Phthirius pubis*. The following drugs are in use but resistance has been noted in recent years, and it is now recommended that different parasiticides should be used in rotation to obtain the optimum response.

Benzyl benzoate

Benzyl benzoate is used mainly for scabies as a 25% emulsion applied to the entire body except the scalp. The application is repeated the following day, and removed a day later by washing. All members of the household should be treated. For pediculosis, the application should be made to the affected areas, and repeated as necessary. The application may be irritant, and should be diluted before use for children.

Carbaryl

Brand names: Carylderm, Derbac, Suleo

Carbaryl is used as a 0.5% alcoholic lotion for the treatment of pediculosis. It is applied to the affected areas, and after 12 hours is removed by washing. The treatment is repeated if required after 1 week. Care should be taken to avoid contact of the drug with the eyes, and asthmatic patients may find the vapour of the lotion disturbing.

Crotamiton

Brand name: Eurax

Crotamiton has antipruritic properties, but it is also effective in scabies. It is applied like benzyl benzoate, and later applications may be useful in controlling the post-treatment itch of scabies.

Lindane

Brand name: Quellada

Lindane, also known as gamma benzene hexachloride, is used like benzyl benzoate as a 1% lotion or cream for scabies and pediculosis, but is now used less frequently as resistant strains of lice have emerged.

Malathion

Brand names: Derbac-M, Prioderm, Suleo-M

Malathion is an organophosphorus insecticide that is widely used in pediculosis, particularly in children, as it is effective against both insects and eggs. It is applied to the scalp or other affected areas as a 0.5% lotion, which is allowed to dry and washed off 12 hours later. A second application is made after a week if necessary.

Permthrin (Lyclear) and **phenothrin** (Full Marks) are new pyrethrin derivatives that function as insect neurotoxins. They are used by local application as solutions in isopropyl alcohol and are effective against head lice and their eggs.

SUNSCREEN PREPARATIONS

Exposure to strong sunlight results in a transient redness of the skin, due to the release of histamine-like substances from the damaged superficial cells. Further exposure leads to a tanning of the skin as the melanin of the basal cells migrates to the superficial cells to provide some protection from further exposure. Sunburn and tanning are caused by the ultraviolet elements of sunshine and radiation with wave-lengths between 310 and 400 nanometres (UVA). UVA is mainly responsible for the erythema of sunburn. Ultraviolet light of the wavelengths of 290–320 nanometres (UVB) causes tanning without marked erythema. An individual's sensitivity to sunlight has been expressed as the minimal erythema dose (MED) which is the time of exposure that will result in a just perceptible redness of the skin after 24 hours. Sensitivity after long exposure to sunlight may be increased by certain drugs such as chlorpromazine and nalidixic acid.

Sunscreen preparations are of two types, those that contain titanium dioxide and zinc oxide which tend to scatter rather than absorb ultraviolet light, and those containing UVL-absorbing compounds. They do not give complete protection, but their activity is expressed as the sun protection factor (SPF). Products with a low SPF give little protection against sunburn but permit tanning, whereas products with a high SPF up to 15 or more offer protection against sunburn with little tanning. Available products include Coppertone (UVB-SPF 23), Piz Buin (UVB-SPF 20), RoC (UVB-SPF 16), Spectroban(UVB-SPF 25), Sun E 45 (UVB-SPF 25) and Uvistat (UVB-SPF 15–30).

Commonsense methods to reduce over-exposure to sunlight include avoiding sunbathing between 12 noon and 2 p.m., when the sun is strongest, adequate clothing after exposure, and the frequent re-application of a sunscreen product. Chronic exposure to strong sunlight is potentially dangerous, as it may lead to the development of skin cancers, of which the incidence has increased dramatically in recent years. Such cancers are of three main types, the most common being the slow-growing basal carcinoma. It appears as white translucent lumps which do not spread, although they may break down and ulcerate. Squamous-cell carcinoma grows more quickly and develops as a hard lump with irregular edges and scaling. Malignant melanoma is the most dangerous, as it grows quickly and may spread. Such melanomas look like moles, but have irregular edges, and are of more than one colour. Ordinary moles are of one shade of brown or black; are smooth in outline and of regular shape; are not inflamed; and not itchy or painful and do not bleed or ooze. Medical advice should be sought if any mole shows signs of activity as it may be a melanoma.

Antiseptics and disinfectants

Definition

The terms antiseptic, bacteriostat, disinfectant, germicide and bactericide are in common use, but are often more easily understood than defined. Strictly speaking, the terms antiseptic or bacteriostat should be applied to substances that inhibit the growth of micro-organisms, and disinfectants, bactericides or germicides are substances that have a definite killing action on such organisms. In practice, these distinctions tend to become blurred, and antiseptics are usually assumed to have a germicidal action. There is a tendency to limit the term antiseptics to substances applied to the body, and to describe as disinfectants those preparations used on equipment and surfaces.

Evaluation of antiseptics

Many attempts have been made to evaluate antiseptic substances and to compare the efficiency of various compounds, but in practice it has proved extremely difficult. Some antiseptics are relatively specific in their action, and are very much more effective against some groups of organisms than others. Other antiseptics are affected by changes in pH, others by the presence of blood or pus.

The position is complicated still further by the fact that some bacteria pass through a stage in the life cycle when 'spores' are formed. These spores are a dormant phase, and usually form when conditions for growth become unfavourable.

Such spores are very resistant to the action of antiseptics, and can survive prolonged exposure, but may develop later when conditions again become favourable. The claims made for any antiseptic product therefore require careful investigation, but the following are among the essential properties that should be possessed by any substance used for its antiseptic properties:

1. wide range of activity in a wide range of strengths;
2. not affected by other substances likely to be present in antiseptic creams, lotions and other products, or by wound exudates;
3. non-irritant and of low toxicity;
4. high degree of penetration and rapidity of action.

Nurses often ask how long an antiseptic or disinfectant solution takes to act, and it can be said at once that no hard-and-fast rules can be given. The killing of bacteria by antiseptics is not an instantaneous process, but takes time. The more bacteria there are to be killed the longer the process. Conversely, when fewer bacteria are present sterilization will be achieved more rapidly.

PHENOLIC ANTISEPTICS
Phenol

This substance is of historical interest, as it was introduced into medicine in 1867 as carbolic acid, and the remarkable results achieved by Lister and his followers in reducing postoperative infection paved the way to the present era of aseptic surgery. Phenol has now been replaced for most purposes by more active and less toxic compounds, but it survives in some mouthwashes and similar preparations.

Cresol

Cresol is chemically related to phenol, and Solution of Cresol with Soap, better known as lysol, was once a widely used disinfectant.

Cresol and related phenols are present in a range of general disinfectant products, usually classified as 'black fluids' and 'white fluids'. Black fluids contain various phenols dissolved in soap solutions; when diluted with water they form white emulsions, and are used to disinfect floors and drains, and for other domestic purposes. White fluids such as *Izal* are emulsions of similar composition but are less liable to stain linen, etc. when used for terminal disinfection.

Chlorocresol

This compound is a more powerful but less soluble derivative of phenol, and is used mainly as a bacteriostat to preserve the sterility of injection solutions. When injections are supplied in multiple-dose containers (i.e. rubber-capped bottles), there is a risk that the unused contents may become contaminated by a faulty technique or the accidental use of an unsterile needle. A preservative is therefore added to such solutions to inhibit bacterial growth, and chlorocresol is used for that purpose in a strength of 0.1–0.2%. Chlorocresol has been used in some instrument storage solutions.

Chlorhexidine

Brand name: Hibitane

Chlorhexidine is a complex phenyl derivative with a powerful bactericidal action against a wide range of organisms that is retained even in very dilute solutions as well as in the presence of blood and other body fluids. But *Pseudomonas* and *Proteus* are resistant, and as with cetrimide, sterilized solutions should be used.

For general antiseptic purposes, chlorhexidine may be used as a 1–2000 solution; for bladder irrigation a 1–5000 solution is effective. For rapid pre-operative sterilization of the skin, a 1–200 solution in 70% alcohol is used.

An aerosol spray product for skin disinfection is also available, which contains a dye to indicate the area treated. Chlorhexidine cream (1%) is also used for obstetric and general antiseptic purposes. Chlorhexidine is present with cetrimide in Hibicet.

Hexachlorophane

Hexachlorophane has a bacteriostatic action against many Gram-positive organisms, even in high dilution, but it is less active against Gram-negative organisms. It is used mainly in soaps and creams, as continued use reduces the bacterial flora in the skin and it is useful in reducing cross-infection. It is also used to prevent neonatal staphylococcal infection and is used after ligation of the cord, and after napkin changes. Hexachlorophane dusting powders should not be applied to mucous membranes or raw surfaces, as absorption of hexachlorophane may occur, and some cases of brain damage have been reported. It is present in Ster-Zac Powder.

Hibicet (Brand name)

Hibicet is a general-purpose antiseptic, and is supplied as a concentrate containing chlorhexidine (1.5%) and cetrimide (15%). While **cetrimide** has some antiseptic properties its range of activity is limited, and it is best regarded as an antiseptic detergent. In Hibicet the advantages of both cetrimide and chlorhexidine are utilized, and the product is characterized by a very wide range of activity and a rapid effect, allied with non-irritant detergent properties.

For general antiseptic purposes, a 1–2000 dilution of Hibicet is used; for the treatment of wounds, hand rinsing, etc., a 1–100 dilution is effective. Hibicet (1–20 in alcohol) can be used for the emergency sterilization of instruments and rubber articles. As with cetrimide and chlorhexidine, contamination and inactivation by *Pseudomonas aeruginosa* may occur and whenever possible, sterilized solutions should be used.

OTHER ANTISEPTICS

Alcohol

Alcohol in the form of methylated spirit has been used for many years as an antiseptic, particularly for skin preparation, but is not very effective or reliable. Isopropyl alcohol has similar general properties and may be used both for pre-operative cleansing of the skin, and for surgical instruments.

Cetrimide

Brand name: Cetavlon

Cetrimide represents a class of substances sometimes referred to as surface-active agents. Such compounds not only have the ability to spread and penetrate easily into tissue crevices, but have some detergent and antiseptic properties.

Solutions containing 0.1% of cetrimide are used for general antiseptic purposes; stronger solutions up to 1% are used for cleaning wounds and burns, and for pre-operative skin preparation.

Cetrimide is a constituent of various creams used for napkin rash and minor abrasions. Cetrimide solutions are often found to be contaminated with *Pseudomonas aeruginosa* and should be supplied as sterilized solutions in screw-capped bottles.

Chlorinated lime

Chlorinated lime, or bleaching powder, is a powerful germicide and deodorant, and has been widely used for general disinfectant purposes and to disinfect excreta. It contains calcium hypochlorite and is used in the preparation of Eusol and for the chlorination of swimming baths.

Eusol

Eusol is a solution of calcium hypochlorite and boric acid, and contains the equivalent of about 0.25% of chlorine. It is used as a general antiseptic wound and ulcer lotion, but the solution soon loses strength, and should not be used when more than 2 weeks old. Eusol has now been largely replaced by stabilized sodium hypochlorite solutions such as **Milton**. The value of these hypochlorite products has been questioned recently. It is claimed that they delay healing, and that their use should be abandoned.

Formaldehyde (formalin)

This powerful germicide is too irritant for general use, but is useful as a 5% solution for the disinfection of apparatus and the preservation of specimens. In association with potassium permanganate it is used for the disinfection of rooms.

Iodine

Iodine is one of the oldest and most effective of antiseptics, and a solution in alcohol has been used for skin preparation. **Povidone-iodine** is now preferred.

Povidone-iodine

Brand names: Betadine, Videne

Iodine can be taken up by various organic substances to form a complex known as an iodophore. In these complexes the iodine is held in a loose combination from which it is slowly liberated when in contact with the skin and mucous membranes. In povidone-iodine, the antiseptic is combined with polyvinylpyrolidine, and the product is used as a 5–10% solution for skin preparation. A 1% solution is used as a lotion or mouthwash.

Iodoform

Iodoform is a lemon-yellow powder with a marked odour and contains iodine in organic combination. It was once used as a wound dressing, but now survives only as the antiseptic constituent of BIPP (bismuth, iodoform and paraffin paste) occasionally used with gauze as a packing for sinuses and abscesses, and in Whitehead's Varnish.

OXIDIZING AGENTS

The chlorine antiseptics owe their action, in part at least to the fact that the hypochlorite finally decomposes to liberate oxygen. A number of other substances are also used as antiseptics by virtue of their oxygen-liberating properties, and the following are in use.

Hydrogen peroxide

Hydrogen peroxide (H_2O_2) is easily decomposed in the presence of oxidizable matter to yield oxygen and water. It is mainly used to treat infected cavities and dirty wounds, as the tissue enzymes cause a rapid release of oxygen, and the gas has the added mechanical action of loosening cell debris in the tissue crevices.

It is also used, when diluted with water, as an antiseptic mouth wash. Solutions of hydrogen peroxide are often described as

'10 volume' or '20 volume' strength. The numbers refer to the volume of oxygen yielded by 1 volume of the solution.

Potassium permanganate

Dark purple crystals which rapidly decompose in contact with organic matter, and have powerful antiseptic and deodorizing properties. A 1–5000 solution is used for suppurating wounds and abscesses, and weaker solutions have been employed for bladder and vaginal irrigation and as a mouthwash.

As the drug rapidly decomposes during use its action is brief, and the decomposition products may cause brown stains on the skin, fabrics and utensils. When potassium permanganate is mixed with formaldehyde solution, there is a very rapid release of formaldehyde gas. The release is made use of in the formaldehyde disinfection of rooms.

Zinc peroxide

A white powder, resembling zinc oxide in appearance, zinc peroxide slowly decomposes to yield oxygen and zinc oxide, and its action therefore resembles that of hydrogen peroxide, but is much more prolonged. It is used as a suspension in water, or as an aqueous cream in the treatment of infected wounds and necrotic ulcers. It is sometimes combined with urea in order to promote granulation.

ANTISEPTIC DYES

A number of synthetic dyes have antiseptic properties, but the therapeutic use of such substances has declined as more active chemotherapeutic drugs have become available for the treatment of infections. The following substances are still in use, but to a steadily diminishing extent and their value is open to question.

Crystal violet (gentian violet)

This dye has powerful but selective antiseptic properties, and is effective chiefly against Gram-positive organisms. A solution containing 0.5% of crystal violet is still used occasionally for pre-operative preparation of the skin but it is not recommended for application to broken skin or mucous membranes.

Proflavine

Proflavine and acriflavine are orange-red dyes with a bacteriostatic action. They were once widely used as a 1–1000 lotion, and proflavine cream (0.1%) is a surviving preparation.

SILVER COMPOUNDS

Silver salts have powerful antiseptic properties, but very few have any therapeutic applications. Silver nitrate solution (1%) was once used extensively as eye-drops as a prophylactic against ophthalmia neonatorum, and in some parts of the USA its use is still mandatory. Solid silver nitrate is used as a caustic to destroy warts.

Silver sulphadiazine (Flamazine §) is used as a 1% cream for the treatment of infected leg ulcers, burns and pressure sores, especially those infected with *Pseudomonas aeruginosa*. The complex is slowly metabolized by tissue exudates, but if the cream is applied extensively, some of the free sulphadiazine may be absorbed systemically.

26

Biological products and immunology

VACCINES, SERA AND RELATED PREPARATIONS

When pathogenic organisms gain access to the body, some of the products of their metabolism, referred to as toxins, pass into the blood. Such foreign substances are known as antigens, and the body defends itself against such antigens by the formation of specific antidotes, termed antibodies or immunoglobulins. Tetanus antitoxin is a well-known example of an antibody preparation. The formation of antibodies in response to infection is termed 'active immunization' and may be naturally acquired or artificially induced.

Natural immunity

Naturally acquired immunity follows recovery from infection, and the degree and duration of the immunity varies with the nature of the invading organism. Thus recovery from diphtheria is accompanied by a high and prolonged degree of immunity, whereas the immunity that follows recovery from tetanus is brief and of low intensity.

A natural immunity may also be acquired from an infection so mild as to escape notice. Such immunity may not be very high in itself, but it sensitizes the reticulo-endothelial system and increases its powers to produce antibodies, and in the event of a subsequent infection the rapid production of antibodies in quantity can cut the infection short. Occasionally, although the patient recovers, the infecting organisms are not killed off, and the individual then becomes a carrier of the disease.

Induced active immunity

The products used to induce active immunity are referred to generally as vaccines. They may be preparations of living attenuated or non-virulent strains of the organisms concerned such as BCG or measles vaccine, or chemically modified and inactivated preparations of the organisms or their toxins or toxoids.

Diphtheria and tetanus vaccines are familiar examples. Vaccines are now available that give protection against a variety of infections, including anthrax, mumps, measles, rabies, rubella, hepatitis, and cholera. These products function as antigens, and stimulate the production of antibodies and other factors of the immune protective system.

In some cases, especially with inactivated vaccines, the response to an initial injection is weak, but it acts as a trigger to the antibody production mechanism, and a second injection, given some days or even weeks later, evokes a powerful response and large amounts of antibodies or antitoxins are produced.

Should a subsequent infection occur, the circulating antibodies can prevent or minimize the development of the disease. The active immunity thus acquired may persist, in some cases for many years, and even if the degree of immunity falls to low levels in time, a further injection rapidly restores the original level of antitoxin.

As with these products there is a definite time-lag between the original injection and the maximum level of antibody, they are of chief value in prophylaxis. In the treatment of established infections products conferring immediate protection are required. Such temporary protection is referred to as passive immunity.

Passive immunity

A transient immunity or protection against certain infections can be obtained by the use of serum which already contains antibodies, which if obtained from human sources are referred to as immunoglobulins. The injection of such a product results in the immediate presence of antibodies in the blood, and before antibiotics were available, such temporary immunity was of considerable value both for treatment and the protection of contacts.

Passive immunity can be very effective, and occasionally lifesaving, but it is a short-term measure, as the immunity thus conferred does not last more than 2–3 weeks and active measures must be taken for extended immunity. Immunological products for passive immunity include diphtheria and tetanus antitoxins, prepared from the blood of immunized horses, but reliance is now placed to a great extent on selected human serum which contains the required immunoglobulins. With these human immunoglobulin preparations, serum-sickness is rare. If an animal-derived product is used, an initial test dose should be given to detect possible sensitivity.

IMMUNOGLOBULINS

Antibodies, also referred to as immunoglobulins, are modified blood proteins that have a direct and specific action against bacterial toxins, or by coating the invading organisms, facilitate their destruction by phagocytosis. This type of antibody-mediated or 'humoral' immunity was once considered to cover all aspects of immunity, but another type now recognized is 'cell-mediated immunity' (CMI).

Cell-mediated immunity is controlled by activated lymphocytes, which originate in the bone marrow, and can be divided into two groups, the B-lymphocytes, and the T-lymphocytes. The B-lymphocytes develop into plasma cells that form antibodies; the immature T-lymphocytes undergo development in the thymus, and acquire antibody-like molecules on the surface, referred to as cell-bound antibodies. These cells, after further maturation in the spleen, circulate in the lymphatic system.

Following infection, phagocytes are attracted to the invading organisms, some of which are engulfed and digested by the phagocytes. Some of the T-lymphocytes are converted into killer-lymphocytes, that also attack the organisms directly. The immunoglobulins (antibodies) bind to the organisms to form an 'immune complex', which in turn combines with special receptor cells of the phagocytes, and increases their ability to destroy the organisms.

Other factors present in normal blood, which in association with antibodies also bring about lysis of the bacterial cells, are referred to generally as 'complement'. Figure 26.1 gives a simplified outline of some aspects of this complex process.

The immunoglobulins are now differentiated to some extent as IgG, IgM, IgA, IgE, etc. IgG is the most abundant of the

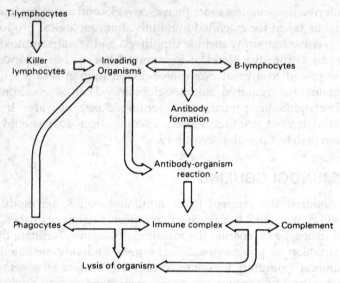

Figure 26.1 Outline of some stages of the immunological attack.

immunoglobulins in the internal body fluids, and is a powerful neutralizer of bacterial toxins, as well as binding with the invading organisms to increase phagocytosis. It easily crosses the placenta, and provides the major line of defence against infection during the first weeks of a baby's life.

IgM is a macroglobulin, as it has a higher molecular weight than the other immunoglobulins, and is a highly active agglutinating and cytolytic agent. It appears in the blood stream as an early response to infection, and is followed later by the emergence of large amounts of IgG. IgM is considered to be the first-line defence in bacteraemia.

IgA is the major immunoglobulin of mucus and other surface secretions. It is synthesized locally by plasma cells, and is largely concerned with the defence of exposed mucous surfaces.

The physiological role of IgE is uncertain, although its serum level may rise markedly during helminth infestations. IgE remains attached to the mast cells for long periods, and it is of considerable interest from the allergic point of view, as the reaginic antibodies of allergic reactions are of the IgE type. It is present in larger amounts in hypersensitive and asthmatic patients, and exposure of the mast cell to the allergic antigen results in the disruption of the mast cell, the release of histamine and other spasmogens, followed by the allergic reaction.

These cell-mediated antibodies are of considerable importance in other ways, as they are concerned with some forms of auto-immunity and in auto-immune disease. When the mechanism by which the body is prevented from developing antibodies that will react with the body's own tissues shows signs of failure, auto-antibodies may be produced, and cause the so-called auto-immune diseases. In some of these conditions the auto-antibody is specific for a certain organ, as in Hashimoto's disease of the thyroid, but generally the reaction is systemic, and pathological changes are widespread.

Systemic lupus erythematosus and rheumatoid arthritis are other diseases in which auto-immune mechanisms may play an important part.

Human normal immunoglobulin injection (HNIG)

Brand names: Kabiglobulin §, Gammabulin §

This product, formerly known as human gamma globulin, is a fraction of pooled adult plasma obtained from at least 1000 individuals, and contains gamma-G globulin and the antibodies normally present in adult human blood. It is used by intramuscular injection to confer temporary protection on children who are unlikely to have developed adequate antibodies of their own against hepatitis A virus and measles. Specific human immunoglobulins obtained from the plasma of immunized individuals, or from patients recovering from an infection are also available for protection against tetanus, rabies, hepatitis B and varicella-zoster.

Human anti-D (Rho) immunoglobulin is used to prevent a rhesus-negative mother from forming antibodies to fetal rhesus-positive blood cells that may pass into the maternal circulation. Such antibodies could produce haemolytic disease in subsequent children. The injection must be given within 72 hours of birth. The usual dose to the mother is 250–500 units by intramuscular injection. It is sometimes given in doses of 250 units.

For replacement therapy in hypogamma-globulinaemia, human normal immunoglobulin (HNIG) for *intravenous* injection is also available as Gamimune-N, Intraglobulin, Sandoglobulin, Endobulin and Venoglobulin §.

IMMUNOSUPPRESSION AND TRANSPLANT SURGERY

It has long been known from early work on skin grafting that the body can recognize foreign tissues, and that grafts are rejected by the cell-mediated immunological response. The problem assumed new importance when organ transplants became possible, and as some cytotoxic agents are now used as immunosuppressants in transplant surgery, it is convenient to refer briefly to such drugs here. By the nature of their action, these drugs also depress the immune defences against infection, so the treatment of immuno-compromised patients is both difficult and complicated.

Azathioprine §

Brand names: Imuran §, Azamune §

Azathioprine is a derivative of mercaptopurine, and has similar cytotoxic properties, but it is mainly used as an immunosuppressant in organ transplant surgery to reduce the risks of rejection of the organ, and facilitate its acceptance and survival. It is given in doses that vary from 1 to 5 mg/kg daily, adjusted to individual requirements, and also depending on the use of other therapy such as the corticosteroids.

Careful control of treatment is essential as myelodepression may be severe. Other **side-effects** are drug fever and liver damage.

Cyclosporin §

Brand name: Sandimmum §

Cyclosporin is a fungal metabolite with a cyclo-polypeptide structure, and the discovery of its remarkable immunological properties added a new dimension to transplant surgery. It acts by inhibiting the proliferation of lymphocytes that is stimulated by the introduction of transplant tissues. It also inhibits the production of regulatory lymphokines such as interleukin-2.

Cyclosporin is highly effective in organ transplantation generally, and in the control of graft-versus-host disease, and is given as a dose of 10–15 mg/kg some hours before transplantation, and continued at that level daily for 1–2 weeks. The dose is then slowly reduced by 2 mg/kg at monthly intervals to a maintenance dose level of 6–8 mg/kg daily. The unpleasant taste can be disguised to some extent by giving the drug mixed with cold fruit juice or other liquid immediately before use. Cyclosporin may also be given by intravenous injection in doses of 3–5 mg/kg daily when oral therapy is not possible.

Side-effects of cyclosporin are usually mild, but some hypertrichosis is common, as well as gastrointestinal disturbances, and tremor, but a dose-related nephrotoxicity is the main **side-effect**. A burning sensation in the hands and feet may occur during the first week of therapy, but unlike other immuno-suppressive drugs cyclosporin is virtually free from myelotoxicity.

Kahan B D 1989 Cyclosporin. New England Journal of Medicine 321: 1725–1738

Diagnostic products

In a few cases, serological products are available which can be used to detect those individuals who lack a natural immunity.

Schick test

This test is occasionally used to detect susceptibility to diphtheria, and is carried out by the intradermal injection of 0.2 ml of a weak solution of diphtheria toxin. A positive reaction is shown by the development of a red area 10–50 mm in diameter. A negative response is not an absolute test of immunity as young children are rarely immune, and the test is used mainly for older children and young adults.

BCG tuberculin test

BCG vaccine is a live attenuated strain derived from *Mycobacterium bovis* which when given by intradermal injection, stimulates the development of a localized hypersensitivity to *M. tuberculosis*. A positive reaction is the development of a papule within 2–6 weeks which progresses to a benign ulcer of about 10 mm in diameter which heals after a few weeks.

A positive reaction indicates that the individual has been

infected at some time with the tubercle bacillus, but it does not distinguish between past infection and present disease, except in young children. A positive reaction in a young child is an indication of an active infection that requires immediate treatment. In adults the diagnostic value of a positive test is of much less significance, but a reaction in a person known to have been a non-reactor is an indication of a new infection.

Vaccines (including toxoids) for active immunization or prophylaxis

The following list of immunological products includes some that are available only from designated laboratories.

Immunological products are quickly inactivated unless properly stored, and as a general rule they should be refrigerator-stored between 2–8°C, unless advised otherwise. They should not be allowed to freeze. Vaccines are often suspensions, and should be well shaken immediately before use to ensure that the proper dose is injected.

Anthrax vaccine. Dose: 0.5 ml by intramuscular or deep subcutaneous injection, repeated at intervals of 3 weeks for three doses, with a final injection after 6 months. Reinforcing doses of 0.5 ml should be given at yearly intervals.

Bacillus Calmette–Guerin vaccine (BCG). Dose: 0.1 ml as a single intradermal prophylactic injection against tuber-culosis. A vaccine prepared from isoniazid-resistant organisms is also available, as well as a special *percutaneous* preparation. The vaccine may lead to keloid formation in some skin areas, and the injection site should be chosen with the cosmetic result in mind.

Cholera vaccine. Dose: 0.5 ml initially by deep subcutaneous or intramuscular injection, followed by 1 ml 4 weeks later. A boosting dose should be given every 6 months if exposure is continuous.

Diphtheria vaccine. Adsorbed vaccine. Dose: 0.2–0.5 ml by intramuscular or deep subcutaneous injection, followed by 0.5 ml after an interval of not less than 4 weeks. Now usually given to children as the triple vaccine (diphtheria, tetanus and pertussis).

Hepatitis A vaccine. A vaccine containing inactivated hepatitis A virus grown in human cells. It is given by intramuscular injection, preferably in the deltoid area, as a three-dose course of 1 ml, the second dose 2–4 weeks later, and the third dose 6–12 months after the initial dose. *Brand name:* Havrix.

Hepatitis B vaccine. A vaccine prepared from inactivated hepatitis B virus antigen, and obtained from yeast cells by recombinant DNA technology. It is given in doses of 1 ml by intramuscular injection, the second 1 month after the first, and the third 6 months after the initial dose. *Brand name:* Engerix B.

Influenza vaccine. Dose: 0.5 ml by deep subcutaneous or intramuscular injection. The virus strains are grown in chick embryo, and the vaccine is contraindicated in those hypersensitive to eggs or feathers. *Brand names:* Fluvirin, Influvac, Fluzone.

Measles vaccine. Now replaced by MMR vaccine.

MMR vaccine. A combined measles, mumps and rubella vaccine, given routinely to children before primary school. Dose: 0.5 ml by intramuscular or subcutaneous injection. It may cause a febrile reaction, and is contraindicated in egg allergy. It is not suitable for prophylaxis after exposure to mumps and rubella, as the onset of immunity is too slow. *Brand name:* MMR-11.

Meningococcal polysaccharide vaccine. Contains one or more of the polysaccharide antigens of *Neisseria meningitidis* A and C. It is used in those countries where the risk of meningitis is high. Dose: 0.5 ml by deep subcutaneous or intramuscular injection. *Brand names:* AC Vax, Mengivae.

Mumps vaccine. A live attenuated virus vaccine that induces protective antibodies in most non-immune individuals. Dose: 0.5 ml by subcutaneous injection. Not intended for children under 1 year of age. Contraindicated in hypersensitivity to eggs or feathers. *Brand name:* Mumpsvax.

Pertussis vaccine. Dose: 0.5 ml by deep subcutaneous or intramuscular injection, repeated after 4 weeks and again after 6 months. It should not be given to children with a history of convulsions. Encephalopathy is a rare complication. It is often given as diphtheria, tetanus and pertussis vaccine.

Pneumococcal vaccine. Contains a mixture of the polysaccharide capsular antigens of *Streptococcus penumoniae*. Dose: 0.5 ml by deep subcutaneous or intramuscular injection. Used when the risk of pneumococcal pneumonia is high, as with patients following splenectomy. Hypersensitivity reactions may occur, and re-vaccination is not recommended. *Brand name:* Pneumovax.

Poliomyelitis vaccine (inactivated). Dose: 0.5 ml by subcutaneous or intramuscular injection, followed by a second dose after 4–6 weeks, and a third dose after 8–12 months. The oral vaccine is preferred.

Poliomyelitis vaccine (oral). It contains three virus types. In infants the first dose should be given at the age of 6 months, the second dose 6–8 weeks later, and the third dose after 4–6 months.

Rabies vaccine. A human rabies vaccine is available for prophylaxis and treatment.

Rubella vaccine. Dose: 0.5 ml by deep subcutaneous injection. If rubella (German measles) is contracted in early pregnancy, there is a risk of damage to the fetus, and rubella vaccine should be given to all girls between the ages of 11 and 14 years, and to other females at risk, provided that they are not pregnant. *Brand names:* Almevax, Ervevax, Rubafax.

Smallpox vaccine. Dose: 0.05 ml by scarification of the skin. It is no longer used routinely.

Tetanus vaccine (tetanus toxoid). Dose: 0.5–1 ml by deep subcutaneous or intramuscular injection, repeated after intervals of 6–12 weeks and 4–6 months.

Typhoid. Three types of typhoid vaccine are now available. The old or whole cell vaccine is given as an initial dose of 0.5 ml by deep subcutaneous or intramuscular injection, followed by a second dose after 4–6 weeks. It has been recommended that the second and any booster dose should be given by intradermal injection in doses of 0.1 ml to reduce side-effects. Another vaccine (Typhim VR) is prepared from the capsular polysaccharides of the organisms, and is given as a single dose of 0.5 ml by deep subcutaneous or intramuscular injection. Subsequent doses can be given at 3-year intervals when exposure is continuous. A live oral vaccine (Vivotif) is given as capsules, one to be taken daily on alternate days for three doses. Protection may persist for 3 years. (*Note.* Capsules should be refrigerator-stored.)

Yellow fever vaccine. Dose: 0.5 ml by subcutaneous injection. Immunity persists for at least 10 years. *Brand name:* Arilvax.

Note. The so-called desensitizing vaccines, used in the treatment of certain allergic conditions, are not true vaccines. They are weak solutions of various protein products known to be associated with allergic reactions, and are referred to on page 432.

Table 26.1 Vaccination schemes, (vaccination against smallpox is no longer used routinely)

Age	Vaccine	Interval
During the first year of life	Diphtheria, tetanus, pertussis and oral polio vaccine (three doses); *Haemophilus* vaccine	The first dose should be given 2 months after birth, the second and third at monthly intervals
1–2 years	Measles, mumps and rubella vaccine; *Haemophilus* vaccine	
School entry	Diphtheria, tetanus and oral polio vaccine; measles, mumps, rubella vaccine if not already given	
10 and 13 years	BCG vaccine	For tuberculin-negative children
	Rubella vaccine	All girls of this age group should receive rubella vaccine; an interval of 3 weeks should elapse between rubella and BCG vaccination
15–19 years	Polio vaccine (oral) Tetanus vaccine	
Adults	Reinforcing doses of polio vaccine Rubella vaccine for susceptible women of child-bearing age	

Vaccination schemes

Vaccination schemes have been designed to give protection during childhood and beyond against many common infections. A standard scheme is outlined in Table 26.1.

Antitoxins and antisera for passive immunization or treatment

Diphtheria antitoxin. Dose: 500–2000 units by subcutaneous or intramuscular injection for prophylaxis; 10 000 –100 000 units by intramuscular or intravenous injection for treatment.

Tetanus antitoxin. Dose: not less than 1500 units by subcutaneous or intramuscular injection for prophylaxis; not less than 50 000 units by intravenous or intramuscular injection for treatment. The use of tetanus antitoxin for prophylaxis has declined because of sensitivity reaction to horse serum. Human anti-tetanus immunoglobulin is preferred; dose: 250 units by intramuscular injection. *Brand name*: Humotet.

27

Diagnostic agents

Some substances are employed in medicine for diagnostic rather than therapeutic purposes. Many of these are used as X-ray contrast agents to outline body cavities and organs, others are used as tests for liver and kidney function and for various other investigations. Serological products used as diagnostic agents are referred to on page 561.

X-ray contrast agents

These are substances of high atomic weight which increase the absorption of X-rays as they pass through the body. As they are relatively opaque to X-rays, they appear as shadows on X-ray films, and are invaluable in outlining various tissues. With the exception of barium sulphate, the substances used as contrast agents are almost invariably complex iodine-containing organic compounds.

Barium sulphate

Barium sulphate is very heavy, dense white powder, used for the visualization of the gastrointestinal tract. It is given as a suspension in water, orally or as an enema, according to the area to be examined, after previous fasting, etc., so that the gastrointestinal tract is empty. When so used, barium sulphate forms a temporary coating of the alimentary tract, and abnormalities can be outlined and detected. Large doses varying from 100–250 g may be given, and it is important to obtain a complete and even coating of the mucosa as otherwise shallow ulcers and similar lesions may escape detection. The double contrast methods that involve the distention of the gastrointestinal lumen by gas (carbon dioxide) has the advantage that gastric folds are opened up for improved visualization. The gas is formed in the stomach by giving citric acid and sodium bicarbonate, after swallowing the barium preparation, and by suitable manipulation of the patient, the anterior and posterior walls of the stomach and the duodenal cap can be visualized. Metoclopramide is sometimes used to reduce stomach transit time, and in all cases the patient should be encouraged to retain the gas during the examination. Basically similar methods are used for the visualization of the large bowel by barium enemas. Proprietary preparations of barium sulphate are represented by Micropaque and Baritop.

IODINE COMPOUNDS

Iodine is highly opaque to X-rays, and the iodine compounds in use are derivatives of various organic acids. Their opacity to X-rays is directly proportional to the iodine content. They fall into three groups, those used orally and concentrated in the gall bladder (for visualization of the biliary tract), those injected into the CSF to detect spinal cord damage, and those used intravenously. The latter can be further divided into the ionic and non-ionic contrast agents. The ionic agents dissociate in solution, with the anion carrying the iodine, and the greater the degree of ionization, the greater is the osmotic pressure of the solution. Ideally, a solution of a contrast agent given intravenously should have the same osmotic pressure or osmolarity as the body fluids, but in practice, most contrast agents have a higher osmotic pressure. That difference is associated with some of the adverse effects of intravenous contrast agents, particularly the sensation of heat that many patients experience, as well as damage to blood cells. The high osmotic pressure may also allow some agents to penetrate the protective blood–brain barrier and cause neurological damage. For that reason, some non-ionic contrast agents have been introduced. At present such agents are very expensive, but have the advantages of a lower osmotic pressure with reduced side-effects, and are better tolerated by poor-risk patients.

The intravenous contrast agents in current use include those for outlining the vascular system (angiography), those for visualization of the urinary tract (urography) and those for examining the liver and bile ducts (choleocystography). Some compounds are suitable for more than one type of investigation. A detailed consideration of contrast agents is beyond the scope of this book, but the notes in Table 27.1 may be useful.

A development in the field of X-ray visualization of the body is the use of nuclear magnetic resonance imaging (MRI) to enhance tissue contrast. The method requires contrast agents of a different type and a compound containing the metal gadolinium, and described as meglumine gadopenetate is available as Magnevist. Gadoteridol (Prohance) is a similar product.

Table 27.1

Type of contrast agent	Brand names
Ionic	Gastrografin, Hypaque, Urografin, Biloscopin, Biligram
Ionic—high osmolar	Uromiro, Biloptin, Cistobil, Myodil, Telepaque (oral)
Ionic—low osmolar	Biligrafin, Conray, Ultravist
Non-ionic low osmolar	Niopam, Amipaque
Angiography	Amipaque, Conray, Hebrix, Niopam, Ultravist
Bronchography	Propylidone
Choleocystography	Cistobil, Biliscopin, Biloptin, Telepaque
Urography	Niopam, Conray, Hebrix, Urografin, Uromiro, Ultravist

ALLERGY TESTS

The full diagnosis of allergic disease depends on the identification of the causative allergen, and skin tests to confirm sensitivity to a suspected allergen are used, particularly where inhalant allergens such as pollens, animal hair and feathers are concerned. Special extracts containing small amounts of the allergens are used as skin test solutions and may be applied as prick tests or scratch tests, but response is variable, and their use is not without risk (p. 432). Patch tests are used to detect the cause of allergic contact dermatitis.

FUNCTIONAL TESTS

Bentiromide

Bentiromide is a derivative of aminobenzoic acid. It is metabolized in the gut by the pancreatic enzyme chymotrypsin to give the free acid, which is absorbed and excreted in the urine. On that account it is used as a test of pancreatic function by measuring the excretion of the drug after a dose of 500 mg. Fluorescein dilaurate has also been used for the same purpose.

Indocyanine green (Cardio green)

When given by intravenous injection, indocyanine green is rapidly eliminated from the circulation, and is used to assess cardiac output and liver function. It is given in doses of 5 mg by a cardiac catheter, and the elimination is assessed photometrically.

Patent blue

Patent blue is used as a 2.5% solution by subcutaneous injection to visualize lymph vessels so that they can be injected with a contrast medium. It is given in a dose of 0.25 ml of the solution after dilution with saline or lignocaine solution.

Phenolsulphonphthalein

Also known as phenol red, phenolsulphonphthalein has been used as a test of renal function. It is given in doses of 6 mg by intramuscular or intravenous injection, and the urine is collected later at intervals. The colour of the urine is then compared with that of a standard solution. Some 25% of the dye is normally excreted in 15 minutes, and over 50% at the end of 1 hour, and any marked delay is an indication of the degree of renal dysfunction.

Sodium aminohippurate

Sodium aminohippurate is given by intravenous injection for the measurement of renal plasma flow in doses to give a plasma concentration of 10–20 micrograms/ml.

Sulphan blue

Sulphan blue has been used to assess the state of the circulation in cases of burns and soft tissue trauma. It is given in doses of 0.25–0.5 ml/kg of a 6.2% solution by slow intravenous injection.

Sulphobromophthalein

This compound is a red dye, and following intravenous injection it is taken up by the liver and excreted in the bile. Normally most of the dye is removed from the blood within 30 minutes, and it has been used for assessing hepatic activity. The dose is 5 mg/kg body-weight, given as a 5% solution by intravenous injection. Samples of blood are taken 45 minutes later and the amount of sulphobromophthalein present in the plasma, normally about 7%, is measured by comparison with standard solutions of the dye. It should not be used in patients with a history of allergy.

The treatment of poisoning

All substances are poisons; there is no such thing as a non-poison. It is the amount that distinguishes a poison from a remedy.

(Paracelsus, 1493–1541)

The increasing use of potent drugs and the widening range of toxic chemicals used for industrial purposes has increased the risk and also the incidence of poisoning. The term 'poison' is a relative one, as many substances not usually regarded as poisons may prove toxic if taken in sufficient dose, or if swallowed by children.

The incidence of poisoning from plants is low, partly due perhaps to more intensive farming, and fewer poisonous plants to collect. Although many cases of suspected laburnum poisoning are admitted to hospital every summer, doubts have been cast upon the need for such admissions, on the grounds that little serious harm has been reported, and that most symptoms are said to subside within 12 hours. It is worth noting that *homeopathic* products are non-toxic even in overdose. *Herbal* remedies, on the other hand, may contain enough pharmacologically active constituents to cause toxic effects in some cases, and poisoning after self-medication with digitalis leaves mistaken for comfrey has also occurred.

READ THE LABEL!

Many cases of accidental poisoning can be traced to careless handling or storage of drugs and chemicals, and every effort should be made to impress on patients, relatives and all users of potentially toxic substances the importance of keeping all such products (including household detergents) under proper control.

With drugs, as with other things of potential danger as well as value, constant vigilance is the only safeguard. No drug should *ever be used from an un-labelled container*, neither should a product be used unless the label is clear and unambiguous, and conveys the required information.

TREATMENT OF POISONING

The primary aim of treatment is the maintenance of vital functions. The identification of the poison is often a secondary matter, as there are very few specific antidotes. Hospital admission is advisable as some poisonous substances have a delayed action that adds to the problems of treatment. A local National Poisons Information Centre should be consulted if necessary, particularly when industrial poisons are concerned.

Respiration

A common cause of death in acute poisoning is the loss of the airway protective reflexes and consequent airway obstruction by the flaccid tongue. Immediate measures include the pulling forward of the tongue, removal of any dentures, and the insertion if available of a oropharyngeal airway. The patient should be turned to a left-side-head-down position to allow any secretion or vomit to drain out of the mouth, and so reduce the risk of pulmonary aspiration. If the poison has been inhaled, the patient should be removed immediately to fresh air.

Many poisons depress the respiration, and assisted ventilation by mouth-to-mouth or Ambu bag may be required; oxygen may also be necessary. Trained personnel should consider endotrachael intubation to maintain the airway and permit mechanical ventilation. Hypotension is also common in severe poisoning, and the patient's head should be kept down while other measures to support vital functions are being instituted. The use of pressor drugs or respiratory stimulants is not recommended.

Emetics and gastric lavage

If the poison has been swallowed, the removal of as much as possible of the poison from the stomach should be considered, but the benefit must be weighed against the risks, bearing in mind the degree of toxicity, and the time lag between poisoning and treatment. Emesis should be considered, and induced if necessary, provided that the patient is fully conscious, and the poison is not corrosive or a petroleum product, by giving Ipecacuanha Mixture (Paediatric) with a glass of water. The adult dose is 30 ml, that for a child of 6–18 months is 10 ml, and 15 ml for older children. A second dose may be given after 20 minutes if necessary. Other methods of inducing emesis have been used, such as mechanical pharyngeal stimulation and the administration of salt, mustard and copper sulphate, but they are now regarded as dangerous or ineffective.

Gastric lavage should be carried out in hospital, but in many cases it is not considered worthwhile unless performed within 4 hours of taking the poison, unless the poison is one that delays gastric emptying, such as the tricyclic antidepressants. The possibility of inhalation of gastric contents and pulmonary complications should be borne in mind, and like emesis, gastric lavage should not be carried out if the poison is a corrosive agent or a petroleum product. In any case, gastric lavage should always be accompanied by the use of activated charcoal, which is a powerful adsorbent of many toxic substances, and a dose of 50 g or more should be given as soon as possible, even before gastric lavage is considered.

The gastric lavage procedure can be outlined briefly as follows:

1. If the patient is unconscious, the airway must be protected by a cuffed endotracheal tube.
2. Pass the largest gastric tube available, followed by 50 g or more of activated charcoal suspended in water.
3. Carry out lavage repeatedly with 300–500 ml of warm water until the returned fluid is free from toxic material.
4. Give further doses of activated charcoal to maintain the adsorptive action in the intestines; it can be repeated until charcoal appears in the faeces.
5. A laxative may be given if necessary to maintain intestinal transit and the elimination of any toxic material not removed by lavage, such as tablets of ferrous sulphate.

Activated charcoal

Activated charcoal has marked adsorptive properties, and is a first-line treatment of poisoning by many substances taken by mouth as it hinders their absorption, and repeated doses of 25–50 g or more can be given as a suspension in water. It has no other action, and is not itself absorbed. Although it should always be given as soon as possible after poisoning, repeated doses may promote the elimination of some drugs even after they have been absorbed, and activated charcoal is valuable in overdose by aspirin, carbamazepine, dapsone, digoxin, barbiturates, phenytoin, quinine and theophylline.

Other measures for the treatment of severe poisoning include forced alkaline diuresis, haemodialysis and haemoperfusion, but they are effective only in poisoning by a limited range of drugs.

Acids: corrosive acids (i.e. hydrochloric acid, spirits of salt, nitric acid, sulphuric acid, oil of vitriol and oxalic acid)

Symptoms. Acids tend to cause more gastric injury than oesophageal damage.

Treatment. Milk or water in quantity. The use of cream of magnesia or sodium bicarbonate to neutralize the acid is no longer recommended. Emetics should not be used and activated charcoal is of no value.

If the poisoning is due to **oxalic acid**, hypocalcaemia may occur after absorption, causing twitching, tetany, convulsions and cardiac arrest.

Treatment. Gastric lavage and/or oral fluid with 10 g of calcium lactate or gluconate to precipitate oxalic acid as the insoluble calcium salt. Control tetany with calcium gluconate 10% (10 ml) intravenously, repeated as needed.

Alkalis (caustic, including caustic potash, caustic soda, soap lyes, strong ammonia, etc.)

Symptoms. Alkalis tend to cause more severe and penetrating tissue damage. Perforation may occur.

Treatment. Water or milk in quantity. The neutralization of the alkali with vinegar, lemon juice or citric acid is no longer recommended.

Antihistamines

Symptoms. Drowsiness, headache, tinnitus, vertigo, uncoordination blurred vision, dryness of mouth, convulsions and coma. Hazardous arrhythmias have occurred with astemizole and terfendadine overdose.

Treatment. Emetics and gastric lavage with sodium bicarbonate solution. If convulsions occur give intramuscular paraldehyde or intravenous thiopentone.

Amphetamine and related central stimulants

Symptoms. Agitation, tremor, sweating, confusion, arrhythmias, hypertension, hyperthermia, convulsions.

Treatment. Gastric lavage (emesis may precipitate convulsions); chlorpromazine i.m. or diazepam i.v. for severe agitation. Intravenous phentolamine or sodium nitroprusside for severe hypertension.

Aspirin and other oral salicylates

Symptoms. Nausea with or without vomiting, dizziness, tinnitus, mental confusion, visual disturbances, profuse perspiration, central nervous system failure and cardiovascular collapse.

Treatment. Gastric lavage with sodium bicarbonate solution. Copious fluids containing dextrose and sodium bicarbonate orally. Alkalize the urine if plasma salicylate level over 600 mg/litre (adults) or 450 mg/litre in children and elderly. Haemodialysis if levels are above 800 mg/litre or 450 mg/litre.

Atropine and related drugs

Symptoms. Dryness of the mouth, thirst, nausea, vomiting, blurring of vision, urinary retention, hyperpyrexia, confusion, hallucinations.

Treatment. Gastric lavage. Peripheral effects reduced by neostigmine injection. Central effects controlled by intravenous diazepam. Physostigmine also used, but repeated doses are required.

Barbiturates

Symptoms. Mild poisoning shown by lethagy and slurred

speech; large doses cause hypotension, bradycardia, respiratory depression, hypothermia and coma. Bullous lesions occur in barbiturate overdose, but are not specific.

Treatment. Gastric lavage and repeated activated charcoal, protect airway and assist ventilation. Forced alkaline diuresis may be required in severe poisoning with phenobarbitone only. Charcoal haemoperfusion is used for those patients with very severe poisoning who do not respond to other treatment.

Benzodiazepines

Symptoms. Drowsiness, ataxia, hypotension, respiratory depression, bradycardia.

Treatment. Gastric lavage. Flumazenil is a drug used in anaesthesia and intensive care to reverse the sedative effects of benzodiazepines. It may be useful in benzodiazepine poisoning. Care is necessary in benzodiazepine dependence, as it may precipitate acute withdrawal symptoms.

Carbon monoxide (including exhaust fumes)

Symptoms. Headache, nausea, giddiness, tinnitus and throbbing of the heart, coma. There may be convulsions and incontinence of urine and faeces. Bright red coloration of the skin and mucosae.

Treatment. Remove patient to fresh air, ensure airway. Take blood sample for carboxyhaemoglobin (COHb) assay, give oxygen until COHb level has fallen below 5%. Hyperbaric oxygen if COHb greater than 20%.

Cyanides (including prussic acid, cherry laurel water, bitter almond oil, etc.)

Symptoms. Characteristic smell of bitter almonds (not detectable by everybody), respiration rapid but becoming slow and gasping, slow imperceptible pulse, glassy protruding eyes, dilated pupils, convulsions, skin clammy and cold. Systemic poisoning from splashes and burns from molten cyanide, which may occur in industry, is relatively slow in onset in most cases.

Treatment. Immediate action imperative. Rescuers should wear protective clothing and breathing apparatus. Break ampoule of amyl nitrite under nose for inhalation; intravenous injections of sodium nitrite (0.3 g in 10 ml water) followed through same needle by sodium thiosulphate (25 g in 50 ml). If available, inject intravenously, and as soon as possible, 20 ml of Kelocyanor, followed immediately by 50 ml of 50% glucose solution. (Kelocyanor contains 1.5% of cobalt edetate.)

Digoxin

The margin between the therapeutic and toxic dose is small. Nausea and vomiting are early symptoms of overdose, with mental confusion and visual disturbances. Pre-existing heart failure may be aggravated with severe arrhythmias; hypokalaemia in chronic overdose; hyperkalaemia in acute overdose.

Treatment. Gastric lavage, atropine by injection for brady-cardia, potassium chloride for hypokalaemia. Intravenous ligno-caine for cardiac arrhythmia. Specific antidote is intravenous Digibind; 40 mg binds 600 micrograms of digoxin.

Ethylene glycol ('anti-freeze')

Symptoms. Burning sensation in the throat, followed by malaise, sweating and vomiting; vertigo, drowsiness, coma, profuse sweating, acidosis, oliguria, anuria or haematuria. Death occurs from uraemia.

Treatment. Gastric lavage with potassium permanganate solution 1–5000, repeated later; calcium gluconate intravenously. Treat for renal failure. Penicillin prophylactically.

Ferrous sulphate and other iron salts

Symptoms. Initially epigastric pain, nausea, vomiting, haematemesis, collapse. Hours to days later, confusion, delirium, convulsions, respiratory and circulatory failure.

Treatment. Immediate i.m. injection of desferrioxamine 1 g in mild poisoning; gastric lavage with desferrioxamine 2 g/litre, leaving some in stomach. In severe poisoning, intravenous desferrioxamine in doses of 15 mg/kg hourly up to 6 g/24 hours. Desferrioxamine-iron complex gives orange-red colour to urine, continue until urine is normal colour or serum iron returns to standard level. X-ray to check all iron tablets removed after lavage. Apparent recovery may be followed by relapse.

Lead

Symptoms. Abdominal pain, vomiting, diarrhoea; ataxia, convulsion, muscular dysfunction. Delirium and coma indicate encephalopathy.

Treatment. Gastric lavage; in severe poisoning treat with chelating agent sodium calcium edetate (Ledclair) intravenously, dose up to 40 mg/kg twice a day for 5 days, repeated if necessary. Penicillamine as follow-up treatment, dose 1–2 g daily before food, continued until urinary lead level falls below 500 micrograms daily. BAL also used, dose 2.5 mg/kg i.m. daily for 10 days or more.

Lithium

Lithium poisoning due to reduced excretion may occur after prolonged lithium therapy, and may be linked with the use of diuretics.

Symptoms. Apathy, muscle twitching, tremor and diarrhoea. In severe poisoning, convulsions, renal failure and coma may occur, and are associated with a lithium plasma level of over 2 mmol/litre.

Treatment is supportive, restoration of electrolyte balance, diazepam intravenously for convulsions. Forced diuresis and dialysis in renal failure.

Nicotine

Present in various horticultural pesticide products. It is one of the most toxic compounds and in severe poisoning death may occur in a few minutes owing to respiratory paralysis.

Symptoms. Giddiness, nausea, vomiting, diarrhoea, confusion, convulsions, respiratory depression and collapse.

Treatment. Gastric lavage with weak potassium permanganate solution; remove contaminated clothing, wash skin. Oxygen, artificial respiration; atropine for bradycardia, intravenous diazepam for convulsions.

Opiates (including morphine, codeine, heroin, dextropropoxyphene etc.)

Symptoms. Preliminary mental excitement followed by headache, dizziness, nausea, 'pin-point' pupils, skin cold and clammy, face cyanosed, respiratory and circulatory depression, pulmonary oedema.

Treatment. Gastric lavage. Naloxone (Narcan) is a specific antagonist of morphine and related alkaloids and also of synthetic narcotic analgesics such as pethidine, methadone, etc. In overdose it is given by intravenous injection in doses of 0.5–2 mg, repeated at intervals of 2–3 minutes according to need up to a total dose of 10 mg. (Check diagnosis if respiratory function does not improve.) Alternatively, naloxone may be given by the intravenous infusion of 2 mg in 500 ml of glucose 5% or sodium choride 0.9%.

Organophosphorus insecticides

Symptoms. Tightness in the chest, headache, nausea, giddiness, anxiety, restlessness. Second-stage symptoms are respiratory distress, sweating, salivation, contraction of pupils, vomiting, abdominal cramps.

Treatment. The organophosphorus insecticides are powerful inhibitors of cholinesterase, so atropine is a specific antidote. It should be given by intramuscular or slow intravenous injection in doses of 1–4 mg repeated every 10 minutes or so until the patient is obviously fully atropinized or improving. Pralidoxime acts as a re-activator of cholinesterase but it is effective only within the first 24 hours of poisoning. It should be given with atropine in doses of 1–2 g by intramuscular or intravenous injection, repeated after 30 minutes if necessary. Emergency supplies are available from many regional distributing centres throughout the UK.

Paracetamol

Symptoms. Vomiting, gastrointestinal haemorrhage, tachycardia, hypotension, liver damage, renal necrosis, hypoglycaemia. With a high blood level of paracetamol the capacity of the liver to metabolize the drug may be overwhelmed, and severe liver damage may occur very rapidly.

Treatment. Gastric lavage, saline purge. Liver damage is caused by the binding of paracetamol or a metabolite to liver cells, and sulphur-containing drugs such as acetylcysteine and methionine have a protective action.

Treatment should be commenced within 15 hours of overdose if plasma paracetamol level greater than 200 mg/litre by the intravenous infusion of 150 mg/kg of acetylcysteine, followed by a further dose of 50 mg/kg over 4 hours, followed by a dose of 100 mg/kg infused over 16 hours. Methionine is also used, after emesis has been induced, in oral doses of 2.5 g 4–hourly for four doses.

Patients taking anticonvulsants, rifampicin and alcohol, and those with glutathione deficiency (anorexics, poorly nourished, HIV positives) are more susceptible to paracetamol poisoning; treat if paracetamol plasma level is half the normal toxic level. Naloxone may also be necessary if the poisoning is due to co-proxamol (paracetamol with dextropropoxyphene) or similar products (see opioids).

Paraquat (pesticide)

Liquid form very toxic; taken up slowly by pulmonary alveolar cells, leading to cell necrosis and pulmonary fibrosis. Corrosive to skin and membranes.

Symptoms. Burning of mouth, nausea, vomiting, later painful buccal ulceration, days later progressive alveolitis and bronchiolitis.

Treatment. Gastric lavage with 300 ml of Fuller's earth suspension 30%, leaving 300 ml in stomach. Activated charcoal 100 g if Fuller's earth not available, magnesium sulphate purge. Oxygen may increase lung damage. Splashes in eyes very irritant; irrigate and instil bactericidal eye-drops.

Petroleum products

Symptoms. Restlessness, coughing and choking of rapid onset, with nausea, vomiting and diarrhoea, drowsiness. Pulmonary congestion and convulsions after high doses, coma. Dyspnoea, cyanosis and pyrexia, especially if inhalation as well as ingestion has occurred; convulsions, coma.

Treatment. In mild cases no active measures need be taken.

No gastric lavage (risk of inhalation). Antibiotics in full doses prophylactically to reduce the risks of bronchopneumonia.

Phenol, creosote and related agents

Symptoms. Phenolic smell in breath and vomit. Burning pain in mouth and stomach which dulls later (local anaesthetic action). Diarrhoea with corrosive intestinal injury, convulsions, respiratory failure. Absorption through skin, leaving painless white patches turning red-brown.

Treatment. Remove contaminated clothing; gastric lavage. Saline purge.

Phenothiazines

Symptoms. Restlessness, cardiac arrhythmias, oculogyric crises, hypotension, parkinsonism, hypothermia, convulsions, respiratory depression.

Treatment. Gastric lavage; intravenous diazepam for convulsions, intravenous benztropine for parkinsonism.

Quinine

Symptoms. Tinnitus, vertigo, deafness, nausea and vomiting. Serious toxic effects are hypotension, cardiac arrhythmias, sudden loss of vision, convulsions and coma.

Treatment Gastric lavage; ECG monitoring; isosorbide dinitrate in loss of sight following retinal artery spasm; possibly also stellate ganglion block. Forced diuresis of doubtful value.

Snake bite

Acute snake bite is rare in the UK.

Symptoms. Local swelling, pain and redness. (If no swelling within 2 hours bite unlikely to contain venom.) Agitation, vomiting, diarrhoea, respiratory failure and collapse.

Treatment. If swelling extends beyond near major joint, give two ampoules of Zagreb antivenom, diluted with sterile saline, by slow intravenous injection. Same dose for children. Risk of allergic reactions – adrenaline injection must be immediately available.

Strychnine

Strychnine is used in certain vermin killers.

Symptoms. Feeling of suffocation, face livid, tetanic convulsions, sweating and exhaustion, rigid abdominal muscles. The jaw muscles are not affected till late (differentiation from tetanus).

Treatment. Short-acting barbiturate intravenously together with muscle relaxants to prevent convulsions. Gastric lavage after convulsions have been controlled. Protect from all possible stimuli. Further doses of barbiturate as required together with muscle relaxants. Oxygen. Recovery is usual if convulsive stage is survived.

29

Drugs and the Law

It has long been accepted that some legal control over the supply, storage and use of poisons is necessary, but with the extensive use of new and increasingly potent drugs, close control is more essential than ever.

DRUGS AND THE LAW

In the UK the manufacture, distribution and use of all medicinal substances is now controlled by the Medicines Act 1968, which combined and replaced several earlier Acts. Some drugs are more liable to misuse than others and are controlled more rigidly by the Misuse of Drugs Act 1971.

The Medicines Act 1968

Before any drug can be marketed in the UK the manufacturer must supply the Committee on Safety of Medicines with detailed information on its safety and proposed use. Approval may then be given for clinical trials, and if the results are satisfactory a Product Licence may be granted. This licence allows the manufacturer to recommend the product only for those conditions for which the clinical trial results were accepted. It may therefore take several years from the discovery of a drug in the laboratory to the marketing of a medicinal product for clinical use.

The Act is also concerned with checking the premises and procedures used to manufacture medicines. This monitoring is carried out by the Medicines Inspectorate, and approval of premises and procedures is required for hospital pharmacy production units as well as commercial pharmaceutical factories and warehouses.

The distribution of medicines is also controlled and here the Act divides products into three categories:

1. General Sales List (GSL) items: a restricted range of simple medicines which may be sold by any retailer.
2. Pharmacy-only medicines (P): those items which may be sold to the public without prescription, but only from a registered pharmacy.
3. Prescription-only medicines (POM): those items which may be sold or supplied to the public in accordance with a prescription issued by a medical practitioner or dentist. This list includes most of the potent drugs in current use.

These categories apply essentially to the supply of medicines directly to the public. In hospital practice it is accepted that any medicine should be prescribed by medical or dental staff. The differentiation into GSL, P and POM does not apply.

All medicines stored on the ward should be in locked cupboards or trolleys and internal, external and reagent preparations should be stored separately. In addition, ward drug trolleys should be immobilised when not in use. A lockable drug refrigerator should also be used for the increasing range of drugs needing storage below 8°C. The keys to these receptacles should be kept on the person of the sister or nurse in charge of the ward, who is also the person responsible for checking and signing orders for pharmaceutical supplies, checking correct storage is used and that stock is rotated regularly.

The Misuse of Drugs Act 1971

Drugs liable to misuse are controlled by the Misuse of Drugs Act 1971, and substances so controlled are usually known as 'Controlled Drugs' or 'CDs'. Under this Act controlled drugs are classified into five groups or schedules. Schedule 5 comprises certain controlled drugs such as codeine and morphine, but which are combined in such small amounts with non-toxic substances that misuse is both difficult and unlikely. Kaolin and Morphine Mixture is an example of a schedule 5 preparation, which may be obtained without a prescription.

Schedule 2 is far more important, as it includes all the drugs subjected to the CD Regulations, i.e. morphine, heroin, cocaine and any related synthetic drugs, but is extended to include amphetamines and other stimulants, and dihydrocodeine injection, all drugs liable to misuse. Schedule 3 includes the less powerful stimulants such as benzphetamine, the barbiturates, except those used for intravenous anaesthesia, the appetite depressants diethylpropion and mazindol, meprobamate, phentermine and pentazocine. These drugs are less likely to be misused, but on rational grounds should not be freely available to the public. Schedule 4 refers to the benzodiazepine group of hypnotics and anxiolytics, Schedule 1 includes hallucinogens and cannabis, which have no therapeutic applications, and are not prescribable. Any individual who requires such a drug for research must first obtain a special licence from the Home Office.

In brief, Schedule 2 and 3 drugs can be supplied only for a particular patient, whose name and address must be specified on the prescription, which must be written in ink, and signed and dated *entirely* by the prescriber personally. In addition, the dose to be taken must be specified, and the quantity to be supplied must be written in both *words and figures*. It is illegal to dispense any prescriptions for Controlled Drugs that do not give this essential information.

Hospital regulation

In hospitals, some relaxation of the strictly legal requirements is usually accepted, as the patient's own case sheet should supply the details of the patient's identity that the Act requires. Storage and record-keeping requirements are as stringent as those applying to Controlled Drugs generally. It should be noted that practitioners are prohibited from prescribing controlled drugs for addicts unless specifically licensed to do so.

Ward stocks of controlled drugs must be ordered in the special book supplied for the purpose, and the order must be signed by the sister or her deputy. The duplicate copies of the orders must be kept by the sister for at least 2 years.

All supplies of the controlled drugs must be signed for when received, and stored away from other drugs in a special locked cupboard, or locked inner compartment of the drugs cupboard, and the key must be kept *on the person* of the ward sister or deputy. No doctor has right of access to ward stocks of any drugs, as the responsibility for their storage and use rests with the sister-in-charge.

A written record should be made of every amount of a controlled drug received by a ward, and a detailed record kept of each dose given. Records of the administration of these drugs should be signed by the nurse who gives the dose, as well as by the nurse who checks the drug and dose.

A running record of stocks of all controlled drugs should be kept, and any wastage or loss must be recorded immediately, counter-signed and reported.

Table 29.1 indicates some of the Controlled Drugs of Schedules 2 and 3 and in general, the restrictions apply to derivatives and preparations of the drugs concerned, but in order to simplify the list, the names of many preparations have been omitted. Any

Table 29.1   Some Controlled Drugs (Schedules 2 and 3)

alfentanil	morphine; its salts and preparations unless diluted below 0.2% morphine or its
amphetamine	equivalent in a base from which the drug cannot be readily extracted
barbiturates	MST Continus
buprenorphine	Narphen
cocaine and its salts and preparations unless diluted below 0.1% cocaine in a base from which the drug	Omnopon
cannot be readily extracted	Omnopon-Scopolamine
codeine for injection	
Cyclimorph	Operidine
dexamphetamine	Opium preparations unless diluted below 0.2%
dextromoramide	morphine in a base from which the drug
diamorphine	cannot be readily extracted
diconal	Palfium
dihydrocodeine for injection	Pamergan preparations
dipipanone	papaveretum
	pentazocine
fentanyl	pethidine
heroin	phenazocine
	phenoperidine
levorphanol	Physeptone
	Rapifen
	Sevredol
methadone	SRM-Rhotard
	Sublimaze
	Temgesic
	Thalamonal

such drugs issued from a pharmacy must bear a label indicating that it is a Controlled Drug.

The strictly legal restrictions governing the use of controlled drugs should be regarded as the minimum, and in most hospitals a greater degree of control is exercised. The actual stock and the recorded stock of such drugs should be checked at frequent intervals, and any loss reported and investigated. Such a system reminds users of the need for care when dealing with potent drugs, and discourages misuse.

THE MEDICINES ACT, PART III

The control of medicinal substances generally has now been extended by the implementation of the Medicines Act, Part III. In effect, this increases the range of products not covered by other controls, so that any substance now in Part III can be sold only on prescription, and under the supervision of pharmacist.

These POM (prescription-only medicines) products include most medicines that few people would wish to buy without medical advice, and represents a further attempt to prevent the misuse of medicines. The list of medicines controlled in this way is too extensive to be given in this book, as it includes many drugs in current use. It is perhaps worthwhile mentioning that in many countries the control of drugs is much more lax than in the UK. In some parts of Europe, for example, antibiotics can be bought freely without prescription!

RESTRICTIONS ON PRESCRIBING

Since 1 April 1985, doctors have not been allowed to prescribe certain drugs under the National Health Service. Restricted products include antacids, laxatives, mild analgesics, cough remedies, expectorants, tonics and vitamins.

In practice, many drugs will continue to be prescribable under the official or non-proprietary name, but not under a brand or proprietary name. Thus if a product such as 'Valium' is required, it must be prescribed as 'diazepam'.

Many non-prescribable products (the so-called 'black list') are simple medicaments that can be easily purchased from any pharmacy; other more sophisticated products remain unprescribable. Special non-branded names have been drawn up for certain mixed products in current use as follows.

Approved names of mixed products:

Co-amilofruse: amiloride and frusemide (Frumil, Lasoride)

Co-amilozide: amiloride and hydrochlorothiazide (Amilco, Hypertane, Moduretic)

Co-amoxiclav: amoxycillin and clavulanic acid (Augmentin)

Co-beneldopa: levodopa and benserazide (Madopar)

Co-careldopa: levodopa and carbidopa (Sinemet)

Co-codamol: codeine and paracetamol (Paracodol)

Co-codaprin: codeine and aspirin (Codis)

Co-dydramol: dihydrocodeine and paracetamol (Paramol)

Co-fluampicil: ampicillin and flucloxacillin (Magnapen)

Co-flumactone: flumethiazide and spironolactone (Aldactide)

Co-phenotrope: diphenoxylate and atropine (Lomotil, Tropergen)

Co-prenozide: oxprenolol and cyclopenthiazide (Trasidex)

Co-proxamol: dextropropoxyhene and paracetamol (Cosalgesic, Distalgesic, Panalgesic)

Co-tenidone: atenolol and chlorthalidone (Tenoret, Tenoretic)

Co-triamterzide: triamterene and hydrochlorothiazide (Dyazide)

Co-trimoxazole: sulphamethoxazole and trimethaprim (Bactrim, Chemotrim, Septrim)

Appendices

Appendix I: Table of drug interactions

Many drug reactions, although undesirable, are of little clinical significance, and occur in but a few patients. They are more likely to occur in those patients mostly at risk, such as the elderly, and others in whom renal and liver function may have deteriorated. In some cases, the potential risks can be anticipated, as the combined use of beta-blockers, antihypertensives and diuretics can be expected to have additive effects. The following table merely gives an indication of the very extensive range of possible drug interactions, and nurses should report all drug reactions that they may observe.

Drug	Drug	Possible effects of combination
ACE-inhibitors	antihypertensives	It should be assumed that the effects of ACE-inhibitors will be enhanced by any other drug with an antihypertensive action, including diuretics
	cyclosporin	Hyperkalaemia
	potassium sparing diuretics	Hyperkalaemia
	levodopa	Increased hypotensive action
	contraceptives	Hypotensive action antagonized
	chlorpromazine	Severe postural hypotension
alcohol	CNS depressants	Depressive action enhanced
	antibacterials	Disulfiram-like reaction with cephamandole, metronidazole, noridazole and tinidazole
	oral anticoagulants	Effects enhanced
	antidiabetics	Effects enhanced by alcohol; flushing with chlorpropramide

Drug	Drug	Possible effects of combination
alcohol (cont'd)	antihistamines	Sedative effects enhanced
	antihypertensives	Effects enhanced
	antipsychotics	Sedative effects enhanced
aminoglycosides	capreomycin cisplatin cyclosporin vancomycin	Increased risk of oto/ nephrotoxicity
	loop diuretics	Muscle relaxants effects enhanced
amiodarone	anticoagulants(oral)	Anticoagulant effects increased
	anti-arrhythmics	Additive effects
	beta-blockers	Increased risk of bradycardia
	calcium channel blockers	
antidepressants (tricyclic)	anti-epileptics	Lower convulsive threshold
	antihypertensives	Hypotensive effects generally enhanced
	antihistamines	Sedative and anticholinergic effects increased
	central depressants	Sedative effects increased
antidiabetics	beta-blockers	Effects enhanced
	diuretics	Effects antagonized
cimetidine	pethidine	Increases plasma concentration
	anti-arrhythmics	Increases plasma concentration
	oral anticoagulants	Effects enhanced
	antipsychotics	Effects enhanced
	beta-blockers	Increases plasma concentration
	calcium channel blockers	Increases plasma concentration
corticosteroids	diuretics	Diuretic action antagonized
	anti-epileptics rifampicin	Increase metabolism and reduce effects of corticosteroid
cyclosporin	aminoglycosides co-trimoxazole amphotericin 4-quinolones	Increase risk of nephrotoxicity
	anti-epileptics rifampicin	Reduce plasma concentration of cyclosporin
	ketoconazole calcium channel blockers progestogen	Increase plasma concentration of cyclosporin

Drug	Drug	Possible effects of combination
digoxin	amiodarone quinine quinidine calcium channel blockers erythromycin	Plasma concentration of digoxin increased
disopyramide	anti-arrhythmics	Increased myocardial depression
	diuretics	Risk of increased toxicity if hypokalaemia occurs
	anti-epileptics rifampicin	Plasma concentration of disopyramide reduced
	erythromycin	Plasma concentration of disopyramide increased
diuretics	NSAIDs	Increased risk of nephrotoxicity; diuretic effects antagonized
	aminoglycosides	Increased risk of ototoxicity
	vancomycin	Increased risk of hyperkalaemia with potassium-sparers
	antidiabetics	Hypoglycaemic effects antagonized
	antihypertensives	Hypotensive action enhanced
	corticosteroids	Increased risk of hypokalaemia
	carbenoxolone contraceptives	Diuretic action antagonized
ergotamine	beta-blockers	Peripheral vasoconstriction increased
erythromycin	oral anticoagulants	Effects of warfarin and nicoumalone increased
	cyclosporin	Plasma concentration of cyclosporin increased
	theophylline	Plasma concentration of theophylline increased
ethosuximide	anti-epileptics	Convulsive threshold lowered
	antidepressants antipsychotics	Toxicity increased without increase in anticonvulsant activity
flecainide	other anti-arrhythmics	Myocardial depression increased
	cimetidine	Increased plasma concentration of flecainide

Drug	Drug	Possible effects of combination
fluconazole	anticoagulants	Effects of warfarin and nicoumalone enhanced
fluvoxamine	anticoagulants	Effects of warfarin and nicoumalone enhanced
griseofulvin	oral anticoagulants	Effects of warfarin and nicoumalone reduced
heparin	aspirin dipyridamole	Anticoagulant effects increased
iron — oral	magnesium trisilicate tetracycline	Absorption of iron reduced
isoniazid	anti-epileptics	Metabolism of some anti-epileptics reduced with an enhanced effect
ketoconazole and similar antifungals	antacids anticholinergics	Reduce absorption
	oral anticoagulants	Effects of warfarin and nicoumalone enhanced
	anti-epileptics	Effect of phenytoin enhanced
	rifampicin	Reduces plasma concentration of antifungals
	cyclosporin	Plasma concentration of cyclosporin increased
levodopa	MAOIs	Risk of hypertensive crisis
	benzodiazepines	Anxiolytic action antagonized
	antihypertensives	Hypotensive action enhanced
lignocaine	beta-blockers anti-arrhythmics	Myocardial depression increased
	diuretics	Effects of lignocaine antagonized
lithium	analgesics ACE-inhibitors	Reduce excretion and increase toxicity of lithium
	fluvoxamine fluoxetine	May cause tremor and convulsions
	diuretics anti-epileptics	May increase neurotoxicity
MAOIs	tricyclic antidepressants	CNS stimulation and hypertension
	antidiabetics	Hypoglycaemic effects enhanced

Drug	Drug	Possible effects of combination
MAOIs (cont'd)	anti-epileptics	Lower convulsive threshold
	antihypertensives	Hypotensive effects enhanced
	sympathomimetics	Risks of hypertensive crisis
methotrexate	aspirin NSAIDs probenecid	Excretion of methotrexate reduced with increased toxicity
methyldopa	alcohol antidepressants beta-blockers calcium channel blockers diuretics nitrates NSAIDs	Enhance hypotensive effects
	corticosteroids contraceptives carbenoxolone	Antagonize hypotensive effects
metoclopramide	analgesics	Absorption increased
	opioid analgesics anticholinergics	Antagonize effects of metoclopramide on gastrointestinal tract
	antipsychotics lithium	Increased risk of extrapyramidal effects
metronidazole	oral anticoagulants	Effects of warfarin and nicoumalone enhanced
	phenytoin	Metabolism of phenytoin inhibited
	cimetidine	Metabolism of metronidazole inhibited
	alcohol	Disulfiram-like reaction
muscle relaxants (tubarine and other non-depolarizing muscle relaxants)	aminoglycosides propranolol verapamil quinidine	Muscle relaxant effects enhanced
	neostigmine	Muscle relaxant effects antagonized
suxamethonium	cyclophosphamide thiotepa lithium	Muscle relaxant effects enhanced
	digoxin	May cause arrhythmias
NSAIDs	ACE-inhibitors diuretics	Hypotensive effects antagonized; diuretic effects

Drug	Drug	Possible effects of combination
NSAIDs *(cont'd)*		antagonized by NSAIDs and nephrotoxicity increased with risk of hyperkalaemia
	lithium	Excretion of lithium reduced
omeprazole	phenytoin warfarin	Anti-epileptic action enhanced; anticoagulant action enhanced
phenindione	aspirin cholestyramine dipyridamole clofibrate	Anticoagulant effects increased
	contraceptives vitamin K	Anticoagulant effects antagonized
phenytoin	aspirin amiodarone metronidazole viloxazine ketoconazole cimetidine sulphinpyrazone	Plasma concentration of phenytoin increased
	contraceptives theophylline cyclosporin digoxin anticoagulants	Metabolism increased by phenytoin
	antidepressants	Convulsive threshold lowered
probenecid	indomethacin naproxen cephalosporins penicillins nalidixic acid acyclovir captopril zidovudine methotrexate	Excretion reduced and plasma concentrations increased by probenecid
procainamide	amiodarone	Procainamide plasma concentration increased
	cimetidine other anti-arrhythmics	Increased myocardial depression
quinidine	amiodarone cimetidine verapamil	Quinidine plasma concentration increased
	diuretics	Toxicity increased in hyperkalaemia
	digoxin	Plasma concentrations of digoxin increased (reduce dose)

Drug	Drug	Possible effects of combination
quinidine *(cont'd)*	oral anticoagulants	Effects of warfarin and nicoumalone increased
	phenobarbitone phenytoin primidone	Plasma quinidine concentration reduced
	muscle relaxants	Relaxant action increased
quinine	cimetidine	Plasma quinine concentration increased
	digoxin	Plasma digoxin concentration increased (reduce dose)
quinolones	antacids	Reduce absorption
	theophylline	Plasma concentration of theophylline increased
	oral anticoagulants	Anticoagulant effects enhanced
rifampicin	antacids	Absorption decreased; rifampicin increases the metabolism and reduces the plasma concentrations of a wide range of drugs
sucralfate	antacids tetracyline	Reduce activity of sucralfate
	warfarin phenytoin	Absorption decreased by sucralfate
sulphinpyrazone	aspirin	Action of sulphinpyrazone antagonized
	oral anticoagulants	Effects of warfarin and nicoumalone enhanced
	antidiabetics	Effects enhanced
	phenytoin	Plasma concentrations of phenytoin enhanced
	theophylline	Plasma concentration of theophylline reduced
sympathomimetics	MAOIs	Risks of hypertensive crisis
	beta-blockers	Risks of severe hypertension
	corticosteroids	Risks in high doses of hypokalaemia
tamoxifen	oral anticoagulants	Anticoagulant effects may be markedly increased
theophylline	ciprofloxacin erythromycin diltiazem	Plasma theophylline levels increased

Drug	Drug	Possible effects of combination
theophylline (cont'd)	verapamil viloxazine contraceptives cimetidine aminoglutethimide rifampicin carbamazepine phenobarbitone phenytoin primidone sulphinpyrazone	Plasma levels of theophylline reduced
	beta-blockers	May cause bronchospasm
thyroxine	oral anticoagulants	Effects of warfarin, phenindione nicoumalone increased
	propranolol	Effects of propranolol reduced
	rifampicin carbamazepine phenobarbitone phenytoin primidone	Metabolism of thyroxine increased
valproate	antidepressants antipsychotics	Convulsive threshold lowered
	aspirin	Effects of valproate increased
	anticonvulsants	May increase toxicity and sedation
vancomycin	aminoglycosides	Increased risk of ototoxicity
	loop diuretics cephalosporins	Increased risk of nephrotoxicity
warfarin	analgesics (NSAIDs) allopurinol alcohol amiodarone choral hydrate cimetidine clofibrates ketoconazole and related antifungals sulphinpyrazone tamoxifen	Anticoagulant effects increased markedly by azapropazone
	many non-penicillin antibiotics rifamycins griseofulvin aminoglutethimide contraceptives sucralfate	Anticoagulant effects reduced

Appendix II: Approved and brand names of drugs

Approved name	Proprietary name	Main action or indication
acarbose	Glucobay	diabetes
acebutolol	Sectral	hypertension
acemetacin	Emflex	arthritis
acetazolamide	Diamox	glaucoma
acetylcholine	Miochol	cataract surgery
acetylcysteine	Fabrol	mucolytic, paracetamol overdose
acipimox	Olbetam	hyperlipidaemia
acitretin	Neotigason	psoriasis
aclarubicin	Aclacin	cytotoxic
acrivastine	Semprex	antihistamine
acrosoxacin	Eradacin	gonorrhoea
actinomycin D	Cosmegen	cytotoxic
acyclovir	Zovirax	antiviral
adenosine	Adenocor	anti-arrhythmic
albendazole	Eskazole	anthelmintic
alclometasone	Modrasone	topical corticosteroid
aldesleukin	Proleukin	cytotoxic
alfacalcidol	Alfa D, One-Alpha	vitamin D deficiency
alfentanil	Rapifen	narcotic analgesic
alfuzosin	Xatral	prostatic hyperplasia
allopurinol	Zyloric, Caplenal	gout
allylestrenol	Gestanin	progestogen
alprazolam	Xanax	antidepressant
alprostadil	Prostin VR	maintenance of ductus arteriosus in neonates
alteplase	Actilyse	fibrinolytic
alverine	Spasmonal	antispasmodic

Approved name	Proprietary name	Main action or indication
amantadine	Symmetrel	parkinsonism
amikacin	Amikin	antibiotic
amiloride	Midamor	diuretic
aminoglutethimide	Orimeten	cytotoxic
amiodarone	Cordarone X	anti-arrhythmic
amitriptyline	Lentizol, Tryptizol	antidepressant
amlodipine	Istin	calcium antagonist
amorolfine	Loceryl	antifungal
amoxapine	Asendis	antidepressant
amoxycillin	Amoxil, Almodan	antibiotic
amphotericin	AmBisome, Amphocil, Fungilin, Fungizone	antifungal
ampicillin	Amfipen, Penbritin	antibiotic
amsacrine	Amsidine	cytotoxic
amylobarbitone	Amytal	hypnotic
ancrod	Arvin	anticoagulant
anistreplase	Eminase	fibrinolytic
apraclonidine	Iopidine	cataract surgery
aprotinin	Trasylol	haemostatic
astemizole	Hismanal	antihistamine
atenolol	Tenormin	beta-blocker
atracurium	Tracrium	muscle relaxant
auranofin	Ridaura	rheumatoid arthritis
azapropazone	Rheumox	antirheumatic
azatadine	Optimine	antihistamine
azathioprine	Azamune, Imuran	immunosuppressive
azelaic acid	Skinoren	acne
azelastine	Rhinolast	rhinitis
azithromycin	Zithromax	antibiotic
aztreonam	Azactam	antibiotic
bacampicillin	Ambaxin	antibiotic
baclofen	Lioresal	muscle relaxant
bambuterol	Bambec	asthma
beclomethasone	Becotide	corticosteroid
beclomethasone	Propaderm	topical corticosteroid

Approved name	Proprietary name	Main action or indication
bendrofluazide	Aprinox, Neo-Naclex	diuretic
benorylate	Benoral	analgesic
benperidol	Anquil	tranquillizer
benzalkonium chloride	Roccal	antiseptic
benzhexol	Artane, Broflex	parkinsonism
benztropine	Cogentin	parkinsonism
benzylpenicillin	Crystapen	antibiotic
beractant	Survanta	neo-natal respiratory distress
betahistine	Serc	Ménière's syndrome
betamethasone	Betnelan, Betnesol	corticosteroid
betamethasone	Betnovate	topical corticosteroid
betaxolol	Kerlone	beta-blocker
bethanechol	Myotonine	smooth muscle stimulant
bezafibrate	Bezalip	hyperlipidaemia
biperiden	Akineton	parkinsonism
bisacodyl	Dulcolax	laxative
bisoprolol	Emcor, Monocor	beta-blocker
botulinum toxin	Botox, Dysport	blepharospasm
bretylium tosylate	Bretylate	cardiac arrhythmias
bromazepam	Lexotan	anxiolytic
bromocriptine	Parlodel	lactation suppressant
brompheniramine	Dimotane	antihistamine
budesonide	Pulmicort, Rhinocort	rhinitis
bumetanide	Burinex	diuretic
bupivacaine	Marcain	anaesthetic
buprenorphine	Temgesic	analgesic
buserelin	Suprefact	prostatic carcinoma
buspirone	Buspar	anxiolytic
busulphan	Myleran	cytotoxic
butobarbitone	Soneryl	hypnotic
cabergoline	Dostinex	inhibition of lactation
cadexomer iodine	Iodosorb	leg ulcers
calcipotriol	Dovonex	psoriasis
calcitonin	Calcitare	hormone

Approved name	Proprietary name	Main action or indication
calcitriol	Rocaltrol	vitamin D deficiency
canrenoate	Spiroctan-N	diuretic
capreomycin	Capastat	antibiotic
captopril	Acepril, Capoten	ACE inhibitor
carbamazepine	Tegretol	epilepsy
carbaryl	Carylderm, Derbac	parasiticide
carbenicillin	Pyopen	antibiotic
carbenoxolone	Bioral, Bioplex	mouth ulcer
carbimazole	Neo-Mercazole	thyrotoxicosis
carbocisteine	Mucodyne	mucolytic
carboplatin	Paraplatin	cytotoxic
carboprost	Hemabate	post-partum haemorrhage
carisoprodol	Carisoma	muscle relaxant
carmustine	BiCNU	cytotoxic
carteolol	Teoptic	glaucoma
cefaclor	Distaclor	antibiotic
cefadroxil	Baxan	antibiotic
cefixime	Suprax	antibiotic
cefodizime	Timecef	antibiotic
cefotaxime	Claforan	antibiotic
cefoxitin	Mefoxin	antibiotic
cefpodoxime	Orelox	antibiotic
cefsulodin	Monaspor	antibiotic
ceftazidime	Fortum	antibiotic
ceftizoxime	Cefizox	antibiotic
ceftriaxone	Rocephin	antibiotic
cefuroxime	Zinacef, Zinnat	antibiotic
celeprolol	Celectol	beta-blocker
cephalexin	Ceporex, Keflex	antibiotic
cephamandole	Kefadol	antibiotic
cephazolin	Kefzol	antibiotic
cephradine	Velosef	antibiotic
cetirizine	Zirtek	antihistamine
chenodeoxycholic acid	Chendol, Chenofalk	gallstones

Approved name	Proprietary name	Main action or indication
chloral hydrate	Noctec, Welldorm	hypnotic
chlorambucil	Leukeran	cytotoxic
chloramphenicol	Chloromycetin, Kemicetine	antibiotic
chlordiazepoxide	Librium, Tropium	tranquillizer
chlorhexidine	Hibitane	antiseptic
chlormethiazole	Heminevrin	hypnotic
chlormezanone	Transcopal	anxiolytic
chloroquine	Avloclor, Nivaquine	antimalarial
chlorothiazide	Saluric	diuretic
chlorpheniramine	Piriton	antihistamine
chlorpromazine	Largactil	tranquillizer
chlorpropamide	Diabinese	hypoglycaemic
chlortetracycline	Aureomycin	antibiotic
chlorthalidone	Hygroton	diuretic
cholestyramine	Questran	bile acid binder
choline theophyllinate	Choledyl, Sabidal	bronchospasm
chymotrypsin	Zonulysin	cataract surgery
cilazapril	Vascase	ACE-inhibitor
cimetidine	Dyspamet, Tagamet	H_2-blocker
cinnarizine	Stugeron	anti-emetic
cinoxacin	Cinobac	antibiotic
ciprofibrate	Modalim	hyperlipidaemia
ciprofloxacin	Ciproxin	antibacterial
cisapride	Alimix, Prepulsid	oesophageal reflux
cisplatin	Neoplatin, Platosin	cytotoxic
clarithromycin	Klaricid	antibiotic
clemastine	Tavegil	antihistamine
clindamycin	Dalacin C	antibiotic
clobazam	Frisium	tranquillizer
clobetasol	Dermovate	topical corticosteroid
clobetasone	Eumovate	topical corticosteroid
clodronate	Bonefos	hypercalcaemia of malignancy

Approved name	Proprietary name	Main action or indication
clofazimine	Lamprene	antileprotic
clofibrate	Atromid S	hyperlipidaemia
clomiphene	Clomid, Serophene	infertility
clomipramine	Anafranil	antidepressant
clonazepam	Rivotril	epilepsy
clonidine	Catapres, Dixarit	hypertension, migraine
clorazepate	Tranxene	anxiolytic
clotrimazole	Canestan	antifungal
cloxacillin	Orbenin	antibiotic
clozapine	Clozaril	antipsychotic
co-dergocrine	Hydergine	dementia
colestipol	Colestid	exchange resin
colfosceril	Exosurf	neonatal respiratory distress
colistin	Colomycin	antibiotic
corticotrophin	Acthar	hormone
cortisone	Cortistab, Cortisyl	corticosteroid
crisantaspase	Erwinase	leukaemia
crotamiton	Eurax	antipruritic
cyanocobalamin	Cytacon, Cytamen	anti-anaemic
cyclizine	Marzine, Valoid	anti-emetic
cyclopenthiazide	Navidrex	diuretic
cyclopentolate	Mydrilate	mydriatic
cyclophosphamide	Endoxana	cytotoxic
cyclosporin	Sandimmun	immunosuppressant
cyproheptadine	Periactin	antihistamine
cyproterone	Androcur, Cyprostat	anti-androgen
cytarabine	Alexan, Cytosar	cytotoxic
dacarbazine	DTIC	cytotoxic
dactinomycin	Cosmogen	cytotoxic
dalteparin	Fragmin	anticoagulant
danaparoid	Orgaran	anticoagulant
danazol	Danol	endometriosis
dantrolene	Dantrium	muscle relaxant
debrisoquine	Declinax	hypertension

Approved name	Proprietary name	Main action or indication
demecarium	Tosmelin	miotic
demeclocycline	Ledermycin	antibiotic
desferrioxamine	Desferal	iron poisoning
desflurane	Suprane	inhalation anaesthetic
desipramine	Pertofran	antidepressant
desmopressin	DDAVP	diabetes insipidus
desoxymethasone	Stiedex	local corticosteroid
dexamethasone	Decadron, Oradexon	corticosteroid
dexamphetamine	Dexedrine	appetite suppressant
dexfenfluramine	Adifax	appetite suppressant
dextromoramide	Palfium	analgesic
dextropropoxyphene	Doloxene	analgesic
diazepam	Atensine, Valium	tranquillizer
diazoxide	Eudemine	hypertension, hypoglycaemic
dichlorphenamide	Daranide	glaucoma
diclofenac	Rhumalgan, Voltarol	antirheumatic
dicobalt edetate	Kelocyanor	cyanide poisoning
dicyclomine	Merbentyl	antispasmodic
didanosine	Videx	antiviral
diethylcarbamazine	Banocide	filariasis
diethylpropion	Tenuate	appetite suppressant
diflucortolone	Nerisone	topical corticosteroid
diflunisal	Dolobid	analgesic
digoxin	Lanoxin	heart failure
digoxin antibody	Digibind	digoxin overdose
dihydrocodeine	DF118	analgesic
dihydrotachysterol	AT10, Tachyrol	hypocalcaemia
diloxanide furoate	Furamide	amoebiasis
diltiazem	Adizem, Britiazim, Tildiem	calcium antagonist
dimenhydrinate	Dramamine	antihistamine
dinoprost	Prostin F2	uterine stimulant
dinoprostone	Prostin E2	uterine stimulant
diphenoxylate	Lomotil	diarrhoea
dipivefrine	Propine	glaucoma

Approved name	Proprietary name	Main action or indication
dipyridamole	Persantin	vasodilator
disodium etidronate	Didronel	Paget's disease
disodium pamidronate	Aredia	Paget's disease
disopyramide	Dirythmin-SA, Rythmodan	cardiac arrhythmias
distigmine	Ubretid	urinary retention
disulfiram	Antabuse	alcoholism
dobutamine	Dobutrex	cardiac stimulant
docusate sodium	Dioctyl	laxative
domperidone	Motilium	anti-emetic
dopamine	Intropin	cardiac stimulant
dopexamine	Dopacard	cardiac surgery
dornase alfa	Pulmozyme	cystic fibrosis
dothiepin	Prothiaden	antidepressant
doxapram	Dopram	respiratory stimulant
doxazosin	Cardura	hypertension
doxepin	Sinequan	antidepressant
doxorubicin	Adriamycin	antibiotic
doxycycline	Nordox, Vibramycin	antibiotic
droperidol	Droleptan	neuroleptic
dydrogesterone	Duphaston	progestogen
econazole	Ecostatin, Pevaryl	antifungal
ecothiopate iodide	Phospholine iodide	glaucoma
edrophonium	Camsilon	diagnostic
enalapril	Innovace	ACE-inhibitor
enflucloxacillin	Floxapen, Stafoxil	antibiotic
enflurane	Enthrane	inhalation anaesthetic
enoxaparin	Clexane	anticoagulant
enoximone	Perfan	heart failure
epirubicin	Pharmorubicin	cytotoxic
epoprostenol	Flolan	bypass surgery
ergotamine	Lingraine	migraine
erythromycin	Erythrocin, Ilotycin	antibiotic
erythropoietin	Eprex, Recormon	anaemia in chronic renal failure
esmolol	Brevibloc	beta-blocker

Approved name	Proprietary name	Main action or indication
estramustine	Estracyt	cytotoxic
ethacrynic acid	Edecrin	diuretic
ethambutol	Myambutol	tuberculosis
ethamivan	Clairvan	respiratory stimulant
ethamsylate	Dicynene	haemostatic
ethosuximide	Emeside, Zarontin	anticonvulsant
etidronate	Didronel	Paget's disease
etodolac	Lodine	arthritis
etomidate	Hypnomidate	i.v. anaesthetic
etoposide	Vepesid	cytotoxic
Factor VIII	Kogenate Monoclate-P	haemophilia A
Factor IX	Mononine	haemophilia B
famciclovir	Famvir	antiviral
famotidine	Pepcid-PM	H_2-blocker
felodipine	Plendil	hypertension
fenbufen	Lederfen	antirheumatic
fenfluramine	Ponderax	appetite suppressant
fenofibrate	Lipantil	hyperlipidaemia
fenoprofen	Fenopron, Progesic	arthritis
fenoterol	Berotec	bronchitis
fentanyl	Sublimaze	analgesic
filgrastim	Neupogen	neutropenia
finasteride	Proscar	prostatic hyperplasia
flavoxate	Urispas	antispasmodic
flecainide	Tambocor	cardiac arrhythmias
fluclorolone	Topilar	topical corticosteroid
fluconazole	Diflucan	antifungal
flucytosine	Alcobon	antifungal
fludrocortisone	Florinef	corticosteroid
flumazenil	Anexate	benzodiazepine antagonist
flunisolide	Syntaris	corticosteroid
flunitrazepam	Rohypnol	hypnotic
fluocinolone	Synalar	topical corticosteroid
fluocinonide	Metosyn	topical corticosteroid

Approved name	Proprietary name	Main action or indication
fluocortolone	Ultralanum	topical corticosteroid
fluorometholone	FML	topical corticosteroid
fluoxetine	Prozac	antidepressant
flupenthixol	Depixol	schizophrenia
fluphenazine	Modecate, Moditen	schizophrenia
flurandrenolone	Haelan	topical corticosteroid
flurazepam	Dalmane	hypnotic
flurbiprofen	Froben	arthritis
fluspirilene	Redeptin	schizophrenia
flutamide	Drogenil	prostatic carcinoma
fluticasone	Cutivate	topical corticosteroid
fluticasone	Flixonase	allergic rhinitis
fluticasone	Flixotide	bronchodilator
fluvastatin	Lescol	hyperlipidaemia
fluvoxamine	Faverin	antidepressant
folinic acid	Refolinon	methotrexate antidote
formestane	Lentaron	cytotoxic
foscarnet	Foscavir	antiviral
fosfestrol	Honvan	cytotoxic
fosfomycin	Monuril	urinary infections
fosinopril	Staril	ACE-inhibitor
framycetin	Soframycin	antibiotic
frusemide	Dryptal, Lasix	diuretic
gabapentin	Neurontin	epilepsy
gallamine	Flaxedil	muscle relaxant
gamolenic acid	Epogam	eczema
ganciclovir	Cymevene	antiviral
gelatin	Gelofusine	blood volume expander
gemeprost	Cervagem	prostaglandin
gemfibrozil	Lopid	hyperlipidaemia
gentamicin	Cidomycin, Genticin	antibiotic
gestrinone	Dimetriose	endometriosis
gestronol	Depostat	endometrial carcinoma
glibenclamide	Daonil, Euglucon	hypoglycaemic

Approved name	Proprietary name	Main action or indication
gliclazide	Diamicron	hypoglycaemic
glipizide	Glibenese, Minodiab	hypoglycaemic
gliquidone	Glurenorm	hypoglycaemic
glutamic hydrochloride	Murispin	achlorhydria
glutaraldehyde	Glutarol	warts
glyceryl trinitrate	Sustac, Tridil	angina
glycopyrronium	Robinul	antimuscarinic
glymidine	Gondafon	hypoglycaemic
gonadorelin	Fertilol	infertility
goserelin	Zoladex	prostatic carcinoma
granisetron	Kytril	anti-emetic
griseofulvin	Fulcin, Grisovin	antifungal
guanethidine	Ismelin	hypertension
guar gum	Guarem, Guarina	diabetes
halcinonide	Halciderm	topical corticosteroid
halofantrine	Halfan	antimalarial
haloperidol	Dozic, Haldol, Serenace	schizophrenia
halothane	Fluothane	anaesthetic
hetastarch	Elohes, Hespan	blood volume expander
hexamine hippurate	Hiprex	urinary antiseptic
hyaluronidase	Hyalase	enzyme
hydralazine	Apresoline	hypertension
hydrochlorothiazide	Esidrex, Hydrosaluric	diuretic
hydrocortisone	Corlan, Efcortelan, Hydrocortistab, Hydrocortisyl, Hydrocortone	corticosteroid
hydroflumethiazide	Hydrenox	diuretic
hydroxocobalamin	Cobalin-H, Neo-Cytamen	anti-anaemic
hydroxychloroquine	Plaquenil	antimalarial
hydroxyprogesterone	Proluton-Depot	progestogen
hydroxyurea	Hydrea	cytotoxic
hydroxyzine	Atarax	tranquillizer
hyoscine butyl bromide	Buscopan	antispasmodic

Approved name	Proprietary name	Main action or indication
ibuprofen	Brufen, Ebufac	arthritis
idarubicin	Zavedos	cytotoxic
idoxuridine	Iduridin	antiviral
ifosfamide	Mitoxana	cytotoxic
imipenem	Primaxin	antibiotic
imipramine	Tofranil	antidepressant
indapamide	Natrilix	hypertension
indomethacin	Imbrilon, Indocid	arthritis
indoramin	Baratol	beta-blocker
inosine pranobex	Imunovir	antiviral
inositol nicotinate	Hexopal	vasodilator
interferon	Intron, Roferon, Wellferon	leukaemia
iopanoic acid	Telepaque	contrast agent
iophendylate	Myodil	contrast agent
iothalamic acid	Conray	contrast agent
ipratropium	Atrovent	bronchodilator
iprindole	Prondol	antidepressant
iron-sorbitol	Jectofer	iron-deficiency anaemia
isocarboxazid	Marplan	antidepressant
isoconazole	Travogyn	candidiasis
isoniazid	Rimifon	tuberculosis
isoprenaline	Saventrine	bronchospasm
isosorbide dinitrate	Cedocard, Vascardin	angina
isosorbide mononitrate	Elantan, Monit	angina
isotretinoin	Isotrex, Roaccutane	acne
isradipine	Prescal	calcium antagonist
itraconazole	Sporanox	antifungal
ivermectin	Mectizan	filariasis
kanamycin	Kannasyn	antibiotic
ketamine	Ketalar	anaesthetic
ketoconazole	Nizoral	antifungal
ketoprofen	Alrheumat, Orudis	arthritis
ketorolac	Toradol	analgesic
ketotifen	Zaditen	anti-asthmatic

Approved name	Proprietary name	Main action or indication
labetalol	Labrocol, Trandate	beta-blocker
lacidipine	Motens	calcium antagonist
lactitol	–	laxative
lactulose	Duphalac, Laxose	laxative
lamotrigine	Lamictal	epilepsy
lansoprazole	Zoton	peptic ulcer
lenograstim	Granocyte	neutropenia
leuprorelin	Prostap	prostatic carcinoma
levobunolol	Betagan	glaucoma
levodopa	Brocadopa, Larodopa	parkinsonism
lignocaine	Xylocaine	anaesthetic
lindane	Quellada	pediculosis
liothyronine	Tertroxin	thyroid deficiency
lisinopril	Carace, Zestril	ACE-inhibitor
lithium carbonate	Camcolit, Phasal	mania
lodoxamide	Alomide	allergic conjunctivitis
lofepramine	Gamanil	antidepressant
lofexidine	Britlofex	opioid withdrawal
lomustine	CCNU	cytotoxic
loperamide	Arret, Imodium	diarrhoea
loratadine	Clarityn	antihistamine
lorazepam	Ativan	tranquillizer
loxapine	Loxapac	antipsychotic
lymecycline	Tetralysal	antibiotic
lypressin	Syntopressin	diabetes insipidus
lysuride	Revanil	parkinsonism
magaldrate	Dynese	antacid
malathion	Derbac, Prioderm	parasiticide
maprotiline	Ludiomil	antidepressant
mebendazole	Vermox	anthelmintic
mebeverine	Colofac	antispasmodic
medroxyprogesterone	Provera	progestogen
mefenamic acid	Ponstan	arthritis
mefloquine	Larium	malaria

Approved name	Proprietary name	Main action or indication
mefruside	Baycaron	diuretic
megestrol	Megace	cytotoxic
melphalan	Alkeran	cytotoxic
menadiol	Synkavit	hypoprothrombinaemia
menotrophin	Pergonal	hypogonadism
mepenzolate	Cantil	antispasmodic
meprobamate	Equanil	tranquillizer
meptazinol	Meptid	analgesic
mequitazine	Primalan	antihistamine
mercaptopurine	Puri-Nethol	cytotoxic
mesalazine	Asacol, Pentasa, Salofalk	ulcerative colitis
mesna	Uromitexan	urotoxicity due to cyclophosphamide
mesterolone	Pro-viron	androgen
metaraminol	Aramine	hypotension
metformin	Glucophage	hypoglycaemic
methadone	Physeptone	analgesic
methocarbamol	Robaxin	muscle relaxant
methohexitone	Brietal	anaesthetic
methotrexate	Maxtrex	cytotoxic
methotrimeprazine	Nozinan	pain in terminal cancer
methoxamine	Vasoxine	vasoconstrictor
methylcellulose	Celevac	laxative
methylcysteine	Visclair	mucolytic
methyldopa	Aldomet	hypertension
methylphenobarbitone	Prominal	epilepsy
methylprednisolone	Medrone	corticosteroid
methysergide	Deseril	migraine
metirosine	Demser	phaeochromocytoma
metoclopramide	Maxolon, Primperan	anti-emetic
metolazone	Metenix, Xuret	diuretic
metoprolol	Betaloc, Lopresor	beta-blocker
metronidazole	Flagyl, Zadstat	anaerobic infections, trichomoniasis

Approved name	Proprietary name	Main action or indication
metyrapone	Metopirone	resistant oedema
mexiletine	Mexitil	cardiac arrhythmias
mianserin	Bolvidon, Norval	antidepressant
miconazole	Daktarin, Dermonistat	antifungal
midazolam	Hypnovel	i.v. anaesthetic
mifepristone	Mifegyne	termination of pregnancy
milrinone	Primacor	severe heart failure
minocycline	Minocin	antibiotic
minoxidil	Loniten	hypertension
misoprostol	Cytotec	peptic ulcer
mitozantrone	Novantrone	cytotoxic
mivacurium	Mivacrom	muscle relaxant
moclobemide	Manerix	antidepressant
molgramostim	Leucomax	neutropenia
mometasone	Elocon	topical corticosteroid
moracizine	Ethmozine	anti-arrhythmic
monosulfiram	Tetmosol	scabies
mupirocin	Bactroban	topical antibiotic
nabilone	Cesamet	anti-emetic
nabumetone	Relifex	arthritis
nadolol	Corgard	beta-blocker
nafarelin	Synarel	endometriosis
naftidrofuryl	Praxilene	vasodilator
nalbuphine	Nubain	analgesic
nalidixic acid	Negram	urinary antiseptic
naloxone	Narcan	narcotic antagonist
naltrexone	Nalorex	opioid dependence
nanadrolone	Deca-Durabolin	anabolic steroid
naproxen	Laraflex, Naprosyn	arthritis
nedocromil	Tilade	anti-asthmatic
nefopam	Acupan	analgesic
neostigmine	Prostigmin	myasthenia
netilmicin	Netillin	antibiotic
nicardipine	Cardene	calcium antagonist

Approved name	Proprietary name	Main action or indication
niclosamide	Yomesan	anthelmintic
nicotinyl alcohol	Ronicol	vasodilator
nicoumalone	Sinthrome	anticoagulant
nifedepine	Adalat, Coracten	calcium antagonist
nimodipine	Nimotop	calcium antagonist
nitrazepam	Mogadon	hypnotic
nitrofurantoin	Furadantin, Macrodantin	urinary antiseptic
nizatidine	Axid	H_2-blocker
noradrenaline	Levophed	hypotension
norethisterone	Primolut N, Menzol	progestogen
norfloxacin	Utinor	urinary tract infections
nortriptyline	Allegron, Aventyl	antidepressant
noxythiolin	Noxyflex	antiseptic
nystatin	Nystan	antifungal
octreotide	Sandostatin	carcinoid syndrome
oestradiol	Climaval	menopausal symptoms
ofloxacin	Exocin, Tarivid	antibacterial
olsalazine	Dipentum	ulcerative colitis
omeprazole	Losec	peptic ulcer
ondansetron	Zofran	anti-emetic
orciprenaline	Alupent	bronchodilator
orphenadrine	Biorphen, Disipal	parkinsonism
oxamniquine	Vansil	anthelmintic
oxatomide	Tinset	antihistamine
oxitropium	Oxivent	bronchodilator
oxpentifylline	Trental	vasodilator
oxprenolol	Trasicor	beta-blocker
oxybutynin	Cystrin, Ditropan	urinary incontinence
oxymetazoline	Afrazine	nasal decongestant
oxymetholone	Anapolon	anabolic steroid
oxypertine	Integrin	tranquillizer
oxytetracycline	Terramycin	antibiotic
paclitaxel	Taxol	cytotoxic
pamidronate	Aredia	hypercalcaemia of malignancy

Approved name	Proprietary name	Main action or indication
pancuronium	Pavulon	muscle relaxant
papaveretum	Omnopon	analgesic
paroxetine	Seroxat	antidepressant
pemoline	Volital	cerebral stimulant
penicillamine	Distamine, Pendramine	Wilson's disease
pentaerythritol tetranitrate	Mycardol	angina
pentamidine	Pentacarinat	leishmaniasis
pentastarch	Pentaspan	blood volume expander
pentazocine	Fortral	analgesic
pentostatin	Nipent	hairy-cell leukaemia
pergolide	Celance	parkinsonism
pericyazine	Neulactil	schizophrenia
perindopril	Coversyl	ACE-inhibitor
perphenazine	Fentazin	schizophrenia
phenazocine	Narphen	analgesic
phenelzine	Nardil	antidepressant
phenindamine	Thephorin	antihistamine
phenindione	Dindevan	anticoagulant
pheniramine	Daneral	antihistamine
phenoperidine	Operidine	analgesic
phenoxybenzamine	Dibenyline	vasodilator
phenoxymethyl-penicillin	Distaquaine V-K, V-Cil-K	antibiotic
phentermine	Duromine, Ionamin	appetite suppressant
phentolamine	Rogitine	phaeochromocytoma
phenylbutazone	Butazolidin	ankylosing spondylitis
phenytoin	Epanutin	epilepsy
phytomenadione	Konakion	hypoprothrombinaemia
pimozide	Orap	schizophrenia
pindolol	Visken	beta-blocker
pipenzolate	Piptal	antispasmodic
piperacillin	Pipril	antibiotic
pipothiazine	Piportil	antipsychotic
piracetam	Nootropil	tics

Approved name	Proprietary name	Main action or indication
pirbuterol	Exirel	bronchodilator
pirenzepine	Gastrozepin	peptic ulcer
piretanide	Arelix	diuretic
piroxicam	Feldene	antirheumatic
pivampicillin	Pondocillin	antibiotic
pizotifen	Sanomigran	migraine
plicamycin	Mithracin	malignant hypercalcaemia
podophyllotoxin	Condyline	penile warts
poldine	Nacton	antispasmodic
polyestradiol	Estradurin	prostatic carcinoma
polygeline	Haemaccel	blood volume expander
polynoxylin	Anaflex	antiseptic
polythiazide	Nephril	diuretic
poractant	Curoserf	neonatal respiratory distress
pravastatin	Lipostat	hyperlipidaemia
prazosin	Hypovase	hypertension
prednisolone	Codelsol, Deltacortril, Deltastab, Precortisyl,	corticosteroid
prednisone	Decortisyl	corticosteroid
prilocaine	Citanest	anaesthetic
primidone	Mysoline	epilepsy
probenecid	Benemid	gout
probucol	Lurselle	hyperlipidaemia
procainamide	Pronestyl	cardiac arrhythmias
procaine-penicillin	Bicillin	antibiotic
procarbazine	Natulan	cytotoxic
prochlorperazine	Stemetil	anti-emetic, vertigo
procyclidine	Arpicolin, Kemadrin	parkinsonism
proguanil	Paludrine	antimalarial
promazine	Sparine	tranquillizer
promethazine	Phenergan	antihistamine
promethazine theoclate	Avomine	anti-emetic
propafenone	Arythmol	cardiac arrhythmias
propantheline	Pro-Banthine	peptic ulcer

Approved name	Proprietary name	Main action or indication
propofol	Diprivan	i.v. anaesthetic
propranolol	Inderal	beta-blocker
propyliodone	Dionosil	contrast agent
protriptyline	Concordin	antidepressant
provastatin	Lipostat	hyperlipidaemia
proxymetacaine	Ophthaine	corneal anaesthetic
pyrantel	Combantrin	anthelmintic
pyrazinamide	Zinamide	tuberculosis
pyridostigmine	Mestinon	myasthenia
pyrimethamine	Daraprim	antimalarial
quinalbarbitone	Seconal	hypnotic
quinapril	Accupro	ACE-inhibitor
ramipril	Tritace	ACE-inhibitor
ranitidine	Zantac	H_2-blocker
razoxane	Razoxin	cytotoxic
remoxipride	Roxiam	schizophrenia
reproterol	Bronchodil	bronchodilator
rifabutin	Mycobutin	tuberculosis
rifampicin	Rifadin, Rimactane	tuberculosis .
rimiterol	Pulmadil	bronchodilator
risperidone	Risperdal	antipsychotic
ritodrine	Yutopar	premature labour
rocuronium	Esmeron	muscle relaxant
salbutamol	Ventolin	bronchospasm
salcatonin	Calsynar, Miacalcic	Paget's disease
salmeterol	Serevent	bronchospasm
salsalate	Disalcid	antirheumatic
selegiline	Eldepryl	parkinsonism
sermorelin	Geref	growth hormone
sertraline	Lustral	antidepressant
silver sulphadiazine	Flamazine	antibacterial
simvastatin	Zocor	hyperlipidaemia
sodium acetrizoate	Diaginol	contrast agent
sodium aurothiomalate	Myocrisin	rheumatoid arthritis

Approved name	Proprietary name	Main action or indication
sodium clodronate	Bonefos, Loron	hypercalcaemia of malignancy
sodium cromoglycate	Intal, Rynacrom	anti-allergic
sodium diatrizoate	Hypaque	contrast agent
sodium fusidate	Fucidin	antibiotic
sodium iothalamate	Conray	contrast agent
sodium ipodate	Biloptin	contrast agent
sodium iron edetate	Sytron	anti-anaemic
sodium metrizoate	Triosil	contrast agent
sodium nitroprusside	Nipride	hypertensive crisis
sodium picosulphate	Laxoberal	laxative
sodium stibogluconate	Pentostam	leishmaniasis
sodium valproate	Epilim	epilepsy
somatropin	Genotropin, Saizen	growth hormone
sotalol	Beta-Cardone, Sotacor	beta-blocker
spectinomycin	Trobicin	antibiotic
spironolactone	Aldactone, Spiroctan	diuretic
stanozolol	Stromba	anabolic steroid
streptokinase	Kabikinase, Streptase	thrombosis
sucralfate	Antepsin	peptic ulcer
sulfametopyrazine	Kelfizine	sulphonamide
sulindac	Clinoril	arthritis
sulphadimidine	Sulphamezathine	sulphonamide
sulphasalazine	Salazopyrin	ulcerative colitis
sulphinpyrazone	Anturan	gout
sulpiride	Dolmatil, Sulpitil	schizophrenia
sumatriptan	Imigran	migraine
suxamethonium	Anectine, Scoline	muscle relaxant
tamoxifen	Nolvadex, Tamofen	cytotoxic
teicoplanin	Targocid	antibiotic
temazepam	Normison	hypnotic
temocillin	Temopen	antibiotic
tenoxicam	Mobilflex	arthritis
terazosin	Hytrin	hypertension
terbinafine	Lamisil	antifungal

Approved name	Proprietary name	Main action or indication
terbutaline	Bricanyl	bronchospasm
terfenadine	Triludan	antihistamine
terlipressin	Glypressin	oesophageal bleeding
testosterone	Virormone	hypogonadism
tetrabenazine	Nitoman	chorea
tetracosactrin	Synacthen	corticotrophin
tetracycline	Achromycin, Tetrabid	antibiotic
theophylline	Nuelin	bronchodilator
thiabendazole	Mintezol	anthelmintic
thiabutosine	Ciba 1906	anthelmintic
thioguanine	Lanvis	cytotoxic
thiopentone	Intraval	i.v. anaesthetic
thioridazine	Melleril	tranquillizer
thymoxamine	Opilon	vasodilator
thyroxine	Eltroxin	thyroid deficiency
tiaprofenic acid	Surgam	arthritis
tibolone	Livial	menopausal symptoms
ticarcillin	Ticar	antibiotic
timolol	Blocadren, Betim	beta-blocker
tinidazole	Fasigyn	anaerobic infections
tinzaparin	Innohep, Logiparin	anticoagulant
tioconazole	Trosyl	antifungal
tobramycin	Nebcin	antibiotic
tocainide	Tonocard	cardiac arrhythmias
tolazamide	Tolanase	hypoglycaemic
tolbutamide	Rastinon	hypoglycaemic
tolmetin	Tolectin	antirheumatic
torasemide	Torem	diuretic
tramodol	Zydol	analgesic
trandolapril	Gopten, Odrik	ACE-inhibitor
tranexamic acid	Cyklokapron	antifibrinolytic
tranylcypromine	Parnate	antidepressant
trazodone	Molipaxin	antidepressant

Approved name	Proprietary name	Main action or indication
treosulfan	–	cytoxic
tretinoin	Retin-A	acne
triamcinolone	Adcortyl, Ledercort	corticosteroid
triamterene	Dytac	diuretic
tribavirin	Virazid	antiviral
triclofos	–	hypnotic
trientine	–	Wilson's disease
trifluoperazine	Stelazine	tranquillizer
trilostane	Modrenal	aldosteronism
trimeprazine	Vallergan	antihistamine
trimetaphan	Arfonad	hypotensive surgery
trimethoprim	Syraprim, Trimopan	antibacterial
trimipramine	Surmontil	antidepressant
triprolidine	Actidil	antihistamine
tropicamide	Mydriacyl	mydriatic
tropisetron	Navoban	anti-emetic
tryptophan	Optimax	antidepressant
tubocurarine	Jexin	muscle relaxant
tulobuterol	Brelomax, Respacal	bronchodilator
urokinase	Ukidan	hyphaemia, embolism
ursodeoxycholic acid	Destolit	gallstones
valproate	Epilim	epilepsy
valproic acid	Convulex	epilepsy
vancomycin	Vancocin	antibiotic
vecuronium	Norcuron	muscle relaxant
verapamil	Cordilox, Univer	angina, hypertension
vigabatrin	Sabril	anticonvulsant
viloxazine	Vivalan	antidepressant
vinblastine	Velbe	cytotoxic
vincristine	Oncovin	cytotoxic
vindesine	Eldisine	cytotoxic
warfarin	Marevan	anticoagulant
xamoterol	Corwin	mild heart failure
xipamide	Diurexan	diuretic

Approved name	Proprietary name	Main action or indication
xylometazoline	Otrivine	nasal decongestant
zidovudine	Retrovir	antiviral (AIDS)
zolpidem	Stilnoct	hypnotic
zopiclone	Zimovane	hypnotic
zuclopenthixol	Clopixol	schizophrenia

Proprietary name	Approved name	Main action or indication
Accupro	quinapril	ACE-inhibitor
Acepril	captopril	ACE-inhibitor
Achromycin	tetracycline	antibiotic
Aclacin	aclarubicin	cytotoxic
Acthar	corticotrophin	hormone
Actilyse	alteplase	fibrinolytic
Acupan	nefopam	analgesic
Adalat	nifedepine	calcium antagonist
Adcortyl	triamcinolone	topical corticosteroid
Adenocor	adenosine	anti-arrhythmic
Adifax	dexfenfluramine	appetite suppressant
Adizem	diltiazem	angina
Adriamycin	doxorubicin	antibiotic
Afrazine	oxymetazoline	nasal decongestant
Akineton	biperiden	parkinsonism
Alcobon	flucytosine	antifungal
Aldactone	spironolactone	resistant oedema
Aldomet	methyldopa	hypertension
Alexan	cytarabine	cytotoxic
Alfa D	alfacalcidol	vitamin D deficiency
Alimix	cisapride	oesophageal reflux
Alkeran	melphalan	cytotoxic
Allegron	nortriptyline	antidepressant
Aller-eze	clemastine	antihistamine
Almodan	amoxycillin	antibiotic
Alomide	lodoxamide	allergic conjunctivitis
Alrheumat	ketoprofen	arthritis
Alupent	orciprenaline	bronchospasm
Alupram	diazepam	anxiolytic
Aluzine	frusemide	diuretic
Ambaxin	bacampicillin	antibiotic
AmBisome	amphotericin	antifungal
Amfipen	ampicillin	antibiotic
Amikin	amikacin	antibiotic

Proprietary name	Approved name	Main action or indication
Amoxil	amoxycillin	antibiotic
Amphocil	amphotericin	antifungal
Amsidine	amsacrine	cytotoxic
Amytal	amylobarbitone	hypnotic
Anaflex	polynoxylin	antiseptic
Anafranil	clomipramine	antidepressant
Anapolon	oxymetholone	anabolic steroid
Androcur	cyproterone	anti-androgen
Anectine	suxamethonium	muscle relaxant
Anexate	flumazenil	benzodiazepine antagonist
Angilol	propranolol	beta-blocker
Angiozem	diltiazem	angina
Anquil	benperidol	tranquillizer
Antabuse	disulfiram	alcoholism
Antepsin	sucralfate	peptic ulcer
Anthranol	dithranol	psoriasis
Anturan	sulphinpyrazone	gout
Apresoline	hydralazine	hypertension
Aprinox	bendrofluazide	diuretic
Apsifen	ibuprofen	arthritis
Aquadrate	urea	ichthyosis
Aramine	metaraminol	vasoconstrictor
Aredia	disodium pamidronate	hypercalcaemia of malignancy
Arelix	piretanide	hypertension
Arfonad	trimetaphan	hypertensive surgery
Arpicolin	procyclidine	parkinsonism
Arpimycin	erythromycin	antibiotic
Arret	loperamide	diarrhoea
Artane	benzhexol	parkinsonism
Arvin	ancrod	anticoagulant
Arythmol	propafenone	cardiac arrhythmias
Asacol	mesalazine	ulcerative colitis
Ascabiol	benzyl benzoate	scabies
Asendis	amoxapine	antidepressant

Proprietary name	Approved name	Main action or indication
AT10	dihydrotachysterol	hypocalcaemia
Atarax	hydroxyzine	tranquillizer
Atensine	diazepam	tranquillizer
Ativan	lorazepam	tranquillizer
Atromid-S	clofibrate	hypercholesterolaemia
Atrovent	ipratropium	bronchodilator
Aureomycin	chlortetracycline	antibiotic
Aventyl	nortriptyline	antidepressant
Avlclor	chloroquine	antimalarial
Avomine	promethazine theoclate	anti-emetic
Axid	nizatidine	H_2-blocker
Azactam	aztreonam	antibiotic
Azamune	azathioprine	cytotoxic
Bactroban	mupirocin	topical antibiotic
Bambec	bambuterol	asthma
Banocide	diethylcarbamazine	filariasis
Baratol	indoramin	beta-blocker
Baxan	cefadroxil	antibiotic
Baycaron	mefruside	diuretic
Becloforte	beclomethasone	corticosteroid
Beconase	beclomethasone	rhinitis
Becotide	beclomethasone	corticosteroid
Bedranol SR	propranolol	beta-blocker
Bendogen	bethanidine	hypertension
Benemid	probenecid	gout
Benoral	benorylate	analgesic
Benoxyl	benzyl peroxide	acne
Benzagel	benzyl peroxide	acne
Berkaprine	azathioprine	cytotoxic
Berkatens	verapamil	angina, hypertension
Berkmycen	oxytetracycline	antibiotic
Berkolol	propranolol	beta-blocker
Berkozide	bendrofluazide	diuretic
Berotec	fenoterol	bronchitis

Proprietary name	Approved name	Main action or indication
Beta-Cardone	sotalol	beta-blocker
Betadine	povidone-iodine	antiseptic
Betagan	levobunolol	glaucoma
Betaloc	metapropolol	beta-blocker
Betim	timolol	beta-blocker
Betnelan	betamethasone	corticosteroid
Betnesol	betamethasone	corticosteroid
Betnovate	betamethasone	topical corticosteroid
Betoptic	betaxolol	glaucoma
Bextasol	betamethasone	local corticosteroid
Bezalip	bezafibrate	hyperlipidaemia
BiCNU	carmustine	cytotoxic
Biliodyl	phenobutiodil	contrast agent
Biloptin	sodium ipodate	contrast agent
Biltricide	praziquantel	anthelmintic
Biophylline	theophylline	bronchodilator
Bioplex	carbenoxolone	mouth ulcers
Bioral	carbenoxolone	mouth ulcers
Biorphen	orphenadrine	parkinsonism
Blocadren	timolol	beta-blocker
Bolvidon	mianserin	antidepressant
Bonefos	clodrinate	hypercalcaemia of malignancy
Botox	botulinum toxin	blepharospasm
Brelomax	tulobuterol	bronchodilator
Bretylate	bretylium	cardiac arrhythmias
Brevibloc	esmolol	beta-blocker
Bricanyl	terbutaline	bronchospasm
Brietal	methohexitone	anaesthetic
Britiazim	diltiazem	angina
Britlofex	lofexidine	opioid withdrawal
Brocadopa	levodopa	parkinsonism
Broflex	benzhexol	parkinsonism
Bronchodil	reproterol	bronchodilator
Brufen	ibuprofen	arthritis

Proprietary name	Approved name	Main action or indication
Buccastem	prochlorperazine	vertigo
Burinex	bumetanide	diuretic
Buscopan	hyoscine butyl bromide	antispasmodic
Buspar	buspirone	anxiolytic
Butazolidin	phenylbutazone	ankylosing spondylitis
Cacit	calcium carbonate	osteoporosis
Calabren	glibenclamide	hypoglycaemic
Calciparine	calcium heparin	anticoagulant
Calcisorb	sodium cellulose phosphate	hypercalciuria
Calcitare	calcitonin	Paget's disease
Calcium Resonium	exchange resin	hyperkalaemia
Calpol	paracetamol	analgesic
Calsynar	salcatonin	Paget's disease
Camcolit	lithium carbonate	mania
Camsilon	edrophonium	diagnosis of myasthenia gravis
Canestan	clotrimazole	antifungal
Cantil	mepenzolate	antispasmodic
Capastat	capreomycin	tuberculosis
Caplenal	allopurinol	gout
Capoten	captopril	ACE-inhibitor
Caprin	aspirin	arthritis
Carace	lisinopril	ACE-inhibitor
Cardene	nicardipine	calcium antagonist
Cardinol	propranolol	beta-blocker
Cardura	doxazosin	hypertension
Carisoma	carisprodol	muscle relaxant
Carylderm	carbaryl	parasiticide
Catapres	clonidine	hypertension
Caverject	alprostadil	prostaglandin
CCNU	lomustine	cytotoxic
Cedocard	isosorbide dinitrate	angina
Cefizox	ceftizoxime	antibiotic
Celance	pergolide	parkinsonism

Proprietary name	Approved name	Main action or indication
Celectol	celiprolol	beta-blocker
Celevac	methylcellulose	laxative
Centyl	bendrofluazide	diuretic
Ceporex	cephalexin	antibiotic
Cervagem	gemeprost	prostaglandin
Cesamet	nabilone	anti-emetic
Cetavlex	cetrimide	antiseptic
Chendol	chenodeoxycholic acid	gallstones
Chenofalk	chenodeoxycholic acid	gallstones
Chloromycetin	chloramphenicol	antibiotic
Choledyl	choline theophyllinate	bronchodilator
Ciba 1906	thiambutosine	leprosy
Cidomycin	gentamicin	antibiotic
Cilazapril	vascase	ACE-inhibitor
Ciloxan	ciprofloxacin	corneal ulcers
Cinobac	cinoxacin	antibiotic
Ciproxin	ciprofloxacin	antibacterial
Citanest	prilocaine	anaesthetic
Claforan	cefotaxime	antibiotic
Clairvan	ethamivan	respiratory stimulant
Clarityn	loratadine	antihistamine
Clexane	enoxaparin	anticoagulant
Climaval	oestradiol	menopausal symptoms
Clinoril	sulindac	arthritis
Clomid	clomiphene	gonadotrophin inhibitor
Clopixol	zuclopenthixol	schizophrenia
Clozaril	clozapine	antipsychotic
Cobalin H	hydroxocobalamin	anti-anaemic
Cogentin	benztropine	parkinsonism
Colestid	colestipol	exchange resin
Colofac	mebeverine	antispasmodic
Colomycin	colistin	antibiotic
Colpermin	peppermint oil	antispasmodic
Combantin	pyrantel	anthelmintic

Proprietary name	Approved name	Main action or indication
Concordin	protriptyline	antidepressant
Condyline	podophyllotoxin	penile warts
Conray	sodium iothalamate	contrast agent
Convulex	valproic acid	epilepsy
Coracten	nifedipine	calcium antagonist
Cordarone X	amiodarone	cardiac arrhythmias
Cordilox	verapamil	angina
Corgard	nadolol	beta-blocker
Corlan	hydrocortisone	local corticosteroid
Coro-Nitro	glycerol trinitrate	angina
Corsodyl	chlorhexidine	antiseptic
Cortistab	cortisone	corticosteroid
Cortisyl	cortisone	corticosteroid
Corwin	xamoterol	mild heart failure
Cosmegen	dactinomycin	cytotoxic
Coversyl	perindopril	ACE-inhibitor
Creon	pancreatin	cystic fibrosis
Crystapen	benzylpenicillin	antibiotic
Curoserf	poractant	neonatal respiratory distress
Cutivate	fluticasone	topical corticosteroid
Cyclogest	progesterone	pre-menstrual syndrome
Cyklokapron	tranexamic acid	antifibrinolytic
Cymevene	ganciclovir	antiviral
Cyprostat	cyproterone	prostatic carcinoma
Cystrin	oxybutynin	urinary spasm
Cytacon	cyanocobalamin	anti-anaemic
Cytamen	cyanocobalamin	anti-anaemic
Cytosar	cytarabine	cytotoxic
Cytotec	misoprostol	peptic ulcer
Daktarin	miconazole	antifungal
Dalacin C	clindamycin	antibiotic
Dalmane	flurazepam	hypnotic
Daneral SA	pheniramine	antihistamine
Danol	danazol	endometriosis

Proprietary name	Approved name	Main action or indication
Dantrium	dantrolene	muscle relaxant
Daonil	glibenclamide	hypoglycaemic
Daranide	dichlorphenamide	glaucoma
Daraprim	pyrimethamine	antimalarial
DDAVP	desmopressin	diabetes insipidus
Decadron	dexamethasone	corticosteroid
Deca-Durabolin	nandrolone	cytotoxic
Declinax	debrisoquine	hypertension
Decortisyl	prednisone	corticosteroid
Deltacortril	prednisolone	corticosteroid
Deltastab	prednisolone	corticosteroid
Demser	metirosine	phaeochromocytoma
De-Nol	bismuth chelate	peptic ulcer
Depixol	flupenthixol	schizophrenia
Deponit	glyceryl trinitrate	angina
Depostat	gestronol	endometrial carcinoma
Derbac	carbaryl	parasiticide
Dermovate	clobetasol	topical corticosteroid
Deseril	methysergide	migraine
Desferal	desferrioxamine	iron poisoning
Destolit	ursodeoxycholic acid	gallstones
Dexedrine	dexamphetamine	appetite depressant
DF118	dihydrocodeine	analgesic
Diabinese	chlorpropamide	hypoglycaemic
Diaginol	sodium acetrizoate	contrast agent
Diamicron	glicazide	hypoglycaemic
Diamox	acetazolamide	glaucoma
Diazemuls	diazepam	anxiolytic
Dibenyline	phenoxybenzamine	vasodilator
Dicynene	ethamyslate	haemostatic
Didronel	disodium etidronate	Paget's disease
Diflucan	fluconazole	antifungal
Digibind	digoxin antibody	digoxin overdose
Dilzem	diltiazem	calcium antagonist

Proprietary name	Approved name	Main action or indication
Dimetriose	gestrinone	endometriosis
Dimotane	brompheniramine	antihistamine
Dimyril	isoaminile	antitussive
Dindevan	phenindione	anticoagulant
Dioctyl	docusate sodium	laxative
Dionosil	propyliodone	contrast agent
Dipentum	olsalazine	ulcerative colitis
Diprivan	propofol	i.v. anaesthetic
Dirythmin-SA	disopyramide	cardiac arrhythmias
Disalcid	salsalate	antirheumatic
Disipal	orphenadrine	parkinsonism
Distaclor	cefaclor	antibiotic
Distamine	penicillamine	Wilson's disease
Distaquaine V-K	phenoxymethyl penicillin	antibiotic
Ditropan	oxybutynin	urinary spasm
Diurexan	xipamide	diuretic
Dixarit	clonidine	migraine
Dobutrex	dobutamine	cardiac stimulant
Dolmatil	sulpiride	schizophrenia
Dolobid	diflunisal	analgesic
Doloxene	dextropropoxyphene	analgesic
Domical	amitriptyline	antidepressant
Dopacard	dopexamine	cardiac surgery
Dopram	doxopram	respiratory stimulant
Doralese	indoramin	prostatic hypertrophy
Dostinex	cabergoline	inhibition of lactation
Dovonex	calcipotriol	psoriasis
Dozic	haloperidol	antipsychotic
Dramamine	dimenhydrinate	antihistamine
Drogenil	flutamide	prostatic carcinoma
Droleptan	droperidol	analgesic
Dryptal	frusemide	diuretic
DTIC	dacarbazine	cytotoxic
Dulcolax	bisacodyl	laxative

Proprietary name	Approved name	Main action or indication
Duphalac	lactulose	laxative
Duphaston	dydrogestone	progestogen
Durabolin	nandrolone	anabolic steroid
Duromine	phentermine	appetite suppressant
Dynese	magaldrate	antacid
Dyspamet	cimetidine	H_2-blocker
Dysport	botulinum toxin	blepharospasm
Dytac	triamterine	diuretic
Ebufac	ibuprofen	arthritis
Ecostatin	econazole	antifungal
Edecrin	ethacrynic acid	diuretic
Efalith	lithium succinate	seborrhoea
Efamast	gamolenic acid	mastalgia
Efcortelan	hydrocortisone	topical corticosteroid
Efudix	fluorouracil	cytotoxic
Elantan	isosorbide mononitrate	angina
Eldepryl	selegiline	parkinsonism
Eldisine	vindesine	cytotoxic
Elocon	mometasone	topical corticosteroid
Elohes	hetastarch	blood volume expander
Eltroxin	thyroxine	thyroid deficiency
Emblon	tamoxifen	cytotoxic
Emcor	bisoprolol	beta-blocker
Emeside	ethosuximide	anticonvulsant
Emflex	acemetacin	arthritis
Eminase	anistreplase	fibrinolytic
Endobulin	immunoglobulin G	antibody deficiency
Endoxana	cyclophosphamide	cytotoxic
Epanutin	phenytoin	anticonvulsant
Epilim	sodium valproate	anticonvulsant
Epogam	gamolenic acid	eczema
Eppy	adrenaline	glaucoma
Eprex	epoetin alpha	anaemia in chronic renal failure
Equanil	meprobamate	tranquillizer

Proprietary name	Approved name	Main action or indication
Eradacin	acrosoxacin	gonorrhoea
Erwinase	crisantaspase	leukaemia
Erythrocin	erythromycin	antibiotic
Esidrex	hydrochlorothiazide	diuretic
Eskazole	albendazole	anthelmintic
Esmeron	rocuronium	muscle relaxant
Estracyt	estramustine	cytotoxic
Estradurin	polyestradiol	prostatic carcinoma
Ethmozine	moracizine	antiarrhythmic
Eudemine	diazoxide	hypertension, hypoglycaemic
Euglucon	glibenclamide	hypoglycaemic
Eumovate	clobetasone	topical corticosteroid
Eurax	crotamiton	antipruritic
Exirel	pirbuterol	bronchodilator
Exocin	ofloxacin	antibacterial
Exosurf	colfosceril	neonatal respiratory distress
Fabrol	acetylcysteine	mucolytic
Famvir	famciclovir	antiviral
Farlutal	medroxyprogesterone	progestogen
Fasigyn	tinidazole	anaerobic infections
Faverin	fluvoxamine	antidepressant
Feldene	piroxicam	arthritis
Femulen	ethynodiol	oral contraceptive
Fenbid	ibuprofen	arthritis
Fenopron	fenoprofen	arthritis
Fentazin	perphenazine	tranquillizer
Fertilol	gonadorelin	infertility
Flagyl	metronidazole	trichomoniasis
Flamazine	silver sulphadiazine	antibacterial
Flaxedil	gallamine	muscle relaxant
Flemoxin	amoxycillin	antibiotic
Flexin	indomethacin	arthritis
Flixonase	fluticasone	allergic rhinitis

Proprietary name	Approved name	Main action or indication
Flixotide	fluticasone	bronchodilator
Flolan	epoprostenol	preserving platelet function in bypass surgery
Florinef	fludrocortisone	corticosteroid
Floxapen	flucloxacillin	antibiotic
Fluanxol	flupenthixol	antidepressant
Fluothane	halothane	inhalation anaesthetic
FML	fluoromethalone	topical corticosteroid
Fortral	pentazocine	analgesic
Fortum	ceftazidime	antibiotic
Foscavir	foscarnet	antiviral
Fragmin	dalteparin	anticoagulant
Framygen	framycetin	antibiotic
Frisium	clobazam	anxiolytic
Froben	flurbiprofen	antirheumatic
Fucidin	sodium fusidate	antibiotic
Fulcin	griseofulvin	antifungal
Fungilin	amphotericin B	antifungal
Fungizone	amphotericin B	antifungal
Furadantin	nitrofurantoin	urinary antiseptic
Furamide	diloxanide furoate	amoebiasis
Galcodine	codeine	antitussive
Galenamox	amoxycillin	antibiotic
Galenphol	pholcodine	antitussive
Gamanil	lofepramine	antidepressant
Garamycin	gentamicin	antibiotic
Gastromax	metaclopramide	anti-emetic
Gastrozepin	pirenzepine	peptic ulcer
Gelofusine	gelatin	blood volume expander
Genotropin	somatrophin	growth hormone
Genticin	gentamicin	antibiotic
Gentran	dextran	plasma substitute
Geref	sermorelin	growth hormone
Gestanin	allyloestranol	progestogen
Glibenese	glipizide	hypoglycaemic

Proprietary name	Approved name	Main action or indication
Glucobay	acarbose	diabetes
Glucophage	metformin	hypoglycaemic
Glurenorm	gliquidone	hypoglycaemic
Glypressin	terlipressin	oesophageal varices
Gopten	trandolapril	ACE-inhibitor
Granocyte	lenograstim	neutropenia
Grisovin	griseofulvin	antifungal
Guarem	guar gum	diabetes
Guarina	guar gum	diabetes
Halciderm	halcinonide	topical corticosteroid
Haldol	haloperidol	schizophrenia
Halfan	halofantrine	antimalarial
Hamarin	allopurinol	gout
Harmogen	oestrone	menopause
Hemabate	carboprost	post-partum haemorrhage
Heminevrin	chlormethiazole	psychosis, hypnotic
Hep-Flush	heparin	anticoagulant
Heplok	heparin	anticoagulant
Hepsal	heparin	anticoagulant
Herpid	idoxuridine	antiviral
Hespan	hetastarch	blood volume expander
Hexopal	inositol nicotinate	vasodilator
Hibitane	chlorhexidine	antiseptic
Hiprex	hexamine hippurate	urinary antiseptic
Hismanal	astemizole	antihistamine
Honvan	fosfestrol	cytotoxic
Humatrope	somatrophin	growth hormone
Humegon	gonadotrophin	infertility
Hyalase	hyaluronidase	enzyme
Hydergine	co-dergocrine	dementia
Hydrea	hydroxyurea	cytotoxic
Hydrenox	hydroflumethiazide	diuretic
Hydrocortistab	hydrocortisone	corticosteroid
Hydrocortisyl	hydrocortisone	corticosteroid

Proprietary name	Approved name	Main action or indication
Hydrocortone	hydrocortisone	corticosteroid
HydroSaluric	hydrochlorothiazide	diuretic
Hygroton	chlorthalidone	diuretic
Hypnomidate	etomidate	i.v. anaesthetic
Hypnovel	midazolam	i.v. anaesthetic
Hypovase	prazosin	hypertension
Hytrin	terazocin	hypertension
Ibular	ibuprofen	arthritis
Idoxene	idoxuridine	antiviral
Iduridin	idoxuridine	antiviral
Ilosone	erythromycin	antibiotic
Imbrilon	indomethacin	arthritis
Imdur	isosorbide mononitrate	angina
Imigran	sumatriptan	migraine
Immunoprin	azathioprine	immunosuppressant
Imodium	loperamide	diarrhoea
Imperacin	oxytetracycline	antibiotic
Imtack	isosorbide dinitrate	angina
Imunovir	inosine pranobex	antiviral
Imuran	azathioprine	immunosuppressant
Inderal	propranolol	beta-blocker
Indocid	indomethacin	arthritis
Indolar	indomethacin	arthritis
Indomod	indomethacin	arthritis
Innohep	tinzaparin	anticoagulant
Innovace	enalapril	ACE-inhibitor
Inoven	ibuprofen	analgesic
Intal	sodium cromoglycate	asthma
Integrin	oxypertine	antipsychotic
Intraval	thiopentone	i.v. anaesthetic
Intron A	interferon	leukaemia
Intropin	dopamine	cardiac stimulant
Iodosorb	cadexomer iodine	leg ulcers
Ionamin	phentermine	appetite suppressant

Proprietary name	Approved name	Main action or indication
Iopidine	apraclonidine	cataract surgery
Ipral	trimethaprim	antibacterial
Ismelin	guanethidine	hypertension
Ismo	isosorbide mononitrate	angina
Isotrate	isosorbide mononitrate	angina
Isotrex	isotretinoin	acne
Istin	amlodipine	calcium antagonist
Jectofer	iron-sorbitol	iron deficiency anaemia
Jexin	tubocurarine	muscle relaxant
Kabikinase	streptokinase	fibrinolytic
Kannasyn	kanamycin	antibiotic
Kefadol	cefamandole	antibiotic
Keflex	cephalexin	antibiotic
Kefzol	cephazolin	antibiotic
Kelfizine	sulfametopyrazine	sulphonamide
Kelocyanor	dicobalt edetate	cyanide poisoning
Kemadrin	procyclidine	parkinsonism
Kemicetine	chloromycetin	antibiotic
Kenalog	triamcinolone	corticosteroid
Kerlone	betaxolol	beta-blocker
Ketalar	ketamine	i.v. anaesthetic
Kinidin	quinidine	cardiac arrhythmias
Klaricid	clarithromycin	antibiotic
Kogenate	Factor VIII	haemophylia A
Konakion	phytomenadione	hypoprothrombinaemia
Kytril	granisetron	anti-emetic
Labrocol	labetalol	beta-blocker
Lamictal	lamotrigine	epilepsy
Lamisil	terbinafine	antifungal
Lamprene	clofazimine	leprosy
Lanoxin	digoxin	heart failure
Lanvis	thioguanine	cytotoxic
Laraflex	naproxen	arthritis
Largactil	chlorpromazine	antipsychotic

Proprietary name	Approved name	Main action or indication
Larium	mefloquine	malaria
Larodopa	levodopa	parkinsonism
Lasix	frusemide	diuretic
Lasma	theophylline	bronchodilator
Laxoberal	sodium picosulphate	laxative
Ledercort	triamcinolone	carticosteroid
Lederfen	fenbufen	antirheumatic
Ledermycin	demeclocycline	antibiotic
Lederspan	triamcinolone	corticosteroid
Lentaron	formestane	cytoxic
Lentizol	amitriptyline	antidepressant
Lescol	fluvastatin	hyperlipidaemia
Leucomax	molgramostim	neutropenia
Leukeran	chlorambucil	cytotoxic
Levophed	noradrenaline	vasoconstrictor
Lexotan	bromazepam	anxiolytic
Librium	chlordiazepoxide	antipsychotic
Limclair	trisodium edetate	ocular lime burns
Lingraine	ergotamine	migraine
Lioresal	baclofen	muscle relaxant
Lipantil	fenofibrate	hyperlipidaemia
Lipostat	pravastatin	hyperlipidaemia
Liskonum	lithium carbonate	mania
Litarex	lithium citrate	mania
Livial	tibolone	menopausal symptoms
Loceryl	amorolfine	antifungal
Lodine	etodolac	arthritis
Logiparin	tinzaparin	anticoagulant
Lomotil	diphenoxylate	diarrhoea
Loniten	minoxidil	hypertension
Lopid	gemfibrozil	hyperlipidaemia
Lopressor	metoprolol	beta-blocker
Loron	sodium clodronate	hypercalcaemia of malignancy
Losec	omeprazole	peptic ulcer

Proprietary name	Approved name	Main action or indication
Loxapac	loxapine	antipsychotic
Ludiomil	maprotiline	antidepressant
Lurselle	probucol	hyperlipidaemia
Lustral	sertraline	antidepressant
Macrobid	nitrofurantoin	urinary infections
Macrodantin	nitrofurantoin	urinary infections
Macrodex	dextran	plasma substitute
Madopar	co-beneldopa	parkinsonism
Magnapen	co-fluampicil	antibiotic
Manerix	moclobemide	antidepressant
Marcain	bupivacaine	anaesthetic
Marevan	warfarin	anticoagulant
Marplan	isocarboxazid	antidepressant
Maxolon	metoclopramide	anti-emetic
Maxtrex	methotrexate	cytotoxic
Mectizan	ivermectin	filariasis
Medrone	methylprednisolone	corticosteroid
Mefoxin	cefoxitin	antibiotic
Megace	megestrol	cytotoxic
Melleril	thioridazine	tranquillizer
Menzol	norethisterone	menorrhagia
Meptid	meptazinol	analgesic
Merbentyl	dicyclomine	antispasmodic
Mestinon	pyridostigmine	myasthenia
Metenix	metolazone	diuretic
Metopirone	metyrapone	resistant oedema
Metosyn	fluocinonide	corticosteroid
Metrodin	urofollitrophin	infertility
Mexitil	mexiletene	cardiac arrhythmias
Miacalcic	salcatonin	Paget's disease
Midamor	amiloride	diuretic
Mifegyne	mifepristone	termination of pregnancy
Minitran	glyceryl trinitrate	angina
Minocin	minocycline	antibiotic

Proprietary name	Approved name	Main action or indication
Minodiab	glipizide	hypoglycaemic
Mintezol	thiabendazole	anthelmintic
Miochol	acetylcholine	cataract surgery
Mithracin	plicamycin	malignant hypercalcaemia
Mitoxana	ifosfamide	cytotoxic
Mivacron	mivacurium	muscle relaxant
Mobiflex	tenoxicam	arthritis
Modalim	ciprofibrate	hyperlipidaemia
Modecate	fluphenazine	antipsychotic
Moditen	fluphenazine	schizophrenia
Modrasone	alclometasone	topical corticosteroid
Modrenal	trilostane	adrenal cortex inhibitor
Mogadon	nitrazepam	hypnotic
Molipaxin	trazodone	antidepressant
Monaspor	cefsulodin	antibiotic
Monit	isosorbide mononitrate	angina
Mono-Cedocard	isosorbic mononitrate	angina
Monoclate-P	Factor VIII	haemophilia A
Monocor	bisoprolol	beta-blocker
Mononine	Factor IX	haemophilia B
Monoparin	heparin	anticoagulant
Monotrim	trimethaprim	antibacterial
Monuril	fosfomycin	urinary infections
Motens	lacidipine	calcium antagonist
Motilium	domperidone	anti-emetic
Motrin	ibuprofen	arthritis
MST Continus	morphine	analgesic
Mucodyne	carbocisteine	mucolytic
Multiparin	heparin	anticoagulant
Muripsin	glutamic hydrochloride	achlorhydria
Myambutol	ethambutol	tuberculosis
Mycardol	pentaerythritol	coronary dilator
Mycobutin	rifabutin	tuberculosis
Mydriacyl	tropicamide	mydriatic

Proprietary name	Approved name	Main action or indication
Mydrilate	cyclopentolate	mydriatic
Myleran	busulphan	cytotoxic
Myocrisin	sodium aurothiomalate	rheumatoid arthritis
Myodil	iophendylate	contrast agent
Myotonine	bethanechol	cholinergic
Mysoline	primidone	epilepsy
Nacton	poldine	antispasmodic
Nalcrom	sodium cromoglycate	anti-allergic
Nalorex	naltrexone	opioid dependence
Naprosyn	naproxen	arthritis
Narcan	naloxone	narcotic antagonist
Nardil	phenelzine	antidepressant
Narphen	phenazocine	analgesic
Natrilix	indapamide	hypertension
Natulan	procarbazine	cytotoxic
Navidrex	cyclopenthiazide	diuretic
Navoban	tropisetron	anti-emetic
Nebcin	tobramycin	antibiotic
Negram	nalidixic acid	urinary antiseptic
Neo-Cytamen	hydroxocobalamin	anti-anaemic
Neo-Mercazole	carbimazole	thyrotoxicosis
Neo-Naclex	bendrofluazide	diuretic
Neotigason	acitretin	psoriasis
Nephril	polythiazide	diuretic
Nerisone	diflucortolone	corticosteroid
Netillin	netilmicin	antibiotic
Neulactil	pericyazine	schizophrenia
Neupogen	filgrastim	neutropenia
Neurontin	gabapentin	epilepsy
Niferex	iron complex	anaemia
Nimotop	nimodipine	subarachnoid haemorrhage
Nipent	pentostatin	hairy-cell leukaemia
Nipride	sodium nitroprusside	hypertensive crisis
Nitoman	tetrabenazine	chorea

Proprietary name	Approved name	Main action or indication
Nitrocine	glyceryl trinitrate	angina
Nitrocontin Continus	glyceryl trinitrate	angina
Nitrolingual	glyceryl trinitrate	angina
Nitronal	glyceryl trinitrate	angina
Nivaquine	chloroquine	antimalarial
Nivemycin	neomycin	antibiotic
Nizoral	ketoconazole	antifungal
Noctec	chloral hydrate	hypnotic
Noltam	tamoxifen	cytotoxic
Nolvadex	tamoxifen	cytotoxic
Nootropil	piracetam	tics
Norcuron	vecuronium	muscle relaxant
Norditropin	somatotrophin	growth hormone
Nordox	doxycycline	antibiotic
Norflex	orphenadrine	muscle relaxant
Norval	mianserin	antidepressant
Novantrone	mitozantrone	cytotoxic
Noxyflex S	noxythiolin	antiseptic
Nozinan	methotrimeprazine	pain in terminal cancer
Nubain	nalbuphine	analgesic
Nuelin	theophylline	bronchodilator
Nystan	nystatin	antifungal
Nytol	diphenhydramine	mild insomnia
Ocusert Pilo	pilocarpine	glaucoma
Odrik	trandolapril	calcium antagonist
Olbetam	acipimox	hyperlipidaemia
Omnopon	papaveretum	analgesic
Oncovin	vincristine	cytotoxic
One-alpha	alfacalcidol	vitamin D deficiency
Operidine	phenoperidine	analgesic
Ophthaine	proxymetacaine	corneal anaesthetic
Opilon	thymoxamine	vasodilator
Opticrom	sodium cromoglycate	allergic conjunctivitis
Optimax	tryptophan	antidepressant

Proprietary name	Approved name	Main action or indication
Optimine	azatadine	antihistamine
Orap	pimozide	schizophrenia
Orbenin	cloxacillin	antibiotic
Orelox	cefpodoxime	antibiotic
Orgaran	danaparoid	anticoagulant
Orimeten	aminoglutethimide	cytotoxic
Orudis	ketoprofen	arthritis
Oruvail	ketoprofen	arthritis
Otrivine	xylometazoline	nasal decongestant
Oxivent	oxitropium	bronchodilator
Palfium	dextromoramide	analgesic
Paludrine	proguanil	antimalarial
Panadol	paracetamol	analgesic
Paraplatin	carboplatin	cytotoxic
Parlodel	bromocriptine	lactation suppressant
Parnate	tranylcypromine	antidepressant
Paroven	oxyrutins	varicose states
Parvolex	acetylcysteine	paracetamol overdose
Pavulon	pancuronium	muscle relaxant
Pecram	aminophylline	bronchodilator
Penbritin	ampicillin	antibiotic
Pendramine	penicillamine	Wilson's disease
Pentacarinat	pentamidine	leishmaniasis
Pentasa	mesalazine	ulcerative colitis
Pentaspan	pentastarch	blood volume expander
Pentostam	sodium stibogluconate	leishmaniasis
Pepcid	famotidine	H_2-blocker
Percutol	glyceryl trinitrate	angina
Perfan	enoximone	heart failure
Pergonal	menotrophin	hypogonadism
Periactin	cyproheptadine	antihistamine
Persantin	dipyridamole	angina
Pertofran	desipramine	antidepressant
Pevaryl	econazole	antifungal

Proprietary name	Approved name	Main action or indication
Pharmorubicin	epirubicin	cytotoxic
Phenergan	promethazine	antihistamine
Phyllocontin Continus	aminophylline	bronchodilator
Physeptone	methadone	analgesic
Picolax	sodium picosulphate	laxative
Piportil	pipothiazine	antipsychotic
Pipril	piperacillin	antibiotic
Piptalin	pipenzolate	antispasmodic
Piriton	chlorpheniramine	antihistamine
Plaquenil	hydroxychloroquine	antimalarial
Plendil	felodipine	calcium antagonist
Ponderax	fenfluramine	appetite suppressant
Pondocillin	pivampicillin	antibiotic
Ponstan	mefenamic acid	arthritis
Potaba	potassium p-aminobenzoate	scleroderma
Praxilene	naftidrofuryl	vasodilator
Precortisyl	prednisolone	corticosteroid
Predsol	prednisolone	corticosteroid
Preferid	budesonide	topical corticosteroid
Pregnyl	gonadotrophin	infertility
Premarin	oestrogen	menopause
Prepidil	dinoprostone	cervical ripening
Prepulsid	cisapride	oesophageal reflux
Prescal	isradipine	calcium antagonist
Priadel	lithium carbonate	mania
Primacor	milrinone	severe heart failure
Primalan	mequitazine	antihistamine
Primaxin	imipenem	antibiotic
Primolut N	norethisterone	progestogen
Pro-Banthine	propantheline	peptic ulcer
Profasi	gonadatrophin	infertility
Progesic	fenoprofen	arthritis
Proleukin	aldesleukin	cytotoxic
Proluton-Depot	hydroxyprogesterone	progestogen

Proprietary name	Approved name	Main action or indication
Prominal	methylphenobarbitone	epilepsy
Prondol	iprindole	antidepressant
Pronestyl	procainamide	cardiac arrhythmias
Propaderm	beclomethasone	topical corticosteroid
Propine	dipivefrin	glaucoma
Proscar	finasteride	prostatic hyperplasia
Prostap	leuprorelin	prostatic carcinoma
Prostigmin	neostigmine	myasthenia
Prostin F2	dinoprost	uterine stimulant
Prostin VR	alprostadil	maintenance of ductus arteriosus in neonates
Prothiaden	dothiepin	antidepressant
Provera	medroxyprogesterone	progestogen
Pro-Viron	mesterolone	androgen deficiency
Prozac	fluoxetine	antidepressant
Pulmadil	rimiterol	bronchospasm
Pulmicort	budesonide	rhinitis
Pulmozyme	dornase alfa	cystic fibrosis
Puri-Nethol	mercaptopurine	cytotoxic
Pyopen	carbenicillin	antibiotic
Questran	cholestyramine	bile acid binder
Rapifen	alfentanyl	narcotic analgesic
Rastinon	tolbutamide	hypoglycaemic
Razoxin	razoxane	cytotoxic
Recormon	epoetin alpha	anaemia in chronic renal failure
Redeptin	fluspirilene	schizophrenia
Refolinon	folinic acid	methotrexate antidote
Regaine	minoxidil	baldness
Relifex	nabumetone	arthritis
Resonium A	exchange resin	hyperkalaemia
Respacal	tolubuterol	bronchodilator
Restandol	testosterone	androgen deficiency
Retin-A	tretinoin	acne
Retrovir	zidovudine	antiviral (AIDS)

Proprietary name	Approved name	Main action or indication
Revanil	lysuride	parkinsonism
Rheomacrodex	dextran	blood volume expander
Rheumox	azapropazone	arthritis
Rhinocort	budesonide	rhinitis
Rhinolast	azelastine	rhinitis
Ridaura	auranofin	rheumatoid arthritis
Rifadin	rifampicin	tuberculosis
Rimactane	rifampicin	tuberculosis
Rimifon	isoniazid	tuberculosis
Rinatec	ipratropium	rhinorrhoea
Risperdal	risperidone	antipsychotic
Rivotril	clonazepam	anticonvulsant
Roaccutane	isotretinoin	severe acne
Robaxin	methcarbamol	muscle relaxant
Robinul	glycopyrronium	antimuscarinic
Rocaltrol	calcitriol	vitamin D deficiency
Roccal	benzalkonium	antiseptic
Rocephin	ceftriaxone	antibiotic
Roferon-A	interferon	leukaemia
Rogitine	phentolamine	phaeochromocytoma
Rohypnol	flunitrazepam	hypnotic
Ronicol	nicotinyl alcohol	vasodilator
Rynacrom	sodium cromoglycate	allergic rhinitis
Rythmodan	disopyramide	cardiac arrhythmias
Sabril	vigabatrin	anticonvulsant
Saizen	somatropin	growth hormone
Salazopyrin	sulphasalazine	ulcerative colitis
Salbulin	salbutamol	bronchospasm
Salofalk	melsalazine	ulcerative colitis
Saluric	chlorothiazide	diuretic
Sandimmun	cyclosporin	immunosuppressant
Sandoglobulin	immunoglobulin	hepatitis
Sandostatin	octreotide	carcinoid syndrome
Sanomigran	pizotifen	migraine

Proprietary name	Approved name	Main action or indication
Saventrine	isoprenaline	bronchospasm
Scoline	suxamethonium	muscle relaxant
Scopoderm	hyoscine	motion sickness
Seconal	quinalbarbitone	hypnotic
Sectral	acebutolol	beta-blocker
Securon	verapamil	angina
Selsun	selenium sulphide	dandruff
Semprex	acrivastine	antihistamine
Serc	betahistine	Ménière's syndrome
Serenace	haloperidol	schizophrenia
Serevent	salmeterol	bronchospasm
Serophene	clomiphene	infertility
Seroxat	paroxetine	antidepressant
Sevredol	morphine	analgesic
Simplene	adrenaline	glaucoma
Sinequan	doxepin	antidepressant
Sinthrome	nicoumalone	anticoagulant
Skinoren	azelaic acid	acne
Slo-Phyllin	theophylline	bronchodilator
Slow-Trasicor	oxprenolol	beta-blocker
Soframycin	framycetin	antibiotic
Solu-Cortef	hydrocortisone	corticosteroid
Solu-Medrone	methylprednisolone	corticosteroid
Sominex	promethazine	mild hypnotic
Soneryl	butobarbitone	hypnotic
Sorbid SA	isosorbide dinitrate	angina
Sorbitrate	isosorbide dinitrate	angina
Sotacor	sotalol	beta-blocker
Sparine	promazine	antipsychotic
Spasmonal	alverine	antispasmodic
Spiroctan	canrenoate	diuretic
Spirolone	spironolactone	diuretic
Sporanox	itraconazole	antifungal
Stafoxil	flucloxacillin	antibiotic

Proprietary name	Approved name	Main action or indication
Staril	fosinopril	ACE-inhibiror
Stelazine	trifluoperazine	antipsychotic
Stemetil	prochlorperazine	anti-emetic
Stesolid	diazepam	anxiolytic
Stiedex	desoxymethasone	topical corticosteroid
Stiemycin	erythromycin	acne
Stilnoct	zolpidem	hypnotic
Streptase	streptokinase	fibrinolytic
Stromba	stanozolol	anabolic steroid
Stugeron	cinnarizine	anti-emetic
Sublimaze	fentanyl	analgesic
Sulpitil	sulpiride	schizophrenia
Suprane	desflurane	inhalation anaesthetic
Suprax	cefixime	antibiotic
Suprecur	buserelin	endometriosis
Suprefact	buserelin	prostatic carcinoma
Surgam	tiaprofenic acid	arthritis
Surmontil	trimipramine	antidepressant
Survanta	beractant	neo-natal respiratory distress
Suscard Buccal	glyceryl trinitrate	angina
Sustac	glyceryl trinitrate	angina
Sustamycin	tetracycline	antibiotic
Sustanon	testosterone	androgen deficiency
Symmetrel	amantadine	parkinsonism
Synacthen	tetracosactrin	corticotrophin
Synalar	fluocinolone	topical corticosteroid
Synarel	nafarelin	endometriosis
Synflex	naproxen	arthritis
Synkavit	menadiol	hypoprothrombinaemia
Syntaris	flunisolide	local corticosteroid
Syntocinon	oxytocin	post-partum haemorrhage
Syntopressin	lypressin	diabetes insipidus
Sytron	sodium iron edetate	anti-anaemic
Tagamet	cimetidine	peptic ulcer

Proprietary name	Approved name	Main action or indication
Tambocor	flecainide	cardiac arrhythmias
Tamofen	tamoxifen	cytotoxic
Targocid	teicoplanin	antibiotic
Tarivid	ofloxacin	urinary tract infections
Tavegil	clemastine	antihistamine
Taxol	paclitaxel	cytotoxic
Tegretol	carbamazepine	anticonvulsant
Temgesic	buprenorphine	analgesic
Temopen	temocillin	antibiotic
Tenormin	atenolol	beta-blocker
Tenuate	diethylpropion	appetite suppressant
Teoptic	carteolol	glaucoma
Terramycin	oxytetracycline	antibiotic
Tertroxin	liothyronine	thyroid deficiency
Tetmosol	monosulfiram	scabies
Tetrabid	tetracycline	antibiotic
Tetralysal	lymecycline	antibiotic
Theo-dur	theophylline	bronchospasm
Thephorin	phenindamine	antihistamine
Ticar	ticarcillin	antibiotic
Tilade	neocromil	asthma
Tildiem	diltiazem	calcium antagonist
Timecef	cefodizime	antibiotic
Timoptol	timolol	glaucoma
Tinset	oxatomide	antihistamine
Tobralex	tobramycin	eye infections
Tofranil	imipramine	antidepressant
Tolanase	tolazamide	hypoglycaemic
Tolectin	tolmetin	antirheumatic
Tonocard	tocainide	cardiac arrhythmias
Topicycline	tetracycline	acne
Topilar	fluclorolone	topical corticosteroid
Toradol	ketorolac	analgesic
Torem	torasemide	diuretic

Proprietary name	Approved name	Main action or indication
Tracrium	atracurium	muscle relaxant
Trancopal	chlormezanone	anxiolytic
Trandate	labetalol	beta-blocker
Transiderm-Nitro	glyceryl trinitrate	angina
Tranxene	clorazepate	anxiolytic
Trasicor	oxprenolol	beta-blocker
Trasylol	aprotinin	pancreatitis
Travogyn	isoconazole	candidiasis
Traxam gel	felbinac	sprains
Trental	oxpentifylline	vasodilator
Tridil	glyceryl trinitrate	angina
Triludan	terfenadine	antihistamine
Trimopan	trimethoprim	antibacterial
Tritace	ramipril	ACE-inhibitor
Trobicin	spectinomycin	antibiotic
Trosyl	tioconazole	antifungal
Tryptizol	amitriptyline	antidepressant
Ubretid	dystigmine	urinary retention
Ukidan	urokinase	hyphaemia, embolism
Ultralanum	fluocortolone	topical corticosteroid
Uniparin	heparin	anticoagulant
Uniphyllin Continus	theophylline	bronchospasm
Univer	verapamil	hypertension, angina
Uriben	nalidixic acid	urinary tract infections
Urispas	flavoxate	cystitis
Uromitexan	mesna	urotoxicity due to cyclophosphamide
Ursofalk	ursodeoxycholic acid	gallstones
Utinor	norfloxacin	urinary tract infections
Utovlan	ethisterone	progestogen
Valium	diazepam	anxiolytic, muscle relaxant
Vallergan	trimeprazine	sedative, pruritus
Valoid	cyclizine	anti-emetic
Vancocin	vancomycin	antibiotic
Vansil	oxamniquine	anthelmintic

Proprietary name	Approved name	Main action or indication
Vascase	cilazapril	ACE-inhibitor
Vasoxine	methoxamine	acute hypotension
Velbe	vinblastine	cytotoxic
Velosef	cephradine	antibiotic
Ventolin	salbutamol	bronchospasm
Vepesid	etoposide	cytotoxic
Vermox	mebendazole	anthelmintic
Vibramycin	doxycycline	antibiotic
Videne	povidone-iodine	antiseptic
Videx	didanosine	antiviral
Vidopen	ampicillin	antibiotic
Virazid	tribavirin	antiviral
Virormone	testosterone	hypogonadism
Visclair	methylcysteine	mucolytic
Visken	pindolol	beta-blocker
Vivalan	viloxazine	antidepressant
Volital	pemoline	hyperkinaesia
Volmax	salbutamol	bronchodilator
Volraman	diclofenac	arthritis
Voltarol	diclofenac	antirheumatic
Welldorm	chloral hydrate	hypnotic
Wellferon	interferon	leukaemia
Xanax	alprazolam	anxiolytic
Xatral	alfuzosin	prostatic hyperplasia
Xuret	metolazone	diuretic
Xylocaine	lignocaine	anaesthetic
Yomesan	niclosamide	anthelmintic
Yutopar	ritodrine	premature labour
Zaditen	ketotifen	anti-asthmatic
Zadstat	metronidazole	trichomoniasis
Zantac	ranitidine	H_2-blocker
Zarontin	ethosuximide	anticonvulsant
Zavidos	idarubicin	cytotoxic
Zestril	lisinopril	ACE-inhibitor

Proprietary name	Approved name	Main action or indication
Zimovane	zopiclone	hypnotic
Zinacef	cefuroxime	antibiotic
Zinamide	pyrazinamide	tuberculosis
Zinnat	cefuroxime	antibiotic
Zirtek	cetirizine	antihistamine
Zita	cimetidine	H_2-blocker
Zithromax	clarithomycin	antibiotic
Zocor	simvastatin	hyperlipidaemia
Zofran	ondansetron	anti-emetic
Zoladex	goserelin	prostatic carcinoma
Zonulysin	chymotrypsin	cataract surgery
Zovirax	acyclovir	antiviral
Zoton	lansoprazole	peptic ulcer
Zydol	tramadol	analgesic
Zumenon	oestradiol	menopausal symptoms
Zyloric	allopurinol	gout

New products that have become available since Appendix II was prepared:

Cedax	ceftibutin	antibiotic
Cozaar	losartan	hypertension
Durogesic	fentanyl	analgesic patches
Eferox	venlafaxine	antidepressant
Eucardic	carvedilol	hypertension
Fludara	fludarabine	cytotoxic
Hivid	zalcatabine	HIV infections
Ikoral	nicorandel	angina
Kefadem	ceftazidime	antibiotic
Micronor HRT	norethisterone	progestogen
Mitofene	diclofenac	NSAID
Norprolac	quinazolide	prolactin inhibitor
Nutrineal PD4	amino acids	peritoneal dialysis
Orgafol	urofollitrophin	infertility
Otex	urea-hydrogen peroxide	ear-drops
Posiject	dobutamine	cardiac support

Prograf	tacrolimus	immunosuppressant
Replenine	Factor IX	haemophilia B
Slozem	diltiazem	angina, hypertension
Vividrin	sodium cromoglycate	nasal allergy
Wellvone	atovanquone	Pneumocystis pneumonia

Appendix III: Weights and measures

Metric system

Nanogram	=	0.001 microgram
Microgram (μg)	=	0.001 mg
Milligram (mg)	=	0.001 g
Centigram (cg)	=	0.01 g
Decigram (dg)	=	0.1 g
Gram (g)	=	1 g
Kilogram (kg)	=	1000 g

The common metric measures of volume are the millilitre (ml), which is almost identical with the cubic centimetre (cc), and the litre (1000 ml or cc).

The British National Formulary gives all doses and formulations in the metric system. The standard dose for mixtures is 10 ml, for linctuses and children's mixtures the dose is 5 ml. Special 5-ml medicine spoons are available, and the use of domestic teaspoons for measuring medicines should be abandoned.

Approximate metric and imperial equivalents

60 mg	=	1 grain
1 g	=	15 grains
28.4 g	=	1 oz
453 g	=	1 lb
1 kg	=	2.2 lb
63.5 kg	=	10 st
28.4 ml	=	1 fl oz
100 ml	=	3.5 oz
500 ml	=	17.5 oz
568 ml	=	1 pint
1000 ml (1 litre)	=	35 oz

Appendix IV: Abbreviations

Abbreviations sometimes used in prescriptions are:

a.c.	ante cibum	before food
aq.	aqua	water
b.d.	bis die	twice a day
c.	cum	with
et	et	and
mitt.	mitte	send
o.n.	omni nocte	every night
p.c.	post cibum	after food
p.r.n.	pro re nata	occasionally
q.d.	quater die	four times a day
q.q.h.	quarta quaque hora	every 4 hours
q.s.	quantum sufficiat	sufficient
s.o.s.	si opus sit	when necessary
stat.	statim	at once
t.d.s.	ter die sumendus	to be taken three times a day
t.i.d.	ter in die	three times a day
ung.	unguentum	ointment

Note: The abbreviations s.c., i.m. and i.v. refer to subcutaneous, intramuscular and intravenous injections.

Appendix V: Glossary

aerobes: Organisms that grow in the presence of oxygen. *See* anaerobes.

agonists: Drugs that bind to a receptor, and initiate or increase a response.

alkaloids: Basic organic substances produced by many plants. Many are pharmacologically active such as atropine, morphine and quinine.

amoebiasis: An infection of the intestines and liver by pathogenic forms of single-cell protozoa, particularly *Entamoeba histolytica*.

anaemia: A deficiency of haemoglobin, the oxygen-carrying constituent of red blood cells. It may occur as a result of a lack of iron, a deficiency of vitamin B_{12} (pernicious anaemia), or as a side-effect of some drugs.

anaphylaxis: A state of severe shock, induced by an antigen–antibody reaction in the tissues. The reaction is linked with the release of spasmogens and inflammatory factors, and may cause severe bronchospasm and collapse.

antagonists: Drugs that bind to cell receptors. They function mainly as blocking agents, and by preventing other substances from interacting with the receptors, they inhibit the normal response.

anaerobes: Organisms that cannot develop in the presence of oxygen. *See* aerobes.

anticholinergics: See antimuscarinics.

antimuscarinics: Drugs that block the action of acetylcholine.

antimycotics: Antifungal agents.

antigens: Substances that stimulate the production of antibodies.

antipyretics: Drugs that lower the body temperature in feverish conditions.

aplastic anaemia: A form of anemia due to complete failure of the bone marrow.

antitussives: Cough depressants and suppressants.

ascariasis: Infestation of nematode worms.

Behçet's syndrome: A disease of unknown cause, with conjunctivitis, mouth and genital ulcers.

Bacteroides: A Gram-negative pathogen. It is normally present in the faeces, but may cause ulceration of the skin and mucous membranes and peritonitis.

bacteruria (bacilluria): The presence of more than 100 000 organisms per ml of freshly voided urine.

beta-lactam: A nitrogen-containing ring that is an essential part of the penicillin and cephalosporin structure. Breakdown of the ring by enzymes results in loss of activity.

beta-lactamases: Enzymes that can break the beta-lactam ring structure of penicillins. They are formed by some penicillin–cephalosporin-resistant organisms.

bio-availability: A term referring to that part of a dose of a drug that reaches the circulation and affects tissues.

bolus: A large initial dose of a drug, given to obtain a rapidly effective blood level.

bradycardia: Slowing of the heart rate.

candidiasis: Infection with the fungus *Candida*. Also known as thrush and moniliasis.

carbonic anhydrase: An enzyme that controls the production of carbon dioxide.

carcinoid syndrome: Due to a tumour of the appendix that may secrete large amounts of serotonin (5HT) and cause severe diarrhoea.

chelating agents: Substances that can combine with and inhibit the activity of certain ions, and promote their excretion as an inactive complex. Desferrioxamine is an example of a chelating agent.

cholinesterases: Enzymes that limit the action of acetylcholine by converting it to choline and acetic acid.

Clostridium: A genus of Gram-positive anaerobic exotoxin-producing organisms, some of which are normally present in the gut. They are often associated with intra-abdominal infections, and tetanus is caused by *Clostridium tetani*.

coliform bacteria: See *Escherichia coli*.

cross-resistance: Some groups of antibacterial agents have a common basic structure; in consequence, a strain of organism that has become resistant to one member of a group may be resistant to others.

cryptococcosis: Infection of the central nervous system by the fungus *Cryptococcus neoformans*.

cycloplegics: Drugs that paralyse the ciliary muscle in the eye, and so facilitate examination.

cytomegalovirus: A virus of the same group as herpes simplex. The cause of AIDS-related pneumonia.

cytotoxics: Drugs that have a destructive effect on cells, and are used in the treatment of cancer.

dermatophytes: Fungi that invade the superficial layers of the skin.

double-blind trial: A method of examining the efficacy of a new drug, by which the response is compared with a similar drug or a placebo. The test is so arranged that neither the doctor nor the patient knows who is receiving the new drug until the end of the trial. The identity of the drug is then disclosed (unless some severe side-effect requires early investigation).

endogenous: Originating within the organism.

endomorphins: A group of centrally acting neuropeptides that act on specific receptors concerned with the perception of pain. Analgesics of the morphine type appear to mimic the action of endomorphins.

endotoxins: Toxic protein products of bacterial metabolism that are stored in the cell wall and released after cell breakdown. *See* Exotoxins.

Enterobacter: A genus of Gram-negative bacteria sometimes associated with infections of the urinary tract.

enterococci: Short-chain Gram-positive organisms normally present in the gut. They may be pathogenic if they invade the urinary tract and other tissues.

enzymes: Proteins that function as catalysts of metabolism, and control the activity of cells. Their action is often highly specific.

erythropoiesis: The production of red blood cells.

Escherichia: A genus of Gram-negative rod-like bacteria, of which *Esch. coli* is the most common. They are normally present in the gut, and are a frequent cause of urinary tract infections. Systematic invasion may also occur.

exogenous: Of external origin, as opposed to endogenous.

exotoxin: Toxic products of bacterial metabolism that are released during cell growth, and may cause systematic infections. *See* Endotoxin.

extrapyramidal side-effects: The extrapyramidal tracts of the central nervous system coordinate and control muscular contraction. Disturbance of that control by drugs may produce many side-effects, including tremor and rigidity.

extravasation: The escape of fluid into surrounding tissues. Extravasation of an irritant drug given intravenously may cause severe tissue damage.

glycosides: Organic substances produced by many plants, consisting of a carbohydrate combined with an active principle, such as digoxin.

gonococcus: A Gram-negative pathogen (*Neisseria gonorrhoeae*) which causes the sexually-transmitted disease gonorrhoea.

Gram-positive and Gram-negative: A term applied to a method for distinguishing between two main groups of bacteria by means of a staining fluid. Gram-positive bacteria have a peptidoglycan-containing cell wall that takes up and retains the stain. Gram-negative organisms have a multi-layer cell wall containing lipoproteins, which does not retain the stain. Name of Danish physician (1853–1938.)

half-life: The time taken for the concentration of a circulating drug to fall by half after absorption and distribution is complete.

hypercalcaemia: An excessively high blood calcium level, mainly caused by bone resorption.

hypercalciuria: An increased urinary excretion of calcium.

hyperglycaemia: An elevated blood-sugar level.

hyperkalaemia: An elevated blood-potassium level.

immunocompromised: A term used to describe patients with an inadequate immune response. The condition may be caused by some potent drugs, by irradiation or by disease that affects the immune system. Such patients are very liable to opportunistic infections by organisms not normally regarded as pathogens.

infarct: An area of tissue of which the blood supply is blocked by a clot.

ischaemia: A deficiency in the blood supply to a part of the body.

metabolism: The general term for the processes that provide energy for body functions. It includes the breakdown of food

Index

E